the

28

——— days ———

Lighter Diet

the

28

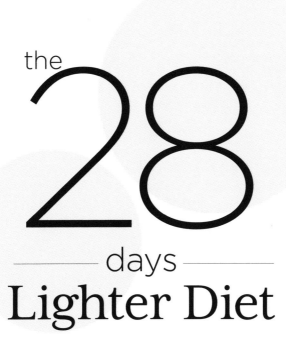

—— days ——
Lighter Diet

Your Monthly Plan to Lose Weight,
End PMS, and Achieve Physical
and Emotional Wellness

Ellen Barrett and Kate Hanley

Guilford, Connecticut
An imprint of Globe Pequot Press

Photos by Arthur Cohen
Text design: Sheryl Kober
Layout: Mary Ballachino
Project editor: Ellen Urban

Library of Congress Cataloging-in-Publication Data is available on file.

ISBN 978-0-7627-8767-8

Printed in the United States of America

10 9 8 7 6 5 4 3 2 1

The health information expressed in this book is based solely on the personal experience of the authors and is not intended as a medical manual. The information should not be used for diagnosis or treatment, or as a substitute for professional medical care.

To all women,

may you harness the power within,
and teach your daughters
and granddaughters
to do the same.

Contents

Introduction

This is the book we wanted to find already written for us in the library, but alas, it did not exist. As health and wellness coaches, we have sensed loneliness and confusion in almost all of our hundreds of female clients with regard to *authentic* reproductive wellness and lasting weight loss. We set out to find answers—through ob/gyns, midwives, naturopaths, chiropractors, traditional Chinese medicine, yoga, hard science, and folk medicine. This book is our way of eradicating the loneliness and confusion that comes from feeling like the only one in the world who snaps at your kids or wants to hide under the covers when you're premenstrual, or from wondering why you can follow the latest diet or exercise plan and only feel wiped out and incompetent when the weight doesn't budge, or comes off only to reappear next month. Our message is simple: *Wake up to the gift inside you.*

As women, we have an omnipresent GPS-like system wired into our beings that offers daily mental, physical, and spiritual guidance. It's called the menstrual cycle, and it affects us all month long, not just during the few days of actual menstruation. Yet, all fitness and diet programs ignore it, as our culture pretty much pretends it isn't there. This infuriates us! We have both learned through our own experiences and studies that when you work *with*, instead of against, your cycle, you find your way to total feminine wellness, and you do it without prescriptions, depriving yourself of delicious food, or killing yourself at the gym.

ELLEN'S STORY

I was an athlete, playing competitive tennis throughout high school and college. In fact, I got my first period at a tennis tournament. I was one of the millions of women duped into thinking I was doing my whole body right by running five miles on the first day of my period. In my fifteen years as a serious athlete, I never once had a coach ask me about my cycle. Looking back now, I find that odd, for my cycle profoundly affected my tennis game. When I was on my period, I was sluggish and self-conscious. Surely my coaches could tell, right?

After graduation I entered the fitness biz, and continued to ignore "Aunt Flo." This is when my body started to really scream. In addition to the two days of debilitating (hunched-over) cramps each month (which I thought were normal), I experienced nausea, night sweats, and an extremely heavy flow. I sought help from my gynecologist, and I recall her quickly walking over to her desk and jotting down a prescription for painkillers—which I never filled—without once looking me in the eye. She shooed me out the door and was off to the next patient in room number three. That same scenario played out again and again at every yearly checkup until I was thirty-two years old.

As I look back, I see how my body took me down. Instead of listening to it, I was defying it month after month with tampons, tennis matches, Jane Fonda aerobics, and a standard American diet (SAD). In my mid-twenties, my body stopped me in my tracks with premenstrual syndrome (PMS) so debilitating that I literally couldn't get out of bed. I called in sick for the first time in my entire life and told my boss I had the flu.

Only when I wanted to start a family did I realize the truth: I've been disrespectful to my feminine nature. I thought I was one of the millions of nonsmoking, nondrinking women who "did everything right," yet I struggled with infertility. Clearly, my body was not a temple! I looked fit on the outside, but inside something was awry, as it took us almost three years to conceive.

Luckily, through a more moderate exercise regime, stress management, and a whole-food diet, my plight proved reversible. While charting the ebb and flow of my energy levels, I began meditating, discovered traditional Chinese medicine, and replaced excessive workouts with long walks in the woods. I also allowed myself quiet time without guilt. Now ladies, here's the miraculous part—not only did I stay slim with much less effort, but I also regained my reproductive wellness and naturally conceived my son at age thirty-seven. This may sound corny, but today I feel I'm growing better, wiser, softer, and happier. Plus, I'm not freaked out about getting older. The 28 Days Lighter Diet program put my body, mind, *and* spirit on the right path.

KATE'S STORY

I got my period for the first time when I was twelve years old. A child of divorced parents, I was visiting my dad for a few weeks when it arrived. I was too embarrassed to tell him about it, so I made do with wadding up toilet paper to serve as makeshift pads until it passed. Not wanting to be uncool, I went right to tampons for my next cycle, and thought it was fabulous that I could wear one tampon the whole day at school and not change it until I got home, so I wouldn't have to carry one in my bag and risk a boy discovering it.

The next decade and a half, I kept on pretty much pretending my period didn't exist. I was enamored of any activity that came my way—softball, soccer, jogging, tennis lessons, bike riding, aerobics, Nautilus machines. I loved them all, because they were the only way to combat my junk food diet and still stay trim (or so I thought). I found a couple Midols and a tampon could carry me through those early period days quite nicely. Funny how I thought that the distended abdomen, wacked-out digestion, sore boobs, and sullenness I experienced the week before each period were "normal."

I discovered yoga in my mid-twenties, which helped me to develop more body awareness and was the first place I learned that perhaps I should modify my activities when I was on my period—namely, abstaining from going upside down in headstand or handstand while I was bleeding. I didn't really understand *why* my teachers advised against it, but the idea of taking it somewhat easy while menstruating resonated with me. *Of course.*

I spent just shy of ten years doing power yoga several times a week, eventually earning my teaching certificate and working as a journalist for magazines including *Yoga Journal* and *Yoga International.* I was also eating salads every day for lunch and thinking I was a model student in the fitness and diet realms. Yet by the time I was twenty-eight, I suffered from ten full days of painful PMS symptoms each month, gaining five pounds in water weight and going up a full cup size. I needed two wardrobes. During these years, I was also plagued by cold sores and migraines.

When I was thirty-four, my fiancé and I moved to Brooklyn, and I had to find a new go-to yoga studio. One fateful day, I tried to go to a power yoga class but was too late to walk in. So I took a walk through the neighborhood, hoping there was another studio around. I stumbled into a restorative class at a studio that specialized in Iyengar yoga (a traditional, slow-paced, conservative school of yoga—you may only do twelve to fifteen poses in a typical class). I had my period at the time, and the teacher gave me a handout with several quiet, supremely relaxing poses in a sequence handed down from India just for menstruating women. I went in the corner with my props and did a completely different class from everyone else. It was a profound aha moment; despite the cramps and sore boobs I'd had when I walked in, my body felt like it was floating on a cloud by the time I walked out. I haven't done a power yoga class since.

That class created an opening in my mind, gradually changing the way I thought of my period—from monthly curse to monthly retreat. It was a paradigm shift, from telling my body what I expected of it when I expected it, to giving it what it needed to function well. Along the way, I also changed the way I exercised, ate, drank, and thought.

I'm so happy to report that, thanks in large part to the 28 Days Lighter Diet, my PMS has been a thing of the past for eight years running. I also conceived naturally (at thirty-six and thirty-eight), and enjoyed pregnancies free of the symptoms we have come to think of as unavoidable—no swelling, varicose veins, constipation, or stretch marks. (Lest you think I'm perfect, it did take me a full three days to birth my daughter! Ugh.)

OUR GOALS

The purpose of this book is to focus on the positive aspects of the female cycle that provide us access to a wide range of abilities and qualities. We aren't going to focus on what you shouldn't do, eat, or think. Instead, we choose to concentrate on proper nutrition, new approaches to fitness, and mind-body practices that will crowd out the habits and beliefs that have nudged us so far out of balance.

We base everything we suggest in this book on the premise that when you give the body what it needs, when it needs it, it will naturally gravitate toward radiant vitality and happiness. Our intention is to raise your awareness of what you need, and when, and then give you plenty of tools so that you can provide it for yourself.

CHAPTER 1

The Problem: Being Out of Touch with Our Cycles

There's a lot of lore floating around the public consciousness about a woman's menstrual cycle—mainly, that it's a monthly curse to be avoided or ignored, if possible, and endured if not. But ladies, ignoring our periods just doesn't make sense. First and foremost, it encourages us to forget that we're cyclical creatures. We're designed to have go-get-'em days and I'm-just-gonna-be-still days, get-your-butt-over-here-and-ravage-me days, and if-you-so-much-as-look-at-me-I'm-gonna-implode days. Remembering that we just aren't built to be the same from day to day is completely validating and comforting—especially on those inevitable days when we feel like a square peg in a round hole.

When we expect to feel and be the same every day, without fail, we set ourselves up for disappointment and feeling like there's something wrong with us when there's nothing wrong whatsoever. We're mutable, flexible, emotional, and dynamic beings, not automatons. When we turn a blind eye on our cycle, we cut ourselves off from ourselves. And that's a lonely place to be, with no access to our innate human-ness.

And this is not just holistic mumbo jumbo we're spouting. Dear old Aunt Flo is the source of an enormous amount of discomfort and even pain among American women of childbearing age: A whopping 85 percent of menstruating women experience PMS (per the American Congress of Obstetricians and Gynecologists).

Take a gander at the symptoms included under the PMS umbrella (also per the ACOG):

- Depression

- Angry outbursts

- Irritability

- Crying spells

- Anxiety

- Confusion

- Social withdrawal

- Poor concentration

- Insomnia

- Increased nap taking

- Changes in sexual desire

- Breast tenderness

- Bloating and weight gain

- Swelling of the hands or feet

- Aches and pains

- Fatigue

- Skin problems

- Gastrointestinal symptoms

- Abdominal pain

Aside from increased nap taking (which sounds pretty darned good), is there anything on this list that sounds tolerable to you, like, "Oh, I'm totally fine and normal, just experiencing some insomnia, pains, anxiety, and depression—just another typical day"? The fact that 85 percent of us—in this country alone—feel this way for several days out of each and every month is not normal. Nor is it okay. As they say down South, *It just ain't right.*

A whopping 85 percent of menstruating women experience PMS.

It gets worse. PMS has a bitchy older sister called premenstrual dysphoric disorder (PMDD) that afflicts between 3 to 8 percent of women of childbearing age (ages fifteen to forty-four), which is as many as five million women in the United States alone. With PMDD, the symptoms of PMS are cranked up in intensity to the point of causing dramatic impact on daily life—missed work, blowout fights with partners, or breakdowns in public.

In a 2010 *Washington Post* article, writer Anne Miller wrote about her PMDD this way: "I swell an entire dress size and try to ban my husband from any room I'm in. Deciding what to eat for dinner so overwhelms me that I've broken down crying in the frozen food section." The treatment? Either the birth control pill or Sarafem, aka Fluoxetine, aka Prozac. Which is not to make light of how hard it is to have PMDD, or bewildering, or upsetting. We can completely understand how, faced with a raging tide of hormonal symptoms every month, it would be tempting to take a pill to make it "go away." Some doctors will suggest dietary changes and/or exercising more frequently, but these are typically sweeping changes intended for consistent application throughout the month, with little regard to working in tandem with the ups and downs of the cycle that's gotten off track.

FACT: When you work with your body consistently and with sensitivity, it responds with an amazing capacity for healing and regeneration.

HOW OUR CYCLES IMPACT OUR LIVES

The negative effects of being out of touch with our cycles extend beyond PMS and the few days a month when we're, you know, actually menstruating. All aspects of our lives are affected, including our overall health and weight, reproductive health, relationships, work, and simply scheduling our busy lives. We can be so much more productive and balanced when we embrace our monthly cycle and use it to our advantage.

Health and Weight

So you already know that 85 percent of women experience PMS. Did you also know that 60 percent of adult women are overweight (according to the CDC)? Ladies, there's a connection between these two statistics. Think about it: Eating anything crunchy, salty, and fried you can get your hands on for two days every month (unless, of course, you tend more toward sweet treats) contributes to those extra pounds you can't seem to budge. They contribute calories, of course, but they also represent a throwing out the window of everything that you know to make you feel better—light workouts, nutritious food, getting to bed at a decent hour—which only perpetuates that "off" feeling. Then, the more out of whack you feel, the easier it is to make bad choices, even when you're no longer in the throes of PMS, the same way it takes you a while to ramp back up into full productivity on Mondays after two days off from work.

Being out of sync with your cycle plays an important role in keeping you in the gray area between true wellness and being sick, which is not totally a bad place to be. After all, who doesn't experience a little insomnia, constipation, or anxiety now and then? But then your particular symptom of choice starts flaring up—your migraines become more frequent, your insomnia grows more insistent, your digestive woes start impacting your activities. When this occurs, the last thing you feel like doing is exercising, and so you give up and just accept that you never feel great.

Reproductive Health

When we maintain a similar level of activity and intensity throughout the month, we take a toll on our finely tuned endocrine system (see chapter 3 for everything you always wanted to know about the symphony of hormones that regulates all the processes in your body!). Forced to work at maximum output without a periodic break, our nervous system gets stuck in a stimulated rut: Our adrenals pump out stress hormones such as adrenaline and cortisol, which then throws our other hormones out of balance, because the three major hormonal systems—the *adrenals* (which produce stress hormones), the *thyroid* (which regulates how energy is produced and consumed throughout the body), and the *sex hormones* (which regulate our cycles and fertility)—work in tandem with each other, like the three legs of a stool. If one of the legs goes off kilter, the other two go wonky, too.

From a biomechanical perspective, going out and running on the first day of your period—when your uterus weighs twice its "normal" weight—can contribute to a tilted or retroverted uterus, which can make for a more difficult passage for a fertilized egg, as well as energetic imbalances that affect your whole body.

Relationships

If you're just soldiering through your PMS without giving yourself some physical and emotional space—despite being grouchy and moody—you are most certainly taking a toll on your closest relationships. Snapping at the kids, picking fights with your partner, or getting offended by your friends' comments are all examples of how your unfulfilled—and completely natural, by the way—need for more solitude can create unnecessary drama in your life. Plus, relationships are our support system. When they are on a roller coaster, so are we.

Work

Imagine scheduling a big presentation, or a meeting to ask for a raise, on a day when all your biological processes are working to make you your most mentally sharp. Now imagine having said presentation landing on the day before or day of your period, when all you want to do is burrow under the covers. Which meeting do you think is going to be more successful?

We know you probably won't be able to call in sick or work from home every first day of your period (it would be awesome if you could; and if you have that flexibility, just try it once—you'll get hooked). But you can have an idea of how you'll be feeling on a week-by-week basis that can help you schedule what you do, and when, at work. Planning your work life with no regard to where you are in your cycle means you're making things more difficult for yourself.

Life

Kate knew it was time to keep closer tabs on her cycle when she and her husband planned their first night away from the kids in four years, and she got her period the morning of their departure.

When you're out of touch with your period, you're flying blind when you're planning your life. Then, boom—a quiet weekend away feels stifling (if you're ovulating), a party trip to Vegas feels like

Reasons to Love Your Period

- It gives you the power of arousal and desire and the ability to decide on a day-to-day basis exactly when you'd like to get it on. If we didn't have monthly cycles, we'd be like deer or other estrous animals, who all come "in heat" at only certain times of the year. (Check out Miranda Gray's book, *Red Moon,* for more information.)

- It's a permission slip from the universe to relax, bow out of obligations, and do exactly as you darn well please one to two days a month.

- The week leading up to your period—otherwise known as PMS—brings your *real* thoughts about things right up to the surface, where they can be expressed, so you can change what needs to be changed and say what needs to be said. The traditional female character traits of "being nice" and "keeping the peace" fly right out the window right on schedule each month, and as long as you honor your feelings and don't try to stuff them down with a bag of chips, you can really harness the power of pre-menstruation to take a stand for what you need.

- It makes life so interesting, giving us access to three major archetypes—Wise Woman, Mother, and Vixen—that we can channel in our behavior, activities, even clothes. It gives us permission to show up differently at different times during our cycle, encouraging us to embrace our wild side, get in touch with our inner wisdom, and focus on getting things done and taking care of others. And it means we don't have to worry about being a Wise Woman, Mother, and Vixen *all* at once. We can space out our various incarnations, and stop trying to be all things to all people, all the time. Phew.

torture (if you're PMS-ing), and a road race becomes a slog (if you've just gotten your period).

FOCUSING ON THE GOOD

Despite the alarming statistics on how our cycles are out of sync and all the ways disconnection from our very nature negatively affects our lives, the point of this book isn't to dwell on the negative. Our goal in these pages is to focus on the positive aspects of the female body: The menstrual cycle is an elaborate, magical process that gives us access to a wide range of abilities and qualities and makes us fluid, mutable creatures.

We aren't going to focus on what you shouldn't do, eat, or think. Instead, we choose to focus on which nutrients to add, new approaches to fitness to explore, and mind-body practices to embrace that will crowd out the habits and beliefs that have nudged us so far out of balance. We base everything we suggest in this book on the premise that when you give the body what it needs, when it needs it, it naturally gravitates toward radiant vitality and happiness. Our intention is to raise your awareness of what you need, and when, and then give you plenty of tools so that you can provide it for yourself.

As a result of getting cozier with your menstrual calendar, your lady parts will thank you, and you'll thank yourself when you slip into your skinny jeans, get regular flashes of insight courtesy of that forgotten feminine power—your intuition—and remember how good it feels to have your mind and body on speaking terms.

CHAPTER 2

A Little "Herstory"

Have you ever longed to stay home from work when you have your period, hanging out in your jammies, talking to your girlfriends on the phone, and just staring into space? That has pretty much been the feminine urge during that time of the month since the dawn of humankind. For thousands of years in cultures all over the world, women spent their periods away from their families and their chores in the company of other women in some form of menstrual hut. (The novel *The Red Tent,* by Anita Diamant, brings the practice to life in a way that will have you composing that e-mail to your boss about how you need to stay home on the first day of your next cycle.)

Now, we're not saying that it was all feather beds and hot baths; in some societies, the customs of menstrual seclusion were downright brutal. And yet, the guiding principle behind the approach to periods was that it was a time to rest, cleanse, be alone, spend time only with other women, get quiet, and dream.

We know that we all feel we have so much to do, but imagine for a minute not only needing to cook and clean up after each meal, but also needing to fetch the water, build the fire to heat it, grow or gather the food, grow your own flax, spin it into thread, make your own clothes, throw your own pots, cure your own meat, make your own cheese. . . . We only *think* we're busy. And yet, in days gone by, despite the incredibly high stakes of all these tasks getting done on a daily basis, women put down their hoes and parked it for a few days each month. This is because they knew that their periods were the time when they were most in need of restoration and the most tuned in to the universe.

THE GOOD OL' DAYS
Do you remember how we used to use a lunar calendar? Well, guess what's synced up with the cycles of the moon, and typically lasts as

long as a lunar month? Yep, the good ol' menstrual cycle. In fact, the word *menstruation* is derived from the Latin word for month, which also means moon. Meaning women's cycles were one of the first ways humans kept time. Think about the power of that during a time when the sun, moon, and stars were our only source of understanding where we were in space and time. When the moon moved into a new phase, the women would bleed.

Generally, women who lived in preindustrial times tended to menstruate with the new moon, because all of our hormones—the ones that regulate sleep as well as reproductive hormones—are influenced by light, and in those days the only nighttime light we experienced came via the moon. When the moon was dark, it triggered menstruation. There is a whole school of thought that you can also restore an off-kilter reproductive system and boost fertility by sleeping in total darkness three weeks out of the month and using a small night-light for one week (look up the book *Lunaception* by Louise Lacey for more information). We ladies were physical reminders of humankind's connection to the natural world and to a higher order. Powerful stuff.

Many creation myths from around the world speak to the supernatural power our ancestors attributed to women and their mysterious cycles:

- In Hinduism, the Great Mother created the universe out of her clotted "substances."

- Native South Americans believed the human race was formed out of "moon blood."

- In Mesopotamia, the goddess Ninhursag made humans out of a mixture of clay and menstrual blood.

- Even the Christian creation myth—that God created Adam out of clay—carries hints of the power given to menstrual blood. The Hebrew word *adamah*, for which Adam was named, actually means "bloody clay."

And why wouldn't ancient man give so much power to menstrual blood? Whenever it ceased flowing and accumulated, it resulted in a baby. That mysterious red stuff had the ability to create life, making it one of the most potent substances on Earth. Period. (Pardon the pun.)

It also had the ability to turn mortals into gods and goddesses. In their 2009 book *Flow: The Cultural Story of Menstruation*, authors Elissa Stein and Susan Kim detail how Taoist emperors, Egyptian pharaohs, and Celtic kings were all believed to have attained their powers by enjoying a cocktail of menstrual blood.

Period blood also made its presence felt in numerous myths, most notably in the story of Demeter, goddess of the harvest, and her daughter Persephone. One day, the young and gorgeous Persephone is out gathering flowers when Hades, the king of the underworld, sees her and instantaneously falls in lust with her. Flowers are symbols of menstrual blood in several different cultures, including India, where young girls who first start their cycles are said to have "borne the flower," and in the Bible (Leviticus 15:24). So Persephone is ripe and foxy, she is symbolically getting her first period and turning into a woman, and Hades can't resist her in that moment—also pointing toward the powerful effect menstrual blood can have (more on this in a moment). Completely overcome, Hades whisks Persephone to the underworld. When Demeter learns her baby is gone, she goes into mourning, and all the crops wither and die as the planet is plunged into winter. Eventually, Demeter manages to convince Hades to allow her darling daughter to return to the surface, but since Persephone ate pomegranate seeds (which are blood-red), she'll have to return for a few days each month to the underworld— just as all women spend a few days each month in the quiet darkness of their period.

And menstruation wasn't just heralded in myth. As Miranda Gray discusses in *Red Moon*, here on good ol' Earth, ancient Greek women held a monthly celebratory ceremony to wash their bloodied clothes and sheets. They weren't partying simply because their periods were over, but because they'd had the opportunity to be cleansed from the inside out and reborn. We can just imagine them rinsing their drapey, goddessy gowns while Aretha Franklin's "You Make Me Feel like a Natural Woman" played in the background.

THE NOT-SO-GOOD DAYS

Gradually, though, a more man-centered view of menstruation began to emerge. Aristotle, much-heralded philosopher and founder of logic and ethics, wrote in the fourth century BC in his book *On the Generation of Animals*—which went on to inspire and inform medical texts as late as the 1700s—"We should look upon the female state as being as it were a deformity." Nice, Aristotle. According to him, women played a passive role in reproduction, merely providing the soft, bloody bed for man's creation—the semen—to magically grow into a human being. He didn't know about or acknowledge the crucial role of a little something called the egg. Nope; women were never more than homemakers in Aristotle's eyes, according to Janice Delaney and her colleagues in *The Curse: A Cultural History of Menstruation.*

Aristotle's teacher, Plato, didn't have a much better grasp on lady parts. He wrote that a woman's womb wandered throughout a woman's body "in every direction." Another famous and influential Greek, Hippocrates ("the father of modern medicine"), was a little closer to the truth. He believed that a woman's period purged her of bad humors, and theorized that the blood she released each month also relieved her of toxins and other causes of disease. His theories eventually led to the practice of bloodletting in both sexes that lasted nearly a whopping two thousand years. According to Stein and Kim in *Flow,* Hippocrates also thought the womb was the source of a woman's emotions, and if it wandered too far, it could cause hysteria. Hey, what man can't understand, he makes up stories about.

Centuries later, in AD 77, Roman philosopher Pliny the Elder cataloged some of the specific evil powers ascribed to menstrual blood in his encyclopedia titled *Natural History.* Here's just a snippet: "Contact with it turns new wine sour, crops touched by it become barren, grafts die, seed in gardens are dried up, the fruit of trees falls off, the edge of steel and the gleam of ivory are dulled, hives of bees die, even bronze and iron are at once seized by rust, and horrible smell fills the air."

In a word: Geez.

But Pliny was just recording the pervading beliefs that held sway in numerous cultures throughout the world and throughout time. Here are a few examples:

The View from the East— Specifically, China

By Laurie Steelsmith, ND, author of *Great Sex, Naturally* and *Natural Choices for Women's Health*

In traditional Chinese medicine, menstrual blood is referred to as "heavenly water," or the "dew of heaven," which is a lot more poetic than our Western view—that it's solely the result of fluctuating levels of estrogen and progesterone—and certainly a far cry from the idea that the arrival of menstrual blood means you are unclean, or, worse, cursed!

Menstrual flow is believed to arise from what's known as your essence—it's vital energy that is passed down from your great-grandparents, grandparents, and parents. Essence is similar to DNA, but it's even more than that. It's also the source of your libido and your innate drive to pass your essence on to offspring. If you are menstruating, it means you have essence in abundance, which is a very good thing indeed. And when you go through menopause, according to the Chinese, it's because you are preserving your essence for yourself, to nurture your own heart and spirit, and to become a source of wisdom for your community.

When you visit an acupuncturist, doctor of traditional Chinese medicine, or naturopath, they will likely ask you about the quantity and quality of your menstrual flow, because it mirrors your overall vital force. It helps us to see where your imbalances and strengths are, by showing us how your yin (quiet, reflective, feminine) and yang (active, outward-focused, and male) energies are working together.

This view of our periods shows us that the menstrual cycle is a dance of yin and yang which is in constant flux; that we have different phases with different attributes; and that it's in our best interests to become aware of and honor where we are. When you become more conscious of your cycle, you enable your body and your mind to work at their best; it shores up your mood, your health, and your overall sense of well-being.

And that is truly heavenly.

- The Maori of New Zealand thought menstrual blood was a super-concentrated concoction of germs.

- The Mae Enga of New Guinea believed contact with a bleeding woman—not just the blood itself—could turn a man's blood black, lay waste to his flesh, drain him of his smarts, and eventually suck the life right out of him.

- The Tinne Indians of the Yukon Territory believed a menstruating woman could turn a manly man into a girlie man.

- The Bible wasn't much better, as Delaney explains in *The Curse*. Leviticus 15:19–33 makes it pretty clear that menstrual blood is supremely yucky, and any woman on her period or man who comes in contact with her, or anything she sat on, is officially "unclean," and to be kept apart from others for seven days.

BRIGHT LIGHTS IN THE DARK AGES

For centuries, the concepts outlined by early Greek philosophers and authors of the Bible pervaded society, and the fact that women hemorrhaged a toxic substance and were ruled by a wandering womb played a large part in keeping us locked in the role of second-class citizens.

Yet there were undertones of girl power in some of the most powerful stories and myths that were created and circulated during this time. Take, for example, the legend of King Arthur that flourished throughout the Middle Ages. In it, the knights of an all-powerful king sought the Holy Grail as the source of ultimate power. That grail was a cup said to have held the wine drunk by the disciples at the Last Supper, and then used to capture Jesus' blood that flowed from his wounds as he died on the cross. Many interpret that cup to symbolize the womb, and the blood in it as a symbol of menstrual blood; the power that King Arthur's knights sought was actually the feminine power of giving life and being connected to the Earth.

Fairy tales, too, refer to menstruation. Think about Snow White; she eats the red part of an apple then falls into a coma, only to be awakened by the kiss of a handsome prince. The apple represents her first period, her coma, the death of her girlhood, and her waking up, her rebirth as a woman. Same for Sleeping Beauty. When she turns fifteen, Sleeping Beauty pricks her finger on a spindle, starts bleeding, and falls asleep for a hundred years. There are messages all around us about the power of the period—the power to transform a girl into a woman, and to put her in touch with the dark side of life where being still, alone, and quiet leads to new life.

We are honored to be playing our part in raising cultural awareness of the power of the feminine cycle. If anything you read in these pages sparks an aha moment for you, please pass the information on to a friend. The more of us who are in tune with our cycles, the better off we'll be.

RECENT TIMES

Even though there were hints of the power afforded women by their monthly cycles out in the collective unconscious, for the most part, menstruation has received a bad rap for the last several hundred years. The notion of our wandering uteruses led to the concept of hysteria, which was first written about in an Egyptian text around 1900 BC, and was frequently diagnosed all the way up to the mid-twentieth century. It was recognized as a disease by the American Psychiatric Association up until 1952, right around the time "PMS" became part of the daily nomenclature. Named for the Greek word for uterus (*hystera*), "hysteria" was the diagnosis given to any woman who experienced so-called "nervous troubles," whether that was irritability, excitability, depression, or downright pissed-off-ness.

And now for the best part: For *centuries,* the treatment of choice for hysteria was for a doctor to use his hands to bring his patient to orgasm. We thank Elissa Stein and Susan Kim, authors of *Flow,* for clueing us in to this practice and its bizarre clinical approach to pleasure. As they write, "It wasn't considered sexual. In a world ruled by a heterosexual, male-oriented notion of sex (i.e., vaginal intercourse in the missionary position), stimulating someone's clitoris was considered therapeutic, and about as racy as bandaging a head wound." One good thing that did emerge from the hysteria hoopla was the birth of the vibrator: In 1883, British physician Dr. J. M. Granville debuted a mechanical "stress reliever." After thousands of years of allowing male doctors to do all the work, it only took a few decades for women to co-opt these medical devices for their own, at-home use, and, boom, the sex-toy industry was born. Thank you, wayward uterus.

Sadly, not all "cures" were so happy. For centuries, women who acted erratically were more likely to be labeled a heretic and tried as a witch than they were to be brought to climax. And by the late 1800s, when hysteria became a full-fledged epidemic among well-to-do American and European women, so did hysterectomies. Uterus giving you mood swings? Take 'er out! In the late 1800s, rates of elective hysterectomies surged—this, despite the fact that the survival rate of the surgery was a mere 50 percent. And it wasn't the ladies clamoring for their parts to be removed; it was husbands checking their wives in for the procedure. As the authors of *Flow* explain, it was "a sort of bizarre reproductive spin on the lobotomy."

Another similarly bizarre but thankfully less deadly cure for the poor, hysteria-prone woman was the rest cure, which, ironically, is close to what was really going on. These women surely needed some time away from the confines of the corset and keeping all their emotions (and organs) under tight wraps. But that led to a fashion of women taking to their daybeds, whiffing smelling salts, and looking as pale as possible. Lying around looking ghastly was the grunge fad of the day in the late 1800s. There were even ads for skin lighteners to add to the deathly pall considered so glamorous. It makes it easier to understand today's tampon commercials—with their bike-riding, mountain-climbing, hurdle-jumping women—when you know they are in response to the idea that women were meant to take to their beds with a bottle of smelling salts in order to cope with the ordeal of their periods.

DAWN BEGINS TO BREAK

Things started to change at the turn of the twentieth century, when the first disposable pad was invented. Before this exciting 1896 development, women used moss, cotton, or rags as homemade pads and tampons. Some historians even suggest that most women on Earth didn't use any kind of "feminine protection" at all—they simply bled into their clothes. (Check out the online resource The Museum of

Menstruation for more bloody details.) Those first pads were daunting contraptions, complete with pins and belts. When you consider the complicated clothing of the day with all their stays and laces, women weren't exactly skipping down the street with freedom. But hey, at least they didn't have to worry about stains.

The first tampons ambled along in the early 1930s. And although we don't think tampons are the best choice for absorbing menstrual flow from a physiological perspective (more on this in chapter 4), we can definitely understand how liberating their arrival was for women at this time. Speaking of liberating, tampons and a woman's right to vote came into being within a year of each other. Coincidence?

The authors of *Flow* tell us that pads lost their belts in 1970 (just in time for the debut of the Equal Rights Amendment), and later in that decade came the first television ads for pads and tampons, which had been banned by the National Association of Broadcasters until 1972. But it wasn't until 1985 that the word *period* was uttered in a TV commercial—by Courteney Cox, no less.

Today, tampon commercials show women taking on the world with no one the wiser that she happens to be bleeding. Some birth control now makes it possible for you to forgo your period altogether.

So we've gone from doing nothing during our periods to doing everything, from building our activities around our cycles to pretending that our cycles don't exist. Buddhists advocate a Middle Path—avoiding extremes to find a happy medium. While we acknowledge all the hardships our periods have exposed women to over the millennia, we also know that completely abolishing it isn't the answer. We also advocate a happy medium of honoring our cycles while still being able to function and thrive in the modern world.

And our final lesson from history: Until very recently, the vast majority of women spent a fraction of the time actively menstruating than we do today. Frequent pregnancies—the average number of children per family was seven to ten as recently as 1800, and that doesn't account for miscarriages and stillbirths—and extended periods of breastfeeding meant women had ten to fifteen years' worth of fewer menstrual cycles than we currently have today. And just as we are having more periods than ever before, we are also pretending they don't exist to such an extent that we are actively exploring doing away with them altogether.

Our cycles carry a rich legacy of power that we deserve to explore and embrace. Furthermore, women have suffered and been persecuted either directly or indirectly because of their cycles, and our making peace with menstruation would go a long way toward healing some of the bad juju that's been aimed at women. The more we know, the more informed our decisions will be; and the more we can model a healthy relationship with our cycles for our daughters, the more positive of an impact we can have on the future of femininity.

> Our cycles carry a rich legacy of power that we deserve to explore and embrace.

CHAPTER 3

Your Exquisite Reproductive System

Mother Nature created a masterpiece when she designed a woman's monthly cycle. The choreography between the glands, hormones, kidneys, red blood cells, the ligaments that support the womb, the uterus, and the ovaries is jaw-dropping. The entire body is involved; even bones are hormone receptors. Ladies, we are physical manifestations of pure genius from head to toe, and this chapter's aim is to enthusiastically enlighten you on our internal awesomeness.

THE ENDOCRINE SYSTEM

Each month, our bodies produce an incredible symphony. While every part of the body has a role in this masterpiece, there is one head honcho that needs its own special shout-out, and that's the endocrine system. It bosses the rest of the body around like nobody's business.

At first glance, the endocrine system is just a group of tiny glands scattered across the head, neck, and torso, but don't let their size fool you. These glands secrete vital hormones into the bloodstream, and these hormones—to put it bluntly—can make or break us. When health is even slightly compromised, the hypothalamus, for example, may send out incomplete information to the pituitary gland, which causes the release of too little or too many (or the wrong formula altogether) hormones. This immediately interferes with the balance of the whole body. Reproductively speaking, an imbalance might manifest as irregular period lengths, overwhelming PMS, early menopause, or infertility. Weight-wise, symptoms of an imbalance could be an inability to drop weight even when you are exercising your day away like a contestant on *The Biggest Loser.*

The almighty endocrine system is precisely why the 28 Days Lighter Diet tackles female reproductive health along with weight

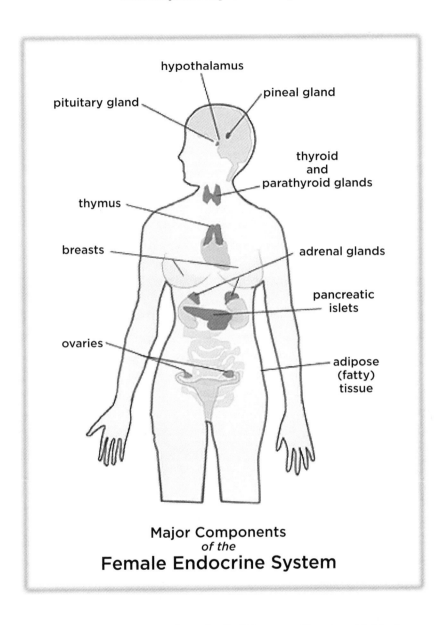

hypothalamus

pineal gland

pituitary gland

thyroid
and
parathyroid glands

thymus

breasts

adrenal glands

pancreatic
islets

ovaries

adipose
(fatty)
tissue

Major Components
of the
Female Endocrine System

management. It governs them both. We avow: Create a highly functional endocrine system and watch your menstrual cycle flow with ease, and, simultaneously, watch the battle of the bulge enter a ceasefire.

FACT: Women experience endocrine system abnormalities more frequently than men. Two of the top endocrine disorders in America are thyroid diseases and osteoporosis, both of which have been labeled "female" disorders, because women are up to eighty times more likely to suffer from them.

The Thyroid

You've probably heard a little something about the butterfly-shaped thyroid gland located in the lower front of the neck. Perhaps a coworker, sister, or neighbor has vaguely said, "I have a problem with my thyroid." In the United States, thyroid problems are increasing at epidemic rates. According to the American Association of Clinical Endocrinologists (AACE), approximately twenty-seven million Americans are currently experiencing a thyroid disorder, and about 50 percent of these people are undiagnosed. Yet with or without a thyroid condition, the truth is that most women don't understand how the thyroid gland affects the body as a whole.

The thyroid manufactures the hormones triiodothyronine (T3) and thyroxine (T4). These hormones influence the metabolism of each and every cell; they help the body use energy, stay warm, and for women, regulate the menstrual cycle. This is precisely why problems with weight and problems with menstruation often go hand in hand. The 28 Days Lighter Diet addresses weight woes and period problems, in huge part, by helping the thyroid function like the all-star it's supposed to be. In our program, we support overall endocrine function through exercise, diet, and lifestyle strategies. There are NO negative side effects. Our solution is not mere weight loss—it's *lasting* weight loss *and* reproductive wellness.

> Our solution is not mere weight loss—it's lasting weight loss and reproductive wellness.

Remember that the endocrine system, including its thyroid, plays a key role in our weight loss and wellness strategy. In upcoming chapters we lay out the steps to a healthy endocrine system, but now, let's dive into the main messengers of the endocrine system: hormones.

Most Weight-Loss Strategies Ignore the Powers of the Endocrine System

Traditional dieting wisdom maintains that losing weight is all about burning more calories than you consume. According to this thinking, eat less and move more, and weight loss is inevitable. (Imagine a loud buzzing sound here.) Wrong! After working with thousands of women over the years, we've watched some women "do everything correctly" but still struggle with weight. "Calories in/out" may be true for a fifteen-year-old, but not necessarily for a forty-five-year-old with a compromised thyroid.

Kate experienced this herself. Two years after having her son, her baby belly wasn't budging, despite her moderate intake of healthful foods. And feeling like she needed a nap every afternoon wasn't exactly inspiring her to amp up her exercise intensity. So she visited a naturopath, who gave her a physical exam, felt her thyroid, listened to an exhaustive list of symptoms, and prescribed one supplement for thyroid support (heavy on the iodine) and a gluten-free diet (gluten can be antagonistic to the thyroid). Two months later, Kate was down eight pounds, she no longer felt like she ran out of gas every afternoon, and she stopped getting hammered by every virus her kids brought into the house. The pounds have stayed off, and she still feels so much better without gluten that she's continued to eat wheat-free—except for rare trips to the coal-fired pizza place with the kids every couple of months.

Hormones 101

Each of the four phases in the menstrual cycle is characterized by unique and identifiable changes in the body, which are the result of hormonal communication between organs. When most of us hear the word *hormones,* we think raging PMS, bodybuilders on steroids, and teenage acne. In fact, hormones reside in all living mammals, all of the time—young or old, male or female. In science, hormones are considered any material that travels through the bloodstream from one organ to another with the purpose of altering that second organ's action. "Hormone" comes from the Greek work *hormone,* which means "to stir up," and they do just that, by:

- Stimulating or inhibiting growth

- Regulating the metabolism

- Controlling the reproductive cycle

- Causing specific food cravings

- Preparing the body for a new phase of life, such as puberty, pregnancy, and menopause

- Triggering sexual arousal

- Influencing mood swings

- Activating a fight-or-flight response

Hormones are always present and always fluctuating. "The only constant in life is change" is especially true with hormones. Acne and PMS aren't signs of hormones as much as they are symptoms of hormonal *fluctuation.* Estrogen rises and falls, progesterone comes and goes. Such is life.

See page 23 for a chart of the monthly hormone dance.

Many clients come to us thinking that women have estrogen and men have testosterone, but it's more complicated than that. Both women and men have an array of hormones, and each sex has both the "masculine" testosterone and the "feminine" estrogen. Yes, men have more testosterone and women have more estrogen—that much is true. The higher levels of testosterone in men lead to denser muscle development. Our higher levels of estrogen give us increased muscle pliability. To be healthy, women should have much less testosterone than men, and men should have less amounts of estrogen, but both genders have both hormones.

However, there are many more hormones than these two well-known players. Menstruating women of the world have a whole mix of hormones circulating in their bloodstream at any given time. Six of these hormones make our "must-know-about" list, as they serve as the main chemical messengers for female reproduction.

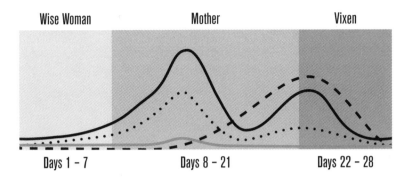

Estrogen	———
Progesterone	— — — —
Testosterone Produced	· · · · · · · · · ·
Testosterone Perceived	~~~~~~~~~~~~~~

1. **Gonadotropin-releasing hormone (GnRH)**
   Produced in hypothalamus
   Surges just before ovulation, responsible for the release of
   FSH and LH hormones
2. **Follicle-stimulating hormone (FSH)**
   Produced by pituitary gland
   Causes monthly ovulation, and also regulates puberty
3. **Luteinizing hormone (LH)**
   Produced by pituitary gland
   Together with FSH, triggers ovulation
4. **Estrogen**
   Produced by the ovaries (mostly)
   Promotes the thickening of the uterine lining

5. **Progesterone**
   Produced by the ovaries and adrenal glands
   Prevents the release of all other eggs for that cycle, causes
   the uterine lining to thicken, and changes the cervical
   position
6. **Testosterone**
   Secreted by the ovaries mostly, but a small amount comes
   from the adrenal glands
   Believed to increase sex drive and help the body build and
   maintain bones and muscles

This chapter touches on hormones in relation to two things: our reproductive system, and women's wellness. Let it be known, however, that just about every coming and going in your body, from the temperature of your nose to the growth of your fingernails, is regulated by these chemical messengers.

THE MONTHLY DANCE

When Ellen first read *Taking Charge of Your Fertility,* you'd have thought she was reading *Fifty Shades of Grey.* She couldn't put the damn book down! Aghast at the words on the page, she thought, *Why am I thirty-three years old and learning about this for the first time?* And, *Nobody I know knows this!!* She really thought menstruation was the five or so days of bleeding that occur each month and nothing else. The cervix changes? Different types of mucus? Whoa . . . A mix of awe and discovery filled her being. The moral of the story, ladies: Don't wait until you are trying to have a baby to understand your body (or, it's never too late to understand your body).

> *Many of us know more about the workings of our car than we do the reproductive cycle.*
>
> —Jeannine Parvati Baker in *Conscious Conception*

Let's start by looking at the organs involved in the menstrual cycle. While hormones are "everywhere," organs are specific locales where specific things happen throughout the month.

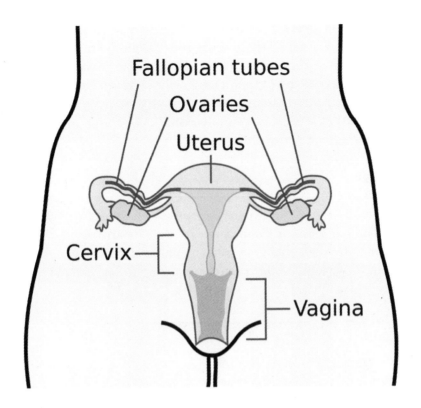

Two Ovaries

The ovaries flank the uterus and are important for two key reasons: 1) They are the source of eggs; and 2) They release estrogen and progesterone, which control the menstrual cycle. Did you know that when a baby girl is born, she already has about 1,000,000 ovarian follicles?

The Uterus and Cervix

These organs sit centrally in the pelvis, at the top of the vagina, supported by strong fibrous structures called ligaments. These ligaments are attached in turn to the bones of the pelvis. They are sufficiently elastic to allow them to stretch considerably during pregnancy and then return to their former size afterwards. The uterus is the womb, or, as the ancient Chinese called it, "the womb palace." The cervix is the opening to the womb.

Two Fallopian Tubes

Ancient Chinese called these tubes the "golden pathways," as they run from the ovaries to the uterus and allow the passage of the egg from the ovary to the uterus. This is where the sperm and egg are most likely to meet! There are little hair-like structures lining the tubes called cilia. With a gentle waving motion, the cilia help to move the egg along its pathway.

The Vagina

This passage leads from the opening of the vulva to the top of the cervix and is crucial in sexual intercourse and childbirth. We are all most familiar with the vagina since it's the one area we can kind of see and definitely touch. The other female reproductive organs are hidden from view. As Miranda in *Sex and the City* said, "What's the big mystery? It's my vagina, not the Sphinx."

THE THREE PHASES OF MENSTRUATION

Phase I (Days 1–7): Menstruation
Low estrogen and low progesterone

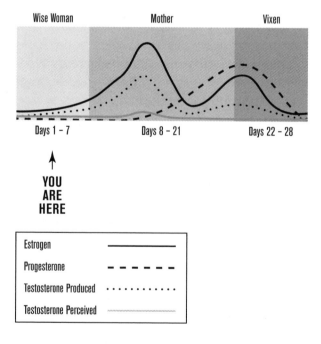

Estrogen	——————
Progesterone	– – – – –
Testosterone Produced	· · · · · · · · · · ·
Testosterone Perceived	~~~~~~~~~~~

Menstruation (your period) is Phase I of the menstrual cycle. Most periods can last from one to eight days, with the average being three to five days. On Day 1, the hypothalamus and the pituitary gland—both of which are situated in the brain—signal the ovaries (both of which are endocrine glands as well as reproductive organs) to stop their production of estrogen and progesterone. That steep decline of estrogen and progesterone signals the uterus to start shedding its lining and results in menstruation.

FACT: Menstrual blood isn't just blood; it's also made up of uterine lining (endometrium), mucus, and toxins exiting the body.

Estrogen and progesterone levels are at their lowest at the onset of menstruation. By Day 2, estrogen starts creeping its way back up, but levels of both hormones are still minuscule throughout this phase. Because of the "double low" hormone combo, other things are happening in the body, too:

- **The Cervix "Drops"**
  It literally moves down, closer to the vagina. It becomes denser, too, making it feel hard. It dilates slightly to allow for menstrual fluid to flow. Some experts believe this positioning is Mother Nature's way of deterring sexual intercourse, as sex can be uncomfortable for many women at this time of the month. (Although plenty of women feel sexy and free now that the premenstrual week is over. We say, whenever you feel like getting it on is a good time!)

- **The Uterus Contracts**
  The uterus has been compared to the moon—it enlarges as the cycle progresses, and during menstruation it shrinks and wanes. Contractions help slough off the lining, kind of like squeezing out a sponge. These contractions contribute to menstrual cramping.

- **Body Temperature Is Low**

   There are two parts to this: One, blood is circulating strongly in your womb area, pulling blood away from the extremities, and two, the lack of hormones affects circulation—a double whammy for body temperature.

Quirks of Phase I

Breath Could Be Stinky. Does anyone have a mint? It's very common to notice bad breath only during your period. This is due to hormones altering the gums, making them more hospitable to bad breath–causing bacteria.

Body Odor Could Be Stinky, Too! Shortly before menstruation, estrogens are at their highest levels in the cycle. Now, the liver has to work hard to break down and eliminate the extra hormones. As a result, it taxes the liver, causing the bad smell coming out of our pores.

Ouch! There's an Increased Sensitivity to Pain. There is an inverse relationship here: When estrogen and progesterone are low, our pain sensitivity is high. Sensitivity to pain is especially obvious on Day 1.

Phase II, Part 1 (Days 8–14): The Mega Phase

Estrogen and FSH rises, testosterone shows up, progesterone lies low

Phase II, a "growth" phase, is all about the estrogen, baby! The increased level of estrogen starts building up the lining of the uterus with a thick blanket of blood vessels that will support a fertilized egg should pregnancy occur. FSH levels rise, causing maturation of several ovarian follicles and the size of the eggs to triple. While the eggs are still positioned inside the ovary, they are very close to "breaking" out.

- **An Egg Is Almost Ready to Release**

   An egg in one of your ovaries is about to reach maturity, quadrupling in size to a whopping .0005 centimeters. Although

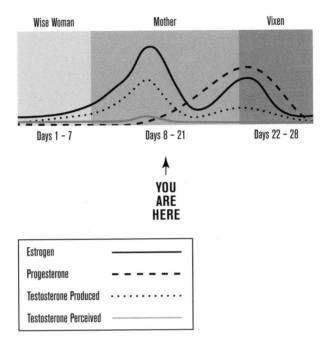

only one egg (usually) fully matures each cycle, somewhere between ten and twenty follicles begin the process of maturation monthly.

- **Cervix Secretes Mucus and Starts to Soften**
  Estrogen lubricates and moistens the vagina for two reasons: The obvious one is to ease sexual intercourse and smooth the passage of any sperm that manage to find their way into the vagina, but it also helps to protect it from infection.

Quirks of Phase II, Part 1

You're Feeling Frisky! Your sex drive is back! Testosterone in women is Mother Nature's way of getting females interested in sex so the species can go on. Plus, increased estrogen makes for happier, more-extroverted moods.

Phase II, Part 2 (Days 15–21): Mega Phase

Estrogen swerves to high point, then dips a bit; testosterone peaks; and progesterone starts its steady ascent

Phase II, Part 2 begins with surges in luteinizing hormone (LH) and follicle-stimulating hormone (FSH) levels. The luteinizing hormone stimulates egg release (ovulation), which usually occurs sixteen to thirty-two hours after the surge begins. The estrogen level peaks smack-dab amidst the surge, and the progesterone level starts to increase. (Pretty awesome coordination, right? It's like Tom Cruise's *Mission Impossible* team.) The cervix is higher and softer (ideal for sexual intercourse). On or around Day 16, estrogen dips, causing a mini-PMS for approximately four days.

Progesterone is produced by the ovaries and works to prepare the body for pregnancy by thickening the lining of the uterus. If pregnancy occurs, the body continues to create progesterone until the placenta has developed to the point that it can take over. If pregnancy does not take place, progesterone levels drop and menstruation occurs.

- **The Ovary Releases an Egg**
  Otherwise known as ovulation! The egg or ovum only lives for a maximum of twenty-four hours without fertilization.

- **The Cervix SHOWs**
  It's soft, high, open, and wet. This is one of the ways women can tell they are in a fertile time of the month.

- **Body Temperature Peaks**
  Aaahhhh, warmth! Body temperature is at its monthly high because of extra thyroid hormones pumping through your veins.

- **Cervical Mucus Is Wet, Slippery, and Sticky**
  Another sign it's your fertile window. The mucus resembles egg whites.

Quirks of Phase II, Part 2

You're Hungrier! Progesterone increases your appetite. A Tufts University study showed that when progesterone levels increase in the female body, so does appetite, by 12 percent.

Phase III (Days 22–28): Pre-Menstruation

Estrogen and testosterone descend while progesterone soars

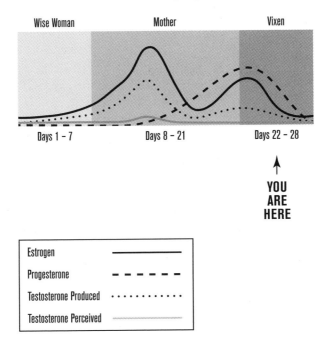

Estrogen	————
Progesterone	— — — — —
Testosterone Produced	· · · · · · · · · · ·
Testosterone Perceived	~~~~~~~~~~~

During Phase III, levels of LH and FSH decrease. The ruptured follicle closes after releasing the egg and forms a corpus luteum, a yellowish mass of endocrine tissue, which produces progesterone. Later in this phase, the estrogen level increases. Progesterone and estrogen cause the lining of the uterus to thicken more. If the egg is not fertilized, the corpus luteum degenerates and no longer produces progesterone, the estrogen level decreases, the lining degenerates and is shed, and a new menstrual cycle begins. Progesterone levels shoot up. This increases after an ovary releases an egg (ovulation) at the middle of the cycle.

- **The Uterus Is Heavy**
  It's thicker, filled with vascular blood vessels, and weighs four times more than it did on the day your period ended.

- **Your Body Is Retaining Water**
  You can thank progesterone for this one. Water retention and swollen breasts are progesterone's way of preparing the body for a growing fetus. Another effect of progesterone that adds to a bloated sensation is the slowing down of food moving through the intestinal tract, so that more nutrients can be "pulled" from the food, improving the well-being of mother and child. (Many women think that bloating is "bad" and a sign of PMS, but actually it should occur—in a moderate, *not* debilitating level—every month.)

Quirks of Phase III

You Crave Solitude. In recent decades, several studies concluded that women are more inner-focused this time of the month and less interested in socializing, thanks to the decline of estrogen.

The decline of progesterone, along with estrogen's already low amounts, causes the uterine lining to break down. And, ta-da! It's Day 1 again, unless of course the egg was fertilized. In that case, you're pregnant and can say good-bye to your period for a while.

GROUNDHOG DAY?

For some women, every cycle is predictably true-blue, making Day 1 feel like déjà vu all over again. Of course, little "blips," like when your period is a day or two early or late, are no big deal, and studies show that things like seasonal shifts in weather, light exposure, and diet can cause alterations to one's flow. However, what about when every cycle is unpredictable? One cycle lasts 15 days, the next is 45 days. Sometimes you experience debilitating PMS, sometimes it's pain-free. What about when you bleed for over a week? Aside from

Favorite Word of the Chapter: Homeostasis

Homeostasis—in Latin, *homeo,* meaning "same," and *stasis,* meaning "condition"—refers to physical balance. When the endocrine system achieves this, the body runs like clockwork.

Okay, so you have a zany menstrual cycle; what now? Well, logic directs us to seek out an ob/gyn. Surely, he or she will solve this problem. So in you go, reporting your symptoms to the good doctor. Most of the time, your gynecologist will pull out her prescription pad and scribble out an order for birth control pills. She may ask if you smoke (because smoking and The Pill are a very bad combo), but somewhere in the conversation, The Pill will be called a "regulator" for cycles run amok. (Let it be known: There are other ways of regulating your cycle.)

being inconvenient, an erratic cycle is worrisome. Something must be askew, right? Not to get too new age-y on you, but the sisterhood of yore called the menstrual cycle "the moon cycle" for a reason. The moon is pretty darn consistent. Here is something to ponder:

Every month the moon transitions from a new moon (phase I) to a waxing moon (phase II, part 1), then to a full moon (phase II, part 2), and finally to a waning moon (phase III) before becoming a new moon once again. This lunar cycle, from new moon to new moon, takes 28 days to complete. Directly related to this is the fact that, on average, a woman's menstrual cycle is 28 days. Coincidence? Nope. We are the only lunar primate on Earth!

THE BIRTH CONTROL PILL

Originally intended to prevent pregnancy, The Pill is now prescribed to women for other reasons, too, such as regulating the menstrual cycle or clearing up acne. Approximately 11.6 million women 15 to 44 years of age use The Pill for contraceptive purposes (NSFG, 2002), and an additional 1.5 million women rely on The Pill for non-contraceptive purposes (Guttmacher Institute, 2011). *That's over 13 million of us!* As a form of birth control, The Pill's aim is to override Mother Nature and stop ovulation. The rationale: If no egg is released, there is nothing to be fertilized by sperm, and the woman cannot get pregnant.

FACT: The FDA regulates birth control medications. It also considers ketchup a vegetable.

Birth control pills contain synthetic (i.e., fake) forms of two female hormones: estrogen and progesterone. These synthetic hormones "flat-line" a woman's natural hormone levels by preventing a mid-cycle estrogen peak. Without the increased estrogen level, the pituitary gland does *not* induce other hormonal processes that normally cause the ovaries to release mature eggs. Meanwhile, synthetic progesterone works to stop the pituitary gland from producing LH, making the uterine lining inhospitable to a fertilized egg.

In a nutshell, we think doctors prescribe The Pill too lightly, and many women think it's no big deal. In our opinion, the cons outweigh the pros *most of the time.*

Birth Control Pills Deplete Nutrients

A study published in *Obstetrics and Gynecology International* in August 2010 showed that women who used hormonal birth control for at least four months had significantly less coenzyme Q10, vitamin E, and total antioxidants than women who did not use hormonal birth control.

Other studies have shown that oral contraceptives can deplete many of the B vitamins, including B6, B12, and folic acid; vitamin C; magnesium; calcium; selenium; and zinc. Nutritional deficiency is a catastrophe in our opinion because it leads to long-term health consequences. And considering many people using birth control have a diet that is far from ideal, the problems associated with nutritional deficiency are compounded.

There Are Scary Side Effects

There is a long list of common side effects with taking birth control pills. The typical ones include nausea, breast tenderness, weight gain, and changes in mood. However, if you take a closer look at the

Safety of The Pill

Let it be known that we support Planned Parenthood and a woman's right to safe and effective birth control. Along with all this Pill-bashing, we want to clarify: We love Gloria Steinem, the women's movement, *Ms.* magazine, and sexual liberation. We just question the true safety of The Pill, and feel that other birth control options should be explored. Family planning is a sensitive issue, one that you must discuss with your partner and your health practitioner.

So yeah, The Pill is effective at preventing pregnancy, but at what cost? *The Pill: Are You Sure It's For You?* by Jane Bennett and Alexandra Pope is a must-read if you want to know all the nitty-gritty details for yourself.

drug index, you'll see a number of "scarier" side effects, including blood clots, heart attack, stroke, gallbladder disease, visual disturbances, and high blood pressure, as well as increased risk of liver, cervical, and breast cancer.

There Is One Ultra-Scary Side Effect

In 2005, the World Health Organization changed their stance on The Pill from "possibly carcinogenic" to "carcinogenic to humans," making the birth control pill a Class 1 carcinogen, same as tobacco and asbestos. This news is terrifying because so many women are unaware of it, and it's also hopeful because it means the WHO is taking a stand. Birth control pills now are what smoking was forty years ago—commonplace and accepted. In the future, maybe the dangers of The Pill will become as obvious as cigarettes are now.

EASTERN WELLNESS CONCEPTS EMBRACED
IN THE 28 DAYS LIGHTER DIET

We like to think we take the best of the West and the best of the East for the best women's wellness plan possible. Western science, like Harvard Medical School, for example, has given us hard-core proof as well as cutting-edge procedures that save lives. Thanks to the

West, we have conclusive research, much of which is cited within the pages of this book. These unshakable physical facts help us to better understand the human body.

But, we love, love, love Eastern medicine just as much. The Eastern way, like the theories found in traditional Chinese medicine, gives us ways of seeing the body that unite us with nature and the universe as a whole. Below are some big Eastern themes we've adopted in this book.

There Is No Beginning or End

Our menstrual cycle is a *cycle*—a circle. Like all circles, there is no real beginning and no real end. For instructional purposes we label the first day of menstruation "Day 1," even though that's not completely accurate. Life, the seasons, the chicken or the egg—these are all cycles. Inhalation or exhalation; what comes first? See what we mean?

Everything Is Connected to Everything

Nothing works in isolation. The reproductive system is a great example of this with its gland-hormone-organ symphony. The body isn't isolated from the mind either. We go to a dermatologist for a skin rash even though the rash is caused by a psychotic lapse (see below).

Once in her life, Ellen got hives. Big red welts appeared on her elbow creases, neck, and upper chest. It's not a coincidence that she was also under extreme pressure at the time; about thirty minutes prior to the breakout, she had a very stressful conversation with a boss. This is a clear-cut example of the mind/body connection at work. It is undeniable how the mind can affect the body, and it works in the other direction as well—the body can affect the mind, too.

Ho-lis-tic (adjective) [hau'listik]
1. analyzing whole system
2. considering all factors when treating illness

Diet, Exercise, and Lifestyle Changes Can Be Curative

Western doctors shy away from using the term *cure*. To cure is to "heal somebody," or "treat illness successfully," or "resolve a problem." When we have an ailment, we don't want to "manage it" or "recover from it" or "take pills forever and pretend it's not there." We want a *cure*. Eastern thought sees health as balance, so the *cure* from any disease is (to put it simply) to return to balance. Sometimes it takes months, sometimes years, but a *cure* is possible.

There's even more great news coming from the East: Not only is a cure possible, but *you* can also play a leading role in your cure by eating, moving, and living in a certain way. Your thoughts and actions can be healing tools. *You* have the power.

CHAPTER 4

The Four Golden Rules

One size doesn't fit all when it comes to diet and exercise plans, and that's true for the 28 Days Lighter Diet program, too. It is eminently customizable to your body on any given day of your cycle. However, there are four universal laws that apply no matter what. We call them the Golden Rules. If you've been through puberty but haven't yet experienced menopause, these are your go-to guidelines for fitness, weight management, and total feminine wellness.

GOLDEN RULE #1: IMPLEMENT A CYCLE-TO-CYCLE SCHEDULING STRATEGY

When you plan week to week, you may be factoring in work responsibilities and daily logistics, but you're probably not considering your female physiology. Your body doesn't know the difference between Wednesday and Sunday, but it certainly knows the difference between ovulation and pre-menstruation. The strenuous spin class that felt so great this Monday at six p.m. can be downright irritating next Monday.

Why? We'll cover this more fully in just a few pages, but during ovulation, you are extroverted and raring to go. Just a week later, during pre-menstruation, your focus turns inward and your uterus grows heavy, meaning you need steady—not strenuous—exercise, and much more time for meditation.

When you go on a diet program that claims you can lose ten pounds in ten days, it doesn't take into consideration that those ten days may fall on a menstrual phase of increased estrogen, which in turn increases water retention and completely sabotages your ability to drop any weight at all, much less ten pounds. The female body changes from week to week, and traditional diet and workout programs never acknowledge this phenomenon, much less take advantage of it.

Put Your Scale into the Cycle, Too

Just say *no* to weighing yourself every day. Even once a week won't give you a truly accurate portrayal. Instead, weigh yourself the same day of each cycle (i.e., every Day 3). You'll get a much more accurate reading, especially if you are tracking weight loss.

We know this to be true: The monthly cycle rarely falls neatly into man-made weekly schedules. So when we stop allowing the calendar to dictate when we perform our wellness activities, we can let our bodies lead the way. By using the menstrual cycle as the foundation from which all things build upon, you'll know exactly what your body and mind need, and exactly the times they'll need it. To start implementing this rule, you'll need to know how long your cycle is (in general), how long each phase is (approximately), and most important, how you feel every step of the way. Prepare to discover this vital information so you can begin putting Golden Rule #1 into effect.

The female body changes from week to week, and traditional diet and workout programs never acknowledge this phenomenon, much less take advantage of it.

The How, What, and When of Your Cycle

The menstrual cycle provides you with a road map to your highs and lows, strengths and vulnerabilities, moods and capabilities. Have you noticed that on certain days, you feel heavier, as if gravity were actually stronger? Or felt that some days you have an abundance of social stamina? Or were impervious to cold one day, only to be shivering in the same conditions a few days later? These are all results of where you are in your cycle. In order to hear the information your body is trying to communicate and give yourself what you need, when you need it, you have to take the time to listen to it. Go get a pen! It's time to start discovering what truly makes you tick.

The Energy Wheel: Know It, Use It, Love It, Live It

For at least one cycle (although we daresay you'll love the info and insight it offers, and will keep going!), from Day 1 to Day 1, chart your energy levels using the handy-dandy Energy Wheel. This is not a diary, so don't write about your secret crushes; instead, write how and what you feel in terms of body/mind/spirit energy.

We've created a sample Energy Wheel below, and there's a blank template for you to use (Appendix A, page 191). There is space for you to jot down specific food cravings, moods, levels of fatigue, workout mode, and so on. Make note of when you are bloated; when you're experiencing back pain, a headache, or breast tenderness; as well as

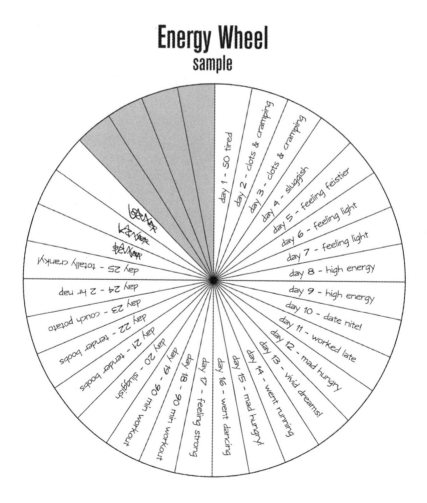

Energy Wheel
sample

day 1 - SO tired
day 2 - clots & cramping
day 3 - clots & cramping
day 4 - sluggish
day 5 - feeling feistier
day 6 - feeling light
day 7 - feeling light
day 8 - high energy
day 9 - high energy
day 10 - date nite!
day 11 - worked late
day 12 - mad hungry
day 13 - vivid dreams!
day 14 - went running
day 15 - mad hungry!
day 16 - went dancing
day 17 - feeling strong
day 18 - 90 min workout
day 19 - 90 min workout
day 20 - sluggish
day 21 - tender boobs
day 22 - tender boobs
day 23 - couch potato
day 24 - 2 hr nap
day 25 - totally cranky!

when you're feeling light and eager to move. Also write down where you're falling on the introverted-extroverted spectrum. This is also a great place to note when you have vivid dreams. You'll likely discover that they accompany specific parts of your cycle each month.

When Kate started tracking her cycles using the Energy Wheel, she was amazed to discover that her first twinges of breast tenderness showed up on Day 22 of her cycle, just like clockwork, even though her cycles lasted between 28 and 30 days. She also noticed that she dreamt a lot more around ovulation and menstruation, and that she could pinpoint her period's arrival by the major energy dip that always came eight to twelve hours before. We may be constantly fluctuating, when you look at it on a day-to-day basis, but month to month, we really do travel a pretty predictable path. Wow.

Kate also loves how using the Energy Wheel on a regular basis really captures what her daily life is like, way better than any planner or journal could. Imagine having a year's worth of Energy Wheels to look back and reflect on; when someone rhetorically asks, *Where does the time go?* you'll be able to grasp your bundle of Energy Wheels and know exactly what that time felt and looked like. Shazam.

Keeping track of how you feel is important on two levels: Noticing how you actually feel on a day-to-day basis helps you to tune in to your experience, and putting it all down on paper gives you objectivity. Both points of view will help you to create the most accurate get-fit plan.

The "data" you collect will help you to understand the inner workings of your body, and how they in turn affect everything from your weight and workout choices to your social interactions and thought processes. From this point forward, you'll be able to work *with* your energy—not against it—as you become sensitive to the subtle and not-so-subtle workings of your hormones, and you'll be better able to hear your intuition.

Wellness Intuition

We've all heard a version of the story where a guy is supposed to get on a certain plane but at the last minute, feeling creeped-out, decides against it. Thirty minutes later, the plane crashes over the

One Caveat: Birth Control Pills

If you are taking birth control pills, your body is held in a state that replicates pre-menstruation (see chapter 7) for most of your cycle. Keep this in mind while journaling. You might not have the same variety of entries as someone not on The Pill, and the length of your cycle will be very predictable. Journal anyway! It will still help you to become more intuitive.

Pacific with no survivors. The guy calls his wife to tell her he's alive and that he didn't get on the plane because it didn't "feel right."

This is an extreme example of intuition at work. Our society expects intuition to come into play only during big moments, such as when we're choosing a mate, or in a life-or-death situation. While these stories are exciting, intuition works for the little moments, too: choosing what workout to do, deciding what to eat, and determining when you should go out or when it's best to catch up on rest.

We think of intuition as making decisions from the inside out—not relying solely on external circumstances, but trusting hunches, gut feelings, and insights that arise seemingly from out of the blue. When you apply your intuition to making fitness, diet, and lifestyle choices, you stop relying on experts or best-selling diet books—which ultimately only disconnect you from your internal experience, and disempower you from making long-term changes—to help you decide, and instead, start trusting your body and your truest self.

There are two steps to following your intuition: taking the time to hear what your inner voice (which resides in the body, not the mind) has to say, and then trusting it enough to heed its advice. It sounds easy enough, yet most of us don't take the time to listen to our bodies, much less use our intuition for wellness purposes. Charting your energy levels throughout your cycle, via the Energy Wheel, will start to change that!

Meditation also helps. And before you get freaked out by the idea of meditating, know that we use the term loosely. We know that just reading the word *meditation* brings up images of sitting cross-legged in a quiet room, chanting *Ommmm* . . . very yogic. It also elicits a touch of guilt, because most everyone in America knows that they'd benefit from a little meditation. So why don't we do it? Why do we clean out our sock drawer, browse the app store, or (Ellen's favorite) take a nap instead?

Well, we actually do meditate. Yep, even you. And it's pretty painless—even fun. We just need to do it more often. Throughout this book, Kate, a bona fide chill-out expert, offers meditation techniques that are doable and pertinent to each phase of your cycle, but here, under Golden Rule #1, we want to emphasize this: *Meditation takes many forms.* Not everyone has to do it like the Buddha. Every moment of your day can be a meditative opportunity.

> *Meditation* (noun): to think or reflect, especially in a calm and deliberate manner.

They say the best things in life are free, and that's certainly true about our favorite ways of meditating.

Ellen's top three:
1. Hike in the woods with just my dog.
2. Knit by myself while listening to classical music.
3. Watch the sun set.

Kate's top three:
1. Spend five minutes in Child's Pose.
2. Sweep.
3. Cook (when I can manage to chase the kids out of the kitchen).

The biggest gift meditation brings is the awareness that no one—not even Dr. Oz—knows what's best for you more than you. *You are the leading expert on YOU.* Yet if you don't take enough time to access your intuition, you doubt your own expertise. This is great news for the guru industry, but bad news for you and your destiny as a vibrant woman of the world! That's why we champion energy charting and meditation—a double whammy for building intuition.

So what does this have to do with your cycle? Well, most weight-loss ventures are based on following outside information. People eat the wrong foods, do the wrong exercises, and basically go against their energy levels for days, weeks, even months at a time. This is not only damaging to the body/mind/spirit, but it's also not sustainable. At some point, your body will crash, and you'll either get sick, or get tired of following someone else's rules, or both. And then you'll gain back all the weight. It's a roller coaster where the end result is feeling like a failure, guaranteed.

On our program, Mother Nature is the guru. In essence, she tells you what to do. We (Ellen and Kate) are merely the messengers, telling you that there's another path you can follow—one that *feels so good,* you'll want to continue it even when the PMS is gone and your weight is perfect. It's a sustainable way of life, not just a diet.

Fitness Should Feel Good

The concept of "No pain, no gain" is so twentieth-century. Losing weight and staying well doesn't have to hurt. (This is hard to believe if you've been brainwashed by *The Biggest Loser.*) When you allow your body to be your guide, exercise always feels good. There is no running on heavy-flow day or bouncing on a trampoline when you feel extra bloated. Because when you're forcing yourself to do a level 10 on the elliptical, or your upper body is so fatigued after a workout that you can't drive your car home from the gym, it's the opposite of true wellness.

Here's when you know exercise has done you well:

- You have more energy *post*-workout than you had *pre*-workout.

- There is no pain or discomfort.

- Your self-talk during exercise is positive and uplifting.

- You lose track of time.

- You don't feel as though you have to "recover" from your workout.

- You are not mad hungry post-workout.

On the 28 Days Lighter path, you know what your body wants. Some days it will crave more intensity, while other days it will need to be mellow. Your cycle leads the way. When we listen to the body's whispers, exercise feels good. *Really* good.

GOLDEN RULE #2: DON'T WORK OUT ON DAY 1 (AND POSSIBLY DAYS 2 AND 3) OF YOUR PERIOD

Every other day of the month, we encourage you to get out there and exercise in some form or another, but there's no spandex allowed on the first day of your period! It's a workout Sabbath. In this chapter, we've created a self-care plan (see pages 114–19 for restorative yoga poses and meditation guidelines) as well as diet and sleep protocols, to incorporate during all of menstruation, not just Day 1. It will help to ease cramps, backaches, and other symptoms that may accompany your period. Here, under Golden Rule #2, our aim is to explain why working out during Day 1 of menstruation is detrimental to your feminine health, and why taking it easy at this point in the cycle is conducive to weight loss.

Your Body Is Already "Working Out"

A woman's basal metabolic rate starts rising by 10 percent during Phase III: Pre-menstruation, and peaks on Day 1. That amounts to burning approximately 150 extra calories a day for a woman whose metabolic output measures 1,500 calories. The bottom line: During your period, your body is hard at work—shedding the uterine lining, cleansing the reproductive system, and readying it for the next ovulatory phase. Your body temperature increases, too, as a result of the additional energy consumption. When you add exercise on top of this built-in "workout," you overtax the whole body/mind/spirit system in three basic ways:

1. Because exercise warms you up (as evidenced by your sweat), when you work out during your period, you run the

risk of overheating your system. While it's good to be warm all cycle long, there is such a thing as *too* warm. Flushed skin, shallow breathing, and dizziness all go along with too much heat.

2. Exercise pulls blood away from the womb—where it is currently needed most—and sends it to the limbs and heart. This could cause overall discomfort and interrupt menstrual flow. (It's the same way digestion pulls blood away from the brain and into the belly, meaning that eating a big meal before a big test could impair your thinking.)

3. It just doesn't feel good. There's a reason that all you want to do on Day 1 is lie on the couch: Your body is tired from the work of menstruation. Ignoring this desire for rest overrides your intuition. It's a subtle form of self-abuse, disconnecting body from spirit.

Your Uterus Is Heavy

Because the uterine lining thickens during Phase III: Premenstruation, it's at its all-time thickest and heaviest on Day 1. That places a lot of strain on the eight slender ligaments that are the only things holding the uterus in place. Put another way, too much jostling on Day 1 could contribute to misalignment of your lady parts. It also just plain doesn't feel good. If your uterus were a baby, Day 1 would be the prime time to swaddle it or carry it around in a sling—not strap it into a jogging stroller or go on a long jaunt.

Normally the uterus leans slightly over the bladder in the center of the pelvis, about one and a half inches above the pubic bone. It is held in this position by muscles, the vaginal wall, and ligaments that attach it to the back, front, and sides of the pelvis. Uterine ligaments are made to stretch to accommodate a growing fetus inside, and to move freely when the bladder or bowel is full. The ligaments and muscles can weaken and loosen, causing the uterus to fall downward, forward, backward, or to either side. A uterus in any of these positions is called *tilted,* or *prolapsed.*

In the Western medicine model, the 20 percent of women who have a prolapsed uterus are generally told, "Your uterus is tipped, but it's perfectly normal and nothing to worry about." Yet these

Surprise! Exercise Bunny (Ellen) Has a Tilted Uterus!

Ellen: My first OB appointment was at the age of eighteen. I had been playing competitive tennis and doing Jane Fonda videos since the dawn of my menstrual cycle at age twelve, so it's no coincidence that the doctor said, "You've got a tilted uterus."

"What does that mean?" I asked.

"Oh, nothing; it's just in the wrong place."

Just in the wrong place? Yikes.

women often have a laundry list of physical and emotional symptoms, from painful periods to infertility, because when reproductive organs shift, they can constrict the normal flow of blood and lymph, the waste-removal medium of the immune system, and disrupt nerve connections. Just a few extra ounces sitting on blood and lymph vessels can have repercussions throughout the different systems in the body.

To protect the alignment of your uterus, it's best to take it easy on the days when your flow is the heaviest. We'll dive more deeply into this subject in chapter 7 (Phase III: Pre-menstruation), but high-impact exercise, and even low-impact exercise (on hard surfaces) can have long-lasting, negative effects.

Your Orientation Is Inward

The magic word for Day 1 is "No." Don't overcommit. Even if it falls on a rockin' Saturday night, stay home and curl up with a good book. We'll give more tips on how to retreat during your period in chapter 5, but here, it's important for you to understand that the reason it's important to take it easy isn't just physical; it's also spiritual.

Day 1 brings with it an inward focus that is difficult to fully define, but it's there nonetheless. It's a powerful time to assess who you are, where you want to go, and what's in the way. You are a quiet force of nature on Day 1—a tsunami of intuitive power. Don't squander this strength with distractions. Stay home, find solitude, relax, and reap the rewards of not *doing,* but *being.*

Honoring the demands of our bleeding, our blood gives us something in return. The crazed bitch from irritation hell recedes. In her place arises a side of ourselves with whom we may not—at first—be comfortable. She is a vulnerable, highly perceptive genius who can ponder a given issue and take her world by storm. When we're quiet and bleeding, we stumble upon solutions to dilemmas that've been bugging us all month. Inspiration hits and moments of epiphany rumba 'cross de tundra of our senses.

—Inga Muscio

Testimonial: Bridget, Age 38

I was a gymnast growing up, and didn't get my period until I was sixteen. By seventeen, I had given up gymnastics and started cheerleading. Given my competitive background, I'd never heard of *not* working out during one's period. In fact, I thought it was recommended. However, I started bleeding so profusely on Day 1 of my period that it became a problem with panty-exposing cheerleading. I couldn't make it through a two-hour game without changing my tampon/pad combo, and had many embarrassing leaks.

After college, when I stopped cheering, my body made the decision for me—I couldn't work out during Day 1 due to a very heavy flow, debilitating cramps, and severe anemia. After two cycles of resting on Day 1, my cramps lessened and my flow evened out. Within a year, I was no longer categorized as anemic. Now I go to work on Day 1 and then return home and relax—no extracurricular activities! My body is better for it, and I'm a happier, less-stressed person overall.

Resting and Weight

So how does a monthly day (or two, or three) of rest affect your weight? It comes down to balance. The female body is innately graceful, gently ebbing and flowing through the month, communicating its needs every step of the way. There is a fine line between invigoration and irritation, and on Day 1 a workout could very easily push the entire 28-day cycle off kilter.

The more you rest on Day 1, the easier the other 27 days of your cycle will be. In terms of weight, that means your PMS will be less extreme, making it less likely that you will binge on chips, cookies, or chocolate. With your seemingly uncontrollable urge to scarf those empty calories gone, your weight won't yo-yo the way it typically does when your PMS is raging.

If you feel your tight abs will turn to flab after only one exercise-free day, hear this: THE UNIVERSE IS GOING TO THE GYM FOR YOU! With the work your body is doing to shed that uterine lining, your workout is automatically checked off your Day 1 to-do list. Let your body do the workout for you, and enjoy the downtime.

If you are still bleeding heavily or suffering any discomfort on Day 2 or Day 3, then continue to honor the no-workout rule and repeat the simple self-care routine we suggest for Day 1 in chapter 6. For most women, the metabolic rate returns to normal, or slightly less than normal, on or around Day 2, but this varies greatly from woman to woman. As always, you need to let your own cycle be your guide.

GOLDEN RULE #3: MINIMIZE TAMPON USE

We've been taught that tampons are cooler and sexier than pads, and that the popular girls use tampons while the rest of us pull up our granny panties and strap on enormous, diaper-like paper products. We'd like to change this stereotype. First, pads have come a long way: There are pads that are ultra-thin, some have "wings" that wrap around the panty to prevent leaks, some are made of soft cotton flannel in vibrant patterns that come clean after a spin through the washer, and some are even shaped especially for thong panties. There are even cool new alternatives to pads, like our favorite, the DivaCup—a silicone cup you wear inside your vagina that stays put, catches the menstrual blood quite nicely, and only needs to be emptied every twelve hours, making it highly convenient. (It also helps you to get in touch with exactly how much you bleed each month, which is probably a lot less than you think.) There is also the Softcup, which is similar in theory to the DivaCup, but is thinner, softer, and disposable—no need to rinse it out in the sink. Think of these products as the diaphragm of menstrual-care products.

But the real reason we maintain that pads (or DivaCups) are cooler than tampons is because they make the body's job of shedding the uterine lining easier—more on this in a moment—and this translates into big-time benefits. Even wearing tampons during the day (changing them frequently, and springing for the organic, non-bleached variety) and switching to pads at night is better than wearing tampons nonstop for the full length of your period.

But before we get to those benefits, let's talk about why pads are friendlier to your body.

More than Blood

Your body sheds more than blood during menstruation; it also sheds the uterine lining. Tampons absorb blood, but other discharge may get blocked from freely flowing out. This material can then be reabsorbed into the body. Menstruation is supposed to flow in one direction: down. When we use tampons, menstruation could go retrograde, meaning that instead of the discharge flowing downward, it goes back up. This is not natural, and the whole point of the 28 Days Lighter program is to align with nature.

All about the Detox

Avoiding tampons also has to do with flow; according to traditional Chinese medicine, menstruation is all about downward flow. Using a tampon is essentially the same as putting a cork in a bottle. It impedes the downward energy, making your body work harder than it needs to, and reducing the effectiveness of this time of detoxification. Now, we ask you, is this a process you want to impede? No. If your body has evolved over millions of years to regularly shed what it doesn't need, by all means, let it. There's no situation that a Diva-Cup can't handle as well—or better—than a tampon. That includes being seen in a bathing suit (chillaxing on a lounge chair rather than swimming laps, naturally).

Toxic Tampons

Dioxin is a by-product of the plastic manufacturing and chlorination processes. It is also one of the deadliest man-made chemicals, second only to radioactive waste. It is found in anything bleached, including paper and tampons. Only tampons that are made from 100 percent organic cotton (and none of the big brands are) are free of chlorine and thus, dioxin.

In the United States, the painful condition of endometriosis (where the lining of the womb grows in other parts of the body) affects up to 20 percent of women of childbearing age. Some of these cases cause severe pain and infertility, but back before 1921 there were only twenty cases of the disease ever recorded in the world (although, granted, issues with lady parts weren't really discussed, much less studied, then). What could have caused this massive surge of disease in a society that has access to the best health care in the world? Hmmm . . .

According to one 2002 study: "Previous work in non-human primates has shown that exposure to dioxin . . . is associated with an increased prevalence and severity of endometriosis." Simply put, when animals are exposed to dioxins, they are significantly more likely to develop endometriosis.

Another 1997 study found that infertile women with endometriosis had detectable levels of dioxin present in their bodies, unlike fertile women without endometriosis.

And it doesn't stop at dioxin! Chemicals in tampons include aluminum, alcohol, pesticides, and additives. Rayon itself is a man-made, artificial fiber that is abrasive. It can actually cut the cervix and vagina, causing more vaginal bleeding and a heavier period. Tampons containing rayon placed in the vagina for any length of time can be a breeding ground for *Staphylococcus aureus,* the germ responsible for toxic shock syndrome (TSS). Although TSS can be caused by other things, tampon usage plays a role in approximately 50 percent of all cases. Manufacturers of tampons say that dioxin in tampons is not at a "detectable" level, but any level is poisonous.

Cigarettes Contain Dioxin, Too

Reason number 1,001 to not smoke: Dioxin is in the rolling paper that surrounds the tobacco in those Marlboro Lights.

It's commonly held in the research world that dioxin is one of the most dangerous chemicals there is, even in seemingly miniscule amounts. Ingesting a tablespoon of it could kill an average-sized adult. Dioxin has been proven to seep into the bloodstream through vaginal skin contact, making it incredibly unsafe in tampons.

GOLDEN RULE #4: SEE YOUR CYCLE AS A GIFT (NOT A CURSE)

"Outsmart Mother Nature" is the tagline for Tampax, the number one–selling brand of tampons in the United States. From what you've read thus far, you can imagine how much this makes us cringe. For one, *outsmarting* Mother Nature is impossible. She brings O'Hare Airport to its knees with a snowstorm. She ruins thousands of acres of crops with drought. She controls the tides and the seasons. We are no match for Her. Go up against Her, and you'll be walloped sooner or later. (It's like outsmarting hunger. Have you tried that? We have, and about an hour after "outsmarting" it, we dove into a box of donuts!)

However, what really bugs us is *why* this Tampax sales pitch works so well . . . because it feeds into, and perpetuates, the notion that our

> *In the red tent, where days pass like a gentle stream, as the gift of Innana courses through us, cleansing the body of last month's death, preparing the body to receive the new month's life, women give thanks — for repose and restoration, for the knowledge that life comes from between our legs, and that life costs blood.*
>
> —Anita Diamant, The Red Tent

Curse to Blessing: The Paradigm Shift

If you missed it when it was at the top of the bestseller lists, or even if you read and enjoyed it then, we highly recommend reading *The Red Tent,* Anita Diamant's work of fiction based on the customs of ancient womanhood in the book of Genesis. It makes us proud to be women. The female characters find singular and communal strength from their menstrual cycles.

menstrual cycle is a curse. The Old English word for monthly bleeding was *bloedsen,* which evolved into our word, "blessing." Isn't that so sweet? Much better than "on the rag" and "the Curse," right?

The menstrual cycle is a gift. It tunes us into ourselves and gives us a more-intimate connection to nature's ebbs and flows. It can be a source of great strength and wisdom. The monthly arrival of our periods forces us to slow down, get quiet, and tap into our intuition. The only reason we perceive it to be a curse is because we continually ignore it and soldier on at our normal, frenetic pace, forcing our bodies to create ever more stronger symptoms in hopes of finally getting us to stop for a day (or more).

The menstrual cycle helps our bodies to stay strong and vital, enables us to create life and give birth, and to enjoy the full spectrum of human abilities. It serves as a portal that connects us more intimately with nature. It truly is a blessing—one we have to own and accept to fully benefit from and appreciate.

WHY WE NEED THESE RULES, NOW MORE THAN EVER

We were each into our thirties before we fully understood the Four Golden Rules, having learned of them slowly through our yoga teachers, acupuncture appointments, holistic journals, personal studies, and off-the-beaten-path retreats. After training hundreds of women, Ellen realized that nobody else knew of these rules either. And Kate, being in the "New Age" inner circle, tried to get stories published that covered the principles behind these Golden Rules, to no avail. They were written off as folklore.

If only we women learned of the Four Golden Rules at puberty! Not only are most of us ignorant of them, but many of us have been doing the *opposite* of them for years, putting in a tampon so we can run five miles, all while grumbling about our periods and their rotten timing. For the most part, we embody the anti-rules. How could we be so off? We're educated women, after all (in the fields of wellness!), with framed diplomas hanging on our walls.

For starters, school is not where women learn about these things. We learn the basics of menstruation from our mothers, sisters, and friends, and where they leave off, the media jumps in. When you are an impressionable twelve-year-old and you see a Tampax commercial where a slim, smiling woman in white shorts rollerblades with a gaggle of cute males, the brainwashing has begun. You want to be like her—she's beautiful, happy, and adored by all. She isn't sidelined by her period. *I should use Tampax,* you think.

If men could menstruate . . . clearly, menstruation would become an enviable, boast-worthy, masculine event: Men would brag about how long and how much . . . Sanitary supplies would be federally funded and free. Of course, some men would still pay for the prestige of such commercial brands as Paul Newman Tampons, Muhammad Ali's Rope-a-Dope Pads, John Wayne Maxi Pads, and Joe Namath Jock Shields —For Those Light Bachelor Days.

—Gloria Steinem

CHAPTER 5

Phase I: Menstruation (Days 1–7) WISE WOMAN

Ah, menstruation, the obvious phase. Day 1—mark it in your calendar. We call it "*my* period," a noun, personal and private, like *my* house and *my* dog. Every woman has her own period, accompanied by her own specific emotions and sensations, and it kind of rules her world for a few days, even when it flows harmoniously. Conscious of it or not, menstruation affects how we move, what we wear, what we do.

So what is a normal, healthy menstrual flow? Does it really matter if there are cramps, back pain, and nausea, as long as the symptoms subside? (That is, until next month when the suffering begins anew.) Our answer is simple: A normal, healthy menstrual flow comes every 28 days, lasts for 3 to 5 days, and *doesn't include pain of any kind.* When a woman's period veers from this aforementioned description, *something is imbalanced.* It might be something very basic, like magnesium deficiency, or it might be something a little complicated, like hypothyroidism. It could be due to a lack of estrogen, or too many of the hormone-like substances called prostaglandins, which are associated with pain and inflammation in the lower abdomen during menstruation.

A normal healthy menstrual flow comes every 28 days, lasts for 3 to 5 days, and doesn't include pain of any kind.

You might be thinking, cramps are no big deal. Ellen suffered much worse and considered herself lucky when, after pregnancy and childbirth, her period became much less dramatic than before. She used to get night sweats and chills, for Pete's sake, so a few hours of mild cramping was a breeze! But it was still not perfect. We want you to set the bar high and aspire for a no-pain period!

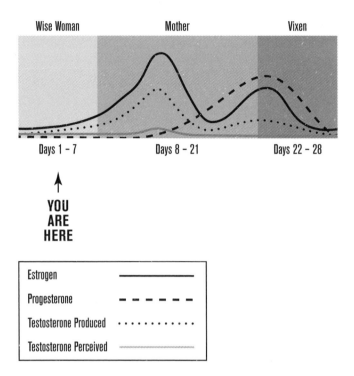

Here's the deal: A woman's period is a major indicator of her state of health. While this may seem foreign coming from a Western medical point of view like ours, it is the way just about every other culture sees things. It's true within Ayurveda, traditional Chinese medicine, and Native American healing models. It's true for Mayan healers and according to the shamans of Africa. In these wellness settings, a "doctor's" consultation with a woman would always contain a detailed view of her menses, considering the blood quality as well as any emotional and physical changes that accompany it. This is another way in which we women are the lucky ones: Mother Nature checks in with us every month and gives us *obvious* feedback regarding our state of being. Monthly guidance!

Speaking of Mother Nature. "*My* period" can't be scheduled like a C-section. It comes when it comes, as in natural childbirth, because something else is in charge. Menstruation is a bodily function that happens with or without our involvement, like digestion or fingernail growing. Our job at this time of the cycle is to get out of the way

Ayurvedic Advice for a Happy Menstruation

By Linda Sparrowe, yoga teacher and author of *The Woman's Book of Yoga & Health* and *Yoga for a Healthy Menstrual Cycle*

Let's get real. If you're like most of us, getting your period every month hardly gives you reason to celebrate, especially if you get PMS the week (or, ugh, two) before it and crazy cramps and heavy flow during it. But yoga and its ancient sister science, Ayurveda, put such a positive spin on the whole experience that you may actually come to appreciate (and even embrace) the wisdom of your whole reproductive system.

In the first place, Ayurveda says that bleeding every month gives us a distinct advantage over men, and it's probably why we live longer than they do. It sounds weird, I know, but that's because Ayurveda believes that your monthly is much more than a way to shed the ol' uterine lining. Think of it as a built-in detox cleanse that you get to do every 25 to 35 days, one in which all the toxins—the sticky, icky stuff Ayurveda calls *ama*—that have accumulated during the month get a free ride out. These toxins can come from anything your body hasn't digested—bad food, stress at work or at home, even any emotions you've shoved down. Of course, if you've taken good care of yourself all month long, your body should have a pretty easy time self-cleansing. But if you've pigged out on junk food, hit the Red Bull a little too hard, functioned with barely any sleep, skipped out on your usual yoga classes, or failed to deal with hurt or angry feelings that cropped up, guess what? It'll be a drag later on in the month.

Here are a few tips from yoga and Ayurveda that work in synchrony with the rest of the advice offered in this book. Add them if they speak to you!

1. Focus on your breath on Day 1. While you're taking it easy on the first day of your period, your body is working really hard to move the menstrual blood (and all the toxins it finds) down and out. You can help it along by focusing on soothing, conscious breaths, with a special emphasis on the exhale. This

type of breathing will encourage what yogis call the *apana vayu*—the downward-moving wind energy. *Apana vayu* (a type of *prana,* or life force) not only governs menstruation and digestion, but it also allows us to let go of what no longer serves us—destructive thoughts or negative emotions.

2. Be selfish. The first day or two should be a time for reflection. This is a perfect opportunity to do a loving-kindness toward yourself, your family, and your friends. It can really help dislodge you from the poor-me attitude your cycle has unleashed. Focusing on your basic goodness—after all, you're beautiful just the way you are—turn it inward and then toward the people you love (even if you're not feeling all that loving toward them right now!). Here's how:

   Sit down comfortably either on a cushion or in a chair. Close your eyes and allow your breath to find its natural rhythm. And then turn your attention to the area around your heart. Breathing in and out of your heart space, repeat the following several times to yourself:

   Loving-Kindness Meditation:
   May I be happy.
   May I be healthy.
   May I be free from harm.

   And now visualize someone in your family, and repeat May s/he be happy, may s/he be healthy, may s/he be free from harm. Repeat the same meditation/prayer with one of your close friends in your heart.

3. Give yourself an Ayurvedic massage. Begin your massage with a loving attitude—toward your body and your mind—and focus your awareness on the task at hand.

   Warm some sesame, almond, or coconut oil and massage a thin coating over your whole body. Use long strokes on your arms and legs—moving from the tips of the toes and fingers in toward the body—and circular movements on your joints. Let the oil soak in and then shower in warm water. No need for soap. If you want to feel even more luxurious and rejuvenated, massage some of the warm oil into your scalp, onto your forehead and temples, and the soles of your feet just before bed. Throw on a pair of cotton socks and call it a night.

4. Give yourself the experience of a sequence of yoga poses designed just for menstruating women.

Sure, I can do a strong practice anytime I like, but I have to say, I love to treat myself to a menstrual sequence at that time of the month. A truly restorative menstrual practice allows me to feel nurtured and supported and, by the end of it, more focused and energized. What's not to love? A moon-time practice includes all kinds of poses—mostly restorative—but what sets it apart is the focus you bring to it: an opportunity to listen deeply, relax completely, and allow your body to work its apana magic.

a) Choose poses that create space between your rib cage and your abdomen. Pay particular attention to your breathing.

b) Leave the standing pose sequences until you have more strength and energy.

c) If your belly feels tight, breathe into that space, softening and releasing. If your chest is constricted, direct your breath there. If you have cramps, allow your breath to flow all the way into your uterus, releasing and relaxing your entire body.

d) A menstrual practice allows you to open the pelvic area, bring space to your abdomen and reproductive organs, and even has a bit of a drying effect on your uterus.

e) Create a practice that will make you feel like a princess—cared for and pampered.

Common Flow Woes Remedy Matrix

By Laurie Steelsmith, ND

In traditional Chinese medicine, a healthy woman has a bright red, clot-free menstrual flow that starts off light, builds to medium, peaks at heavy, then tails off again through medium and light. If your flow doesn't follow this, your body may be sending you clues that it needs you to do things differently. This remedy matrix offers the traditional Chinese medicine perspective on what your flow is trying to tell you, and how you can help bring it back into balance.

Symptom	Traditional Chinese Medicine Perspective on Possible Causes	Remedy
Light periods, with flow that is dull (not bright red); fatigue during period; pale skin.	Blood deficiency	Eat more iron-rich foods, such as meat, greens, and beets (see page 72). Think and worry less (prioritize relaxation).
Brown blood throughout the period and/or clots and/or scanty periods; period-related insomnia; feeling hot or sweaty during period.	Yin deficiency	Slow down. Eat cooling foods, such as cucumbers and melon. Minimize spicy foods. Prioritize quiet time.
Spotting before or after period; long cycle and heavy periods; fatigue during period; can't get warm, or have cold hands and feet during period.	Yang deficiency	Seek out more stimulation. Socialize more often. Implement more vigorous exercise. Eat more spicy foods.

and allow Mother Nature to work her magic through us. So sit back. Relax. You are a mere witness. This phase is *passive.*

Here's the rub: Our action-oriented Western mentality has conditioned us to always *do something.* This clashes drastically with what we really need to do in Phase I, which is to *be still.* As we learned in chapter 2, our ancestors respected this time of the month by retreating from daily chores and activities. Today, with our hectic lifestyles, most women have lost this feminine Sabbath. We want you to rise above the norm, to Wise Woman stature, and keep the Sabbath alive.

THE PHASE I ARCHETYPE: WISE WOMAN

For ages, women were uncertified doctors and natural pharmacists. Barred from reading books and from formal schooling, they learned from each other and from deep observation of nature and experience. They passed on knowledge from woman to woman and from mother to daughter as midwives, herbologists, and witches. People called them Wise Women. They understood that the physical and spiritual were one, and that respecting Mother Nature was the road to authentic health.

We can all be our own Wise Woman, especially during Phase I, as there is a sense of otherworldly wisdom that inhabits all females during this time, if only we are open to it. You might not know how wise you really are because modern living has distracted you, by directing your attention away from the intelligence that lies within. Nonetheless, wisdom *does* reside within you, and menstruation is a time for acknowledging it.

THE WISE WOMAN ACTION PLAN

Picture this: A woman is curled up in front of a fireplace. Maybe she's reading a book, petting her cat, or taking a nap. She's wrapped in a blanket with a cup of tea by her side. The hustle and bustle of the world outside her window is none of her concern. She is "here now," content. Ladies, this is what Phase I should feel like. Cozy and warm. It's a time to be gentle with yourself. Once you begin to bleed, traditional Chinese medicine says that you are most energy-deficient and most vulnerable, because the body is under strain. We don't want to add to the strain by working out, overeating, or overworking.

Move, Part 1—Be Still

Stillness and warmth are the two reoccurring themes in this phase, and in the Wise Woman Action Plan. Our protocol for Move is *don't*. Just be still—at least for the first half of this phase. Then, just like the moon, we want your amount of movement to wax, by peacefully increasing your activity level in little increments over the last 4 or 5 days of the phase. This will require a keen mind/body connection, and also an important paradigm shift. Instead of looking at exercise as fitness, look at fitness as a piece of whole self-healing. In this case, *less is more.*

> *During the monthly period (48–72 hours), complete rest is advisable.*
>
> —Geeta Iyengar, yoga guru

Here is where we are intentionally vague. Days 1, 2, and/or 3 will look different for every woman. Those with debilitating cramps or other symptoms may need an all-out "sick day" from work or school, staying home curled up in bed or lounging on the couch watching HGTV. Others may go about their day but exclude extra exertion. That translates as doing the bare minimum. Do you *have* to go to the PTA meeting? Can you go straight home from work and forgo picking up the dry cleaning? Only fulfill the urgent obligations and then return to *home, sweet home.* Even at home we encourage you to make adjustments. If you usually cook for the whole family, can you order take-out delivery, or put someone else in charge of it for a few nights? Maybe you have the luxury of working from home, so you can stay in your PJs all day.

Some women have told us, "Oh, I go running on Day 1, and it minimizes my cramps," or, "I heard exercise on Day 1 is good for you." To this we respond with one phrase: Step back, gaze at the big picture, and look at how Mother Nature *always* seeks balance. Night follows day. Winter follows summer. Roots grow down as the tree trunk grows up. In order for you to be vibrant all cycle long there's got to be yin to the yang. Once you get synced in to this routine of moving for three phases and then mellowing out during just this

Ellen's Dog Gives Her a Pass on Day 1

Ellen: My dog is an energy reader and therefore knows when I'm on low-energy Day 1. The only time of the month she doesn't campaign for her long midday walk is when I'm on my period. She gives me a free pass and is suddenly very content with a backyard romp without me.

part of Phase I, you will find yourself feeling fit and fab. You self-regulate, and the work/rest rhythm will become more and more obvious month after month on our program. The *rest* will make you more productive and efficient in the *work*.

Move, Part 2—Wise Woman Yoga
During the later half of Phase I, after heavy bleeding has stopped—which could be on Day 3, 4, or 5 (and only you know)—we still want you to *be still*, but now, we want you to find that sense of stillness by hanging out in a few yoga poses. We call this twenty-minute routine "Wise Woman Yoga." Our goal is to massage and rejuvenate the abdominal organs, as well as to soothe the nervous system. We'll accomplish this with gentle spine twists, forward bends, and easy hip openers. Keywords: gentle and easy. It's done entirely on the floor (no standing), and all of the poses are passive once you get into them, so we want you to relax. You should be able to hold them for a dreamy three minutes each.

Wise Woman Yoga
Wide-Knee Child's Pose (Salamba Balasana)—Hold for 3 minutes
How to do it: From a kneeling position, bring your big toes to touch behind you as you spread your knees apart. Fold forward, allowing your forehead to rest on the ground (if it doesn't comfortably reach, grab a couch cushion or your firmest pillow and place it under your torso and head). Extend your arms comfortably forward and relax.
What it does: This pose releases lower back tension and helps to calm the nervous system.

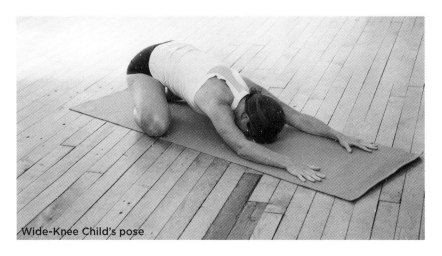

Wide-Knee Child's pose

Upright Bound Angle (Baddha Konasana)—Hold for 3 minutes

How to do it: From a seated upright position, bend your knees, bringing the soles of your feet together and pulling your feet toward your hips. Drop your knees out to the sides as you press the soles of your feet together. Bring your feet as close to your pelvis as you

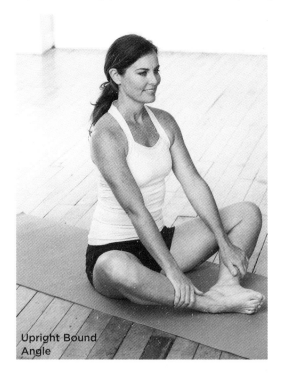

Upright Bound Angle

comfortably can by grasping your shins, ankles, or big toes. Always keep the outer edges of the feet on the floor.

What it does: This pose stretches the hips, bringing increased blood flow to the pelvic area.

Seated Spinal Twist (Marichyasana III)—Hold for 3 minutes each side

How to do it: From a seated upright position, extend your left leg long and bend your right knee, planting the right foot on the floor as close to the hips as possible. Inhale and lengthen your torso, then exhale and twist it to the right. Place the right hand on the floor behind you, as you either hug your right knee with your left arm or bring the left arm to the outside of the right knee. Repeat on the other side.

What it does: This pose stretches the lower back as well as relieves abdominal congestion.

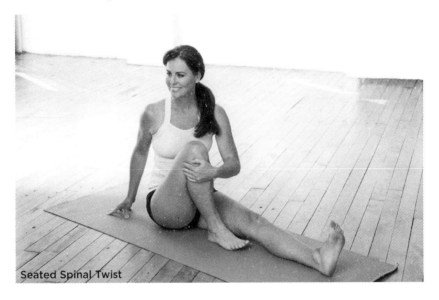
Seated Spinal Twist

Seated Forward Bend (Paschimottanasana)—Hold for 3 minutes

How to do it: Sit on the floor with your legs straight in front of you. Inhale and lengthen your torso, feeling the rib cage lift off the hip bones slightly; then, as you exhale, lean forward over your legs. Be sure to keep your spine straight (no rounding).

What it does: This pose stretches the lower back and the hamstrings.

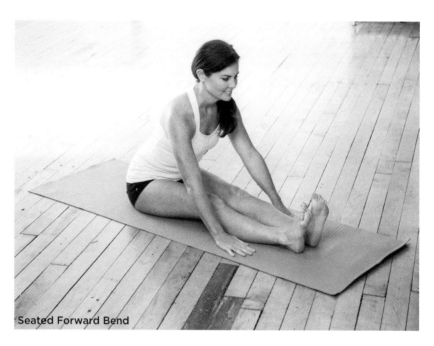

Seated Forward Bend

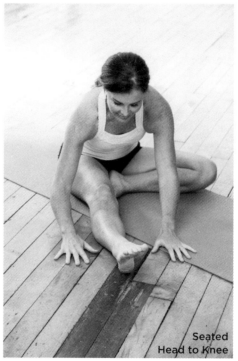

Seated
Head to Knee

Seated Head to Knee (Janu Sirsasana)—Hold for 3 minutes each side
How to do it: Sit on the floor with your legs straight. Bend your left knee, drawing the left sole of the foot in to touch the inside of the right upper thigh. The left knee should rest on the floor (if it doesn't, place a rolled-up towel under the upper thigh so the leg can rest comfortably). Exhale and turn the torso to the right, lining up the center of your chest with the right knee. Inhale and lengthen the torso. On the following exhale, lean the torso forward over the extended leg. Repeat on the other side and hold for another 3 minutes.
What it does: This pose stretches the hamstrings and releases tension in the lower back.

As you approach the end of the Wise Woman Phase, there will be an energy surge, where you find yourself feeling more inclined to tackle chores and be productive. You may opt to take a stroll through the park, do some gardening, and get more physical in informal ways. Great! Use your inner Wise Woman and assess for yourself. The Phase I Move protocol is loose and not clearly defined, leaving room for you to be your own guide. Let it be known, though, that the other three phases have greater specification and don't encourage "days off," so appreciate it while you can!

Nourish—Eat Warm
The foods and beverages you intake during menstruation should be room temperature or slightly warmer. Ice cubes are outlawed. Ice cream, too. According to traditional Chinese medicine, your body has to work extra hard to heat up cold water, so make sure your water is room temperature or warmer as well. The actual temperature of your food matters, especially at this time of the month, and it's not just about the temperature; some foods have warming properties, so warm and warming foods are ideal for the Wise Woman.

Traditional Chinese medicine classifies food according to its energetic effects rather than its nutrient components. Certain foods are viewed as warming while others are seen as cooling. Raw food, in general, is the most cooling for the body, requiring more energy to digest than food that has been cooked. Because our body is already working hard on menstruation, when the body has to direct a lot of energy to digestion, it can (and often does) get overwhelmed. Eating warm and warming foods do not add to the workload, or stress the body, as much as cooling foods.

Of course, coming from a purely Western medical perspective, this sounds silly. We've never really looked at food as warming or cooling. Trust us, and try this out for yourself. You'll see, instantly, how cool foods affect menses. It may cause blood clots to appear in the menstrual flow or increase cramping sensations. It may temporarily halt the flow for a short time, too.

Instead of having cold cereal with milk, have warm oatmeal with walnuts. If you are noshing on a salad for lunch, take it out of the refrigerator at 9 a.m. so it is room temperature by the time you eat it, or maybe switch to soup for a few days. We showcase many warming dinner options in chapter 8, like our Quinoa Stir-Fry on page 149.

Warming Foods

Asparagus	Ginger (fresh)
Basil	Ginseng
Chives	Leeks
Cinnamon sticks	Millet
Cloves	Mustard greens
Coriander	Quinoa
Fennel	Rosemary
Garlic	Scallions

Warm doesn't mean hot. Spicy and overly hot foods, like many Mexican dishes that use jalapeños or Asian cuisine that uses chili peppers, act a lot like cold foods in that they add to the workload of our already strained body, directing blood away from the womb. Overeating does this too, so eat small, warm meals that are not too hot or spicy, and not cold or chilled, during Phase I.

Live, Part 1—Use a Hot-Water Bottle

There are two components to Wise Woman *Live*. The first is quite honestly the easiest, cheapest, lowest-drama way to help ease menstrual cramps and back pain—using a hot-water bottle on your belly. Just fill the bottle with the hottest water you can muster up, then

No Baths during Phase I

This saddens us to say because we loooove baths, but no baths allowed during Phase I, or at least during the bleeding part of Phase I. Baths may disrupt menstrual flow. According to traditional Chinese medicine, women that submerge in water could stifle the shedding process, which could lead to problems now or later. (A great time for soaking in the tub is Phase III, Pre-menstruation.)

place on your lower abdomen, exactly on top of the uterus. You can do this all day long (not just at night when you are lying down) by placing it in your lap or between your lower back and your chair back at your desk chair. To avoid depletion while you are bleeding, keep your feet warm, too; don't walk around barefoot on cold floors. The same theory applies—the hot-water bottle minimizes the workload for the body at this time of the month.

Hot-water bottles are our preferred form of heat. Heating pads are okay, but two things bug us about heating pads: First, you can't fall asleep with a heating pad as easily and as safely as you can with a hot-water bottle. And second, the electric currents that run through the heating pad (and electric blankets) aren't the greatest things to press up against your body, especially your womb palace! You may have those warmers that you throw in the microwave, too. We don't trust microwaves—the radiation they emit can't be good for you.

Live, Part 2—Thirty to Sixty Minutes More Sleep per Day

The second part of the Wise Woman Live action plan is slumber. Now is the time to sleep more, and by more, we mean about thirty to sixty minutes more than what you typically do. If you usually get eight hours a night, seek eight and a half to nine hours during Phase I. Sleeping obviously doesn't burden the body—quite the opposite; it recharges the body—so take a nap, turn in earlier, and/or sleep in later. If you are paying attention, you might notice feeling more "sleepy" during Phase I anyway, or perhaps you have noticed that during Phase I, you sleep more soundly, like a "rock."

> *Sleep makes people calmer, more alert, less fearful—just plain happier, or so I see around me and in me. I am sure that if this great nation were to concentrate on getting more sleep, we would be a happier, more confident people, and that by itself would be a major achievement.*
>
> —Ben Stein

You might be about to throw in the towel with this "more sleep" stuff, mumbling to yourself, "More sleep? Yeah, right . . . don't you think I would if I could?" We know that most of America is sleep-deprived (sigh), and we're well aware that during menstruation, many women sleep less because they are uncomfortable during the night due to menstrual cramping and other pains. Studies show most women in Phase I get less REM-stage sleep (the kind that helps us feel refreshed) because of disruption due to their periods. All the more reason to seek out more zzz's, ladies!

Sleep deprivation is directly related to weight gain. Studies show that the less we sleep, the more we eat. Sleeping regulates hormones too, so a lack of sleep can send your estrogen and progesterone on a roller-coaster ride from hell.

All Month Long: Be an Iron (Wo)man

Iron deficiency, also known as anemia, is the most common single nutrient-deficiency disease *in the world,* and women account for at least 85 percent of this deficient population. Are you feeling tired? Weak? Do you have pale skin? Do you always feel cold? These are all symptoms of low iron levels.

We lose iron every month in our menstrual flow, so it is one of the minerals we need to replenish *aggressively.* Menstruating women generally require about 15 mg of iron per day. (Women who are pregnant should be consuming double that—about 30 mg per day.) Most women today get a mere 6 mg/day. Oh, we've got work to do, ladies!

So let's first minimize our iron depletion by avoiding over-the-top, strenuous exercise. It is unnecessary and potentially harmful. (Of course, if your passion is doing ultra-marathons, or your

A Dreamy Trick to Help You Get More Zzzs

While you're lying in bed, wishing you were asleep already, there's something super simple you can do to help yourself settle down enough to actually drift off. Place one hand on your heart and the other hand on your solar plexus—the soft spot just beneath where your ribs meet in the center of your chest. Stay here a minute or two until you feel more relaxed, then move the hand that's on your heart to your belly, just beneath your belly button. Stay here until you feel yourself getting sleepy, verrrry sleepy. . . .

What you're doing here is a little acupressure, which is DIY acupuncture that uses your fingers instead of needles. The energy pathway (or meridian) known as the conception vessel (CV) runs right down the front of your torso, and this is your most primal energy. By resting the hands on key points along the CV and gradually moving them lower, you're soothing that energy and drawing it down, away from your head, making you less likely to churn out stress-inducing thoughts. It's like singing your inner self a lullaby.

livelihood is as a CrossFit trainer, this may not be possible or desirable.) Exercise should be invigorating, not irritating. A second way to minimize our iron depletion is to stop with the "starvation" dieting. Seriously restricting calories tends to restrict iron consumption as well, and sets our bodies up for major problems, not just iron deficiency. The third way to minimize our iron depletion is to regulate our menstrual cycles, so periods don't come too soon or last too long in duration. (Luckily, you're already working on that by reading this book!) Last but not least, the fourth way to minimize our iron depletion is to get ample amounts of vitamin C.

Only 15 percent of the iron we consume is absorbed by our bodies. If you consume 15 mg of iron per day, your body is actually only absorbing about 2.25 mg of iron. Vitamin C can help the body better absorb iron, so iron and vitamin C go hand in hand. We have recipes in chapter 8 that offer a perfect one-two punch of iron and vitamin C. Be sure to check out Chicken and Broccoli over Almond Rice on page 152, and Blueberry and Walnut Smoothie on page 143.

It is ideal to get your iron from food, not supplements. We recommend avoiding synthetic forms of iron that are commonly found in pharmaceutical products. (There are whole-food supplements that fare a bit better.) The synthetic ones have been shown to cause constipation and have an inconclusive track record (i.e., the jury is still out on whether they even boost iron levels). As a high school and college athlete, Ellen, and just about every girl on her college tennis team, was iron-deficient. She was perennially given iron supplements. Clearly, they didn't work because, at the six-month mark, when her iron levels were retested, she was at the same low level. (FYI, it wasn't until Ellen graduated and no longer succumbed to a grueling tennis schedule that she saw some improvement in her iron levels.)

As we mentioned, chapter 8 is loaded with recipes that happen to be great iron suppliers, but just so you know, iron is everywhere—in meats, in vegetables, and even in herbs. Seaweeds, like kelp and blue-green algae, are fantastic sources of organic, dietary iron. Here are a few lists for your information:

Natural Food Sources of Iron

Very good	Good
(Eat at least one serving of one of these every day)	(Make these part of your regular rotation)
Kidney and lima beans, chickpeas and lentils	Pine nuts, cashews, almonds, (1 cup)
Clams, mussels, oysters, or shrimp (3 oz. serving)	Dark chocolate (3 squares)
Cooked spinach or Swiss chard (1 cup)	Dried apricots (½ cup)
Pumpkin seeds (1 ounce, about 140 seeds)	Quinoa, oatmeal, rice (1 cup cooked)
Beef, lamb, or liver (3 oz. serving)	Beets
Seaweed, spirulina, blue-green algae	Dried prunes or raisins (¼ cup)

Herbal Teas that Provide Iron

Dandelion Root
Nettle
Red Raspberry Leaf

In addition, cooking in a cast-iron skillet will lend your food some added iron, which is why we recommend investing in one of these black beauties. It does require some maintenance (see page 134 for more information), but a well-tended iron skillet will last you a lifetime.

When iron levels are sufficient, you'll know it. You'll feel it and see it with stronger energy levels, a glowing complexion, and no longer needing a sweater on summer days. (No more cold toes, either!) Mentally, you'll be able to focus for longer periods of time. Restoring iron in your system could take a few months, or even a year. It depends on two things: 1) How deficient you are to begin with; and 2) how heavy your periods are. The 28 Days Lighter Diet program seeks to "even out" imbalances within your cycle that contribute to anemia, like when periods lasts for six or more days, or when cycles are very short (causing you to bleed more often). There is one caveat—fibroids. Many heavy periods are caused by uterine fibroids. If you are suffering from fibroids, we encourage you to schedule an appointment with your doctor (and don't leave that office without a game plan!).

READY, SET, FLOW FOR DAYS 1–7

- On Day 1 (and possibly Days 2 and 3): Just say *no* to formal workouts on Day 1 (and possibly Days 2 and 3). Be still.

- All phase long: Get an extra thirty minutes to two hours of downtime every day. This means curling up with a good book, staying home, and saying *no* to invitations and houseguests.

- On Days 3–7 (approximately): Do Wise Woman Yoga (exercises are illustrated on pages 64–66) every day.

- All phase long: Eat warm and warming foods. Avoid cold and cooling foods, and especially ice cubes and frozen desserts. Also, avoid hot and spicy foods.

An ideal menu for a Wise Woman is filled with warm, iron-rich meals:

> Breakfast: Almost Eggs Florentine (page 140)
> Lunch: Lentil Soup (page 155)
> Dinner: Chicken and Broccoli over Almond Rice (page 152)

- All phase long: Avoid overeating by eating small meals throughout the phase. A simple bowl of soup is a perfect portion for a Wise Woman.

- On Days 1 and 2 (approximately): Use a hot-water bottle on your belly as often as possible. This may be only in the evening, but perhaps you can use it during the day, too, whenever your work life allows.

- On Days 1–5: Get thirty to sixty minutes more sleep per day. Do this by turning in earlier, lingering in bed longer, or napping during the day.

- All cycle long: Be an iron woman. Aim for 15 mg/day in your food, not from supplements.

The Top Three Habits of the Highly Successful Wise Woman

1. Rest as much as possible on Day 1.
2. Invest in and use an iron skillet all month long.
3. Eat warm and warming foods during the entire Phase I.

We know that many of you struggle with Phase I because you feel menstruation sets you back career-wise, workout-wise, or even in your love life. Instead of a setback, think of Phase I as a Sabbath. After three weeks of hustle, you get to reward yourself with a bit of R&R. One phase isn't necessarily harder than another—they're all just different, and place different demands on your body and your life. The Wise Woman knows that the universe is working for us, even when we are taking time off.

CHAPTER 6

Phase II: Mega Phase (Days 8–21) MOTHER

Welcome to the Mega Phase! Sounds good, doesn't it? "Look out world, it's mega me!" These next two weeks are all about life at full speed, in full color. You have energy to spare, focus galore, and a special shot of pixie dust that makes even the most daunting project or longest list of tasks easily doable. In Mega Phase, you're livin' large.

In this second phase of your cycle, you're at your energy peak, so it's important that you concentrate on covering new ground, and you aren't merely doing the bare minimum. After all, you're at your best right now—you want to take advantage of it! The three major things that are going to help you thrive right now are: plenty of physical motion, sufficient protein intake, and an increased outward focus on friends, family, and colleagues.

These next two weeks are about *growth* and *circulation*, both within the body and out in the world. Inside your body, your uterine lining thickens (growth) and ovulation occurs (circulation). In the first week,

> The three major things that are going to help you thrive right now are: plenty of physical motion, sufficient protein intake, and an increased outward focus on friends, family, and colleagues.

the fast-climbing estrogen levels put you in a jovial mood and help your womb fluff its pillows and feather its nest in anticipation of a fertilized egg rolling its way (or not, depending on your goals and actions). Your uterus right now is like an Italian grandma, preparing for the family to come over for dinner. It's busy creating a hospitable environment, cooking, totally focused on tending to its loved ones. There's so much exciting work to be done now, all in the name of the greatest things: love, life, family, creativity, and putting your best efforts into things that are meaningful to you.

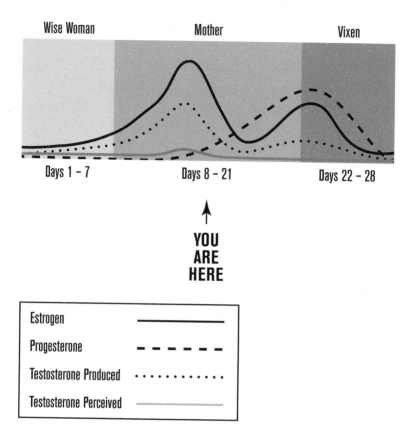

Wise Woman	Mother	Vixen
Days 1 – 7	Days 8 – 21	Days 22 – 28

**↑
YOU
ARE
HERE**

Estrogen	————
Progesterone	– – – – –
Testosterone Produced	· · · · · · · · · · ·
Testosterone Perceived	～～～～～～～～～

In the second week of Mega Phase, follicle stimulating hormone (FSH) peaks, causing your ovaries to cue a couple of eggs to begin to ripen. The eggs are located within the tip of long, hair-like appendages called follicles. One egg will grow the most, and its follicle will swell to the point that the end bursts, and voila, the egg is released into the Fallopian tube. (This is why some women experience a little pain and perhaps some spotting, known as *Mittelschmerz*, which means "middle pain," in their abdomen during ovulation.)

To top it off, progesterone rises now, keeping the uterine landscape nice and fertile. Hormones are in abundance, and they are churning throughout the body. If you don't experience Mittelschmerz, you might have no inkling of the intricate workings of your reproductive system at this point in time, but it's there nonetheless, as evidenced by these two monthly "miracles."

Ovulation Makes a Woman More Injury-Prone—True or False?

By Katy Bowman, MS

Some research indicates that women athletes are more likely to incur an injury during the pre-ovulatory phase of their menstrual cycle. For years, the theory has been that cycling hormones created excessive joint laxity. But upon further investigation, studies have not supported the "hormone" theory.

What could be going on? When looking at studies it is important to consider the group being tested. Most research, in this case, looks at college-aged females. While fluctuating hormonal levels might make sense, there could be, perhaps, something simpler going on: regular old fatigue.

Anytime your body does anything—in this case, begin the cycle of ovulation—the body requires more energy. These studies show the outcomes of physically straining the body, already fatigued from the college lifestyle (little sleep, stressful studying, not-as stressful partying, and questionable dietary intake), with vigorous exercise. A more simple explanation is that the body is too fatigued during pre-ovulation to cut and jump. To decrease potential injury during your cycle, be aware of your body's needs when it comes to energy input (good food!) and rest.

Your hormones have cranked up the intensity and, ladies, it's time for you to do it, too. You've wiped the slate uterus clean and here you are, light and free—reborn. It's the spring and summer of the cycle. Most women feel awesome in Phase II, and if you followed the Phase I plan, you are rested and rejuvenated. Say bon voyage to stillness—it's time for action.

In Phase I, we retreat physically. In Phase III (which you'll learn more about in chapter 7), we retreat mentally and emotionally. In this phase, the Mega Phase, there's no retreating happening, in any way, shape, or form. We put ourselves out there and go for it. (As Ellen likes to say, "It's the yang to the yin.") How do muscles get stronger? How do bones get denser? How do relationships become stronger? How does your career trajectory rise higher? *Effort. Action. Doing stuff!* We're all about growing and circulation now. And since Mega Phase is twice the length of the other phases, we've got two whole weeks of hustle and bustle to capitalize on. (We think it's twice the fun, too, as we get to push ourselves a little and play a lot!)

PHASE II ARCHETYPE: MOTHER

A mother is the ultimate in feminine power. We've all heard the story of the mother who lifts an entire automobile off her child who is trapped underneath. Her enormous love gives her superhuman strength. The Mother archetype is a combination of Wonder Woman and Oprah. Sure, physical power is spotlighted, but equally important are all of the qualities attributed to the feminine, like love, compassion, and kindness.

Labor and childbirth have been well documented as (to put it lightly) tough.

Ellen had a twenty-eight-hour labor with her son, Luca, that involved tears of pain, puking, and diarrhea, all at the same time.

Kate had a seventy-two-hour endurance-fest—complete with fevers, multiple nights spent timing contractions, and a couple shots of whiskey—with her daughter, Lil. Then, her son Teddy came so fast he would have been born in the back of a cab had she not insisted the driver take Sixth Avenue instead of the route suggested by his GPS.

As all mothers can attest: *Labor is not for sissies.* Labor is for mothers. The Mother Action Plan, like labor, is not for sissies either! You want to lose five pounds? To end PMS? You want a raise? You want more friends? A flat belly? Well, you're not going to reach those goals by sitting at home on your Pottery Barn couch all month long. Now's the time for . . . *Effort. Action. Doing stuff!*

Even if you are not a mother and have no intention of having kids anytime soon, or ever, you are still the mother of your life and your happiness. You'll stay up nights, wake up early, cook your food, do your dishes, and never, ever stop thinking about yourself and your happiness. This Mega Phase is all about harnessing the strength, love, and faith of mothers and using these qualities to get the life you want.

THE MOTHER PLAN

One of the most important things to do during this phase is to get moving. Just about every kind of exercise promotes muscle and bone growth and lymphatic and blood circulation. To support all that growth in your muscles, you need plenty of protein. And all those good-feeling endorphins and energy you'll produce while working out are the perfect fuel for socializing—also known as interpersonal circulation. Vitamin E intake helps with blood circulation. See where we are going with this? Growth and circulation . . . your mantra for the next fourteen days!

Move, Part 1—Move like a Banshee

"The only valid excuse for not exercising is paralysis," says Moira Nordholt, the founder of Feel Good Guru, and while it's funny, it's so true (unless you're in Phase I), especially now in Phase II. We know you know that exercise increases the metabolic rate, helps circulation, improves blood-sugar regulation, and is one of the healthiest things you can do to find and maintain your ideal weight, prevent or manage PMS, and thrive all around. Your doctors have told you this. Your friends have told you this. *Cosmopolitan* magazine has told you this. You know already! What you may not know is that there are two kinds of exercise: formal and informal.

Formal exercise—the kind you do at the gym, which we'll get to in a moment—is mandatory for Mother, but the informal kind, aka, "non-exercise activity," is equally vital. We're talkin' taking the stairs, lifting the twenty-pound bag of dog food into and out of your car, walking to the post office, taking the trash out to the curb. In other words, be like most mothers—"work out" even when you're not working out. You should be "up and at 'em" during Phase II, active in general, not just during your workout.

Our ancestors, distant and not-so-distant, were masters of non-exercise activity. Their bodies were in constant motion. They didn't do aerobics or take tennis lessons. They shucked corn, churned butter, and walked for miles and miles, carrying water on their heads. From prehistoric times right up to the mid-twentieth century, our ancestors were in motion from sunup to sundown. Of course,

How Many Miles?

The average person's stride length is approximately 2.5 feet long. That means it takes around 2,000 steps to walk one mile. Ten thousand steps is about five miles.

Getting more non-exercise activity requires a mini paradigm shift. You need to start seeing and seeking out opportunities to move, because the status quo is much too sedentary. Here's a simple quiz:

You are jonesin' for a coffee and happen to be driving by a drive-through Starbucks. You choose:
   A. the drive-through, thinking, "I won't have to get outta my car!"
   B. to park and walk inside, thinking, "I want to dress my coffee myself."

It snowed last night and your walkway isn't cleared. You:
   A. yell up to your husband to do it; you don't want to put on snow boots.
   B. pick up the shovel and do it yourself. It'll only take a few minutes.

You are taking your child to the park. You:
   A. bring a book and sit on the bench.
   B. lace up your Converse sneakers and proceed to go up and down the slide a billion times.

"B" is the correct answer for all three of the quiz questions (in case you didn't know!). How does your brain work? Do you need to rewire it to gravitate toward action and, as Kate's grandmother likes to call it, "pep"?

sometimes the amount of "toil" was too much and not ideal in terms of wellness, but the point is that they were active.

The human body is engineered to move, not to sit still, and definitely not to hunch over a desk for eight hours a day. This is one of many reasons why modern life is not natural, for men and women alike. Ellen tells a story of when she went to replace her garage door. She requested a manual one, the kind you have to bend down, engage your abs, and pull open yourself. No electricity, no codes. Her goal was to just keep things simple. The garage door salesman said no one had asked for a manual door in "forever," and didn't have one to sell her. Just think: With a door that you have to open yourself, you sneak in some activity every time you need to get into your garage, and even that action has disappeared for most of America. We push a button instead of using brawn.

During Phase II, we want you to find ways of using the proverbial manual garage door. Maybe it's by riding your bike to work and leaving your car at home. Maybe it's by getting on your hands and knees and scrubbing the kitchen floor yourself instead of paying someone to do it. Maybe it's by replacing your desk chair with an exercise ball, or by organizing a walking meeting, instead of a "slouching" meeting over the phone.

A 2004 study published in *Medicine and Science in Sports and Exercise* showed the variation between 200 men and women in regards to steps taken per day. The men in the survey took an average of 7,192 steps each day, while the women in the survey took an average of 5,210 steps. This upsets us so much. First, we "lost" to the boys. (Joke.) And second, according to a lifestyle index, 5,000 to 7,499 steps per day is considered *low activity*, so 5,210 is "unacceptable," says Ellen!

Move, Part 2—One Daily 30-Minute Minimum Formal Workout

Schedule a bona fide 30- to 60-minute workout every single day of Phase II. That's fourteen days in a row of donning the workout clothes and busting it out. Running, Zumba, yoga class, Pilates session? All good. The ideal duration is 30 to 60 minutes, but the type of workout and its level of intensity are up to you to decide.

You know how the contestants on *The Biggest Loser* always look so tortured while working out? That's because they are! "Exercise is torture" is a primary belief for them because 1) They partake in someone else's workout preference; and 2) the level of intensity is all wrong / too much / borderline insane. We want you to enjoy and be happy with your workouts, because when you actually look forward to them, you'll do them, and it's only by doing them that you'll become fit for the long haul.

> We want you to enjoy and be happy with your workouts, because when you actually look forward to them, you'll do them, and it's only by doing them that you'll become fit for the long haul.

Exercise, in all its forms, promotes circulation, and circulation (remember, it's one of our two themes in Phase II) keeps things percolating—energizing your thyroid, your reproductive organs, and your metabolism. Your lymphatic system works directly with your cardiovascular system to keep blood and lymphatic fluid moving and flushing toxins out of the body. The lymphatic system also carries immune cells throughout the body to help defend against infections. But your lymphatic system doesn't have a pump the way the circulatory system has the heart. The only way to move lymph is to *move*.

Here's Ellen's Mega Phase workout journal:

Day 8: Hike with Roxy—60 minutes
Day 9: Hatha yoga class—75 minutes
Day 10: 10 Sun Salutations—30 minutes
Day 11: Hatha yoga class—75 minutes
Day 12: Ran a 5K race for charity—35 minutes
Day 13: Hike with Roxy—60 minutes
Day 14: 10 Sun Salutations—30 minutes
Day 15: At-home exercise DVD—30 minutes
Day 16: Power walk with pal—60 minutes
Day 17: Ashtanga yoga class—90 minutes
Day 18: Mini hike with Roxy—30 minute
Day 19: Bike ride to and from yoga studio for restorative yoga class—2 hours
Day 20: 10 Sun Salutations—30 minutes
Day 21: Power walk with pal—60 minutes

The Do-Anywhere Perfect and Complete Workout—
Sun Salutations

Sun Salutations are genius. Someone or something very awesome must have created them thousands of years ago in India. These twelve or so poses, linked in a series, lengthen and strengthen the main muscles of the body and flex the spine, all while distributing energy (aka, circulation) throughout the system. The low lunge stretches the muscles of the upper and inner thighs, brings energy into the hips, while also stimulating what Eastern medicine calls the stomach, spleen, and liver meridians. Sun Salutations are lovingly weight-bearing, so they help use, build, and maintain solid bone density. Five—or more, if you are so inclined—Sun Salutations can be a complete workout in and of itself, or a great start to your active day.

The cycle goes as follows:

1. Start in **Mountain Pose,** standing tall with arms by your sides. Inhale and sweep arms out to the sides and up. Exhale and swan-dive with a flat back into **Standing Forward Bend,** with fingertips on the floor outside your feet in line with your toes.

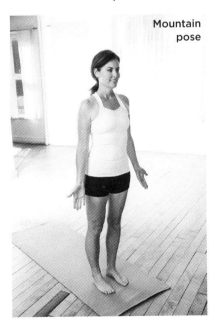

Mountain pose

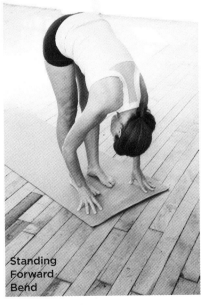

Standing Forward Bend

2. Exhale and step the left foot way back and lower the left knee and top of the left foot to come into a **Low Lunge (arms down)**.

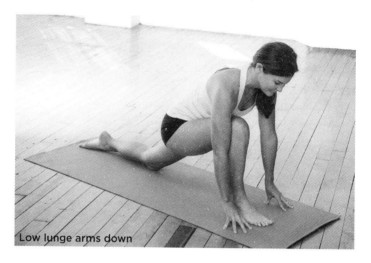

Low lunge arms down

3. Inhale and **lift the arms up in Low Lunge** and stay for five breaths, then exhale and lower the arms, bringing the fingers to the floor outside the front foot.

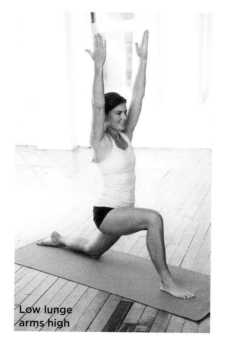

Low lunge arms high

4. Inhale and step the right foot back into **Plank Pose** (both palms are planted directly under the shoulders, arms and legs straight, head, shoulders, hips, and ankles forming one long incline).

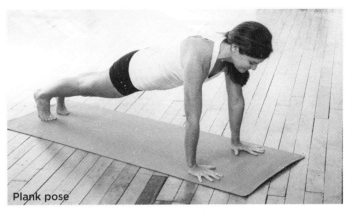

Plank pose

5. Exhale as you bend elbows straight back to lower down into **Chaturanga Dandasana,** with legs straight or knees on the ground, or you can lower down into Modified Chaturanga Dandasana.

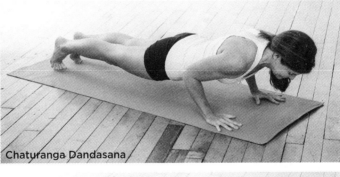

Chaturanga Dandasana

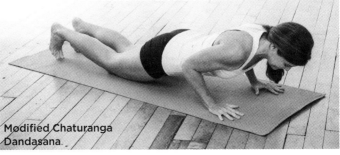

Modified Chaturanga Dandasana

6. Bring your hips to the ground and press your hands into the floor to lift the chest into **Cobra Pose,** strengthening the lower back.

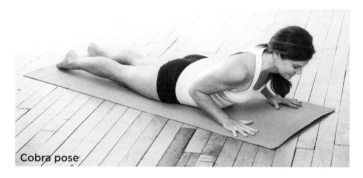

Cobra pose

7. Exhale and lift the hips up to come into **Downward-Facing Dog Pose,** lengthening the hamstrings, calves, and torso, while strengthening the upper body.

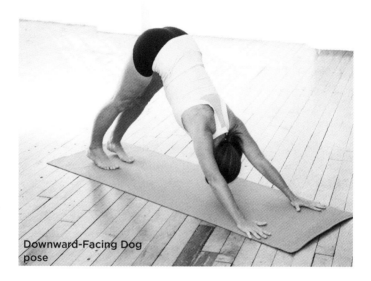

Downward-Facing Dog
pose

8. After five breaths, inhale and step the right foot forward into a **Low Lunge** on the other side.

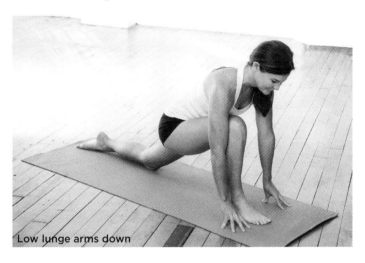

Low lunge arms down

9. Inhale and **lift the arms in Low Lunge** for five breaths.

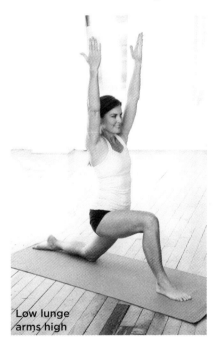

Low lunge arms high

10. On the fifth exhalation, lower the arms, and on the inhalation, step the back foot forward to meet the front one. Lift the chest and exhale; fold into **Standing Forward Bend.**

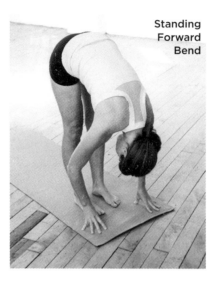

Standing Forward Bend

11. On the next inhalation, lift the arms, leading from the sternum, and come up to standing (bend the knees if the lower back is tight or weak) and reach both arms up and slightly back into a **Standing Back Bend.**

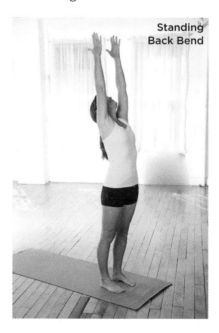

Standing Back Bend

12. Exhale and return to **Mountain Prayer Pose with hands in Namaste** (hands in prayer position at the chest).

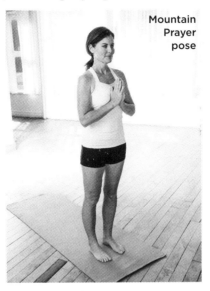

Mountain
Prayer
pose

Linger in Mountain Pose for five breaths and feel the effects wash over you. Notice the energy circulating within you and feel your body's heat. We encourage repeating this for at least five rounds, or for 15 to 30 minutes.

After your Sun Salutations, spend a few minutes in a **Supported Shoulder Stand,** with a block underneath your sacrum.

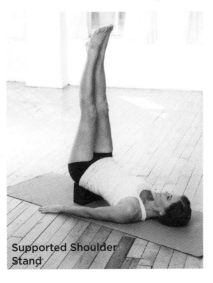

Supported Shoulder
Stand

How to do it: To come into Supported Shoulder Stand, lie on your back with your knees bent and feet flat on the floor. Push into the floor with your feet, lift your hips, and place the block under the back of your pelvis. Bend your knees into your chest, then straighten your legs. Press the palms into the floor, and concentrate on lifting your chest, elongating your neck, but don't let your chin fall toward your chest.

What it does: Getting your legs above your heart promotes the circulation of blood and lymph from the lower half of the body. And pressing your chin toward your chest and reaching your chest toward your chin massages the thyroid, bathing it in fresh blood and promoting its optimal function. Stay at least 1 minute and as long as 5.

Nourish: Be Protein-centric

Protein is a building block. We are literally made of it; our heart, brain, liver, kidneys, and lungs are composed of tissue made from protein. Protein is present in every cell in the human body. It's a crucial, natural compound and responsible for *growth.*

According to the Centers for Disease Control and Prevention, the recommended dietary allowance for protein for menstruating women is 46 grams. This is a highly debated figure, as there are many theories out there regarding how much protein we should consume. Many protein devotees and athletic trainers recommend more than 100 grams per day! Like calories, we don't want you to count protein amounts. That would be too mechanical, and could potentially take away from the enjoyment of eating. (French women who "don't get fat" would never count protein grams!) We do want you to be protein-centric, and make protein the focal point of every single meal and snack during Mega Phase, because the more you exercise, the greater your protein needs will be, and since you are moving like a banshee these days, you'll need ample amounts. Here's our strategy:

Eat Whole

Here's a little secret: Every whole food, even sugar in its natural, unprocessed state, has protein. Whole fruit. Whole veggies. Even whole wheat. It's the processing that strips away the protein, fiber, and other nutrients, so the less processed food you eat, the more likely your diet will be protein-centric.

Ginger Tea

Ginger is a circulation superstar, and homemade ginger tea made from fresh ginger is a yummy way to get your energy flowing.

Ingredients:
4 to 6 thin slices raw ginger
1½ to 2 cups water
Lemon slice (optional)
1 to 2 Tbsp honey (optional)

Peel the ginger and slice thinly to maximize the surface area. This will help you make a very flavorful ginger tea. Boil the ginger in water for at least 10 minutes. For a stronger tea, allow to boil for 20 minutes or more, and use more slices of ginger. Remove from heat by pouring into a mug. Add lemon slices and honey to taste.

Be Atypical

Chicken, beef, and fish are typical. Everyone knows they are protein-rich. Sadly, however, many people think animal flesh is the *only* way to get protein. That's simply not true. You don't have to eat meat at all, and certainly not at every meal. Here are non-meat examples of high protein:

- 1 large egg: 6 grams

- ½ cup almonds: 8 grams

- ¼ cup pumpkin seeds: 8 grams

- ¼ cup flax seeds: 8 grams

- 1 cup milk: 8 grams

- 1 cup cooked quinoa: 8 grams

- 8-ounce container of yogurt: 11 grams

- 1 cup beans: 16 grams

Switch to Protein-centric Grains

Oats and quinoa are our kind of grains! They are loaded with nutrients and—ta-da—protein! Our Tart Cherry Granola, Good Morning Oatmeal, and Quinoa Stir-Fry featured in chapter 8 are downright perfect for Mega Phase. Remember, protein is a steady fuel source as well as a building material, and grains—being easily digestible and usually loaded with fiber—are a home run when you're a Mother.

Live—Circulate

Get out there. Socialize. Say yes to invitations. Stay late at work. It's not about being an extrovert as much as it's about building relationships, having experiences, and making headway in your career or in your passions. Now's the time! Carpe diem! No need to conserve your energies in Phase II—physical, social, or otherwise. What does this have to do with ending PMS and dropping ten pounds? Everything, because it's part of the cycle.

Let's go back to the Mother archetype. Does a mom ever have an eight-hour day? No, she has a twenty-four-hour day, seven days

Mega Phase Is a No-TV Phase for Ellen

Ellen: This happened unconsciously, but I noticed that during my Mega Phase, I didn't watch TV. There are two reasons for this phenomenon: One, I was busy outside of the house, leaving early and returning home late. And two, when I was inside the house, I was on the phone, playing "bad guys" with my son, or otherwise engaged. This happened naturally. When you are full of energy and experiencing an extroverted surge, TV is boring.

a week! (We get feisty when talking motherhood.) Don't go straight home from work. Organize a play date with your kids. Have a date night with your husband. Meet your girlfriends at a cafe for tea and chitchat. In Phase I, you are too low-energy to circulate, and in Phase III, you'll be "socially short-fused," so do it now. When the other phases come around, you'll be satiated and guilt-free. Most important, you will have invested in your relationships, building emotional strength and interpersonal power.

All Month Long, Part 1—Nurture Your Thyroid
The thyroid affects weight, fertility, the menstrual cycle, and the theme of Phase III—circulation. We touched on the powers of the thyroid a bit in chapter 3, but here we'll take things into a proactive realm, answering the question "What can we do, without drugs or doctors, that'll get—and keep—our thyroid in top shape?"

The first, and probably the most important, action to take when it comes to thyroid health is to *ingest sufficient iodine* into your body. Iodine is the mineral associated with the thyroid, and it regulates estrogen production in the ovaries, making it a crucial component to women's health. The recommended daily allowance (RDA) for iodine is 150 mcg/day, but many health advocates (including us) believe that figure is too low, especially for women, who have iodine stores in ovary and breast tissues, so we urge you to aim for 220mcg/day, by eating iodine-rich foods like seaweeds, seafood, nuts, and

We Are Not into Soy

You may notice that in all of our recipes in chapter 8, soy is absent. That's because we *never* use soy. Let it be known that many studies have concluded that soy injures the thyroid. Researchers have identified that the isoflavones in soy products act as anti-thyroid agents, and can suppress thyroid function, thus causing or worsening hypothyroidism. Soy acts like a hormone in the body as it is a phytoestrogen, so it can upset the balance of hormonal systems.

We're Not Crazy about Gluten, Either

Kate and Ellen have slightly differing opinions on this, but when Kate's post-baby weight was still firmly attached to her middle after two years, she went to see an ND (naturopathic doctor). Her amazing doctor gave her a good old-fashioned physical exam and said Kate's thyroid was palpable—which isn't typical, and is an indicator that it's not functioning well. The ND suggested that Kate give up gluten, which is antagonistic to the thyroid, for three weeks so she could see how different she felt without it, and take one thyroid supplement that contained plenty of iodine.

After three weeks, Kate tried eating whole wheat (a dark-chocolate-dipped, whole-wheat biscotti, to be exact) and was shocked to discover that that little bit of wheat was enough to make her constipated for three days. Three days! Needless to say, Kate was inspired to stick with the gluten-free lifestyle (finding gluten-free beer made it much easier to take), and discovered some great things along the way. First, being gluten-free required her to reach for whole foods more often, since the "convenient" options of sandwiches, pizza, and pasta were out. Second, she stopped falling asleep while putting her daughter to bed at eight o'clock every night. Third, she lost eight pounds of stubborn, jiggly belly weight. (Ellen knows how challenging it can be to be 100 percent gluten-free, both socially and economically, so she recommends opting for organic wheat products, as they will not have GMOs, and minimizing gluten intake overall—not cutting it out completely. We explain gluten a bit more on page 160 in chapter 8.)

vegetables. With our nutrient-rich diet strategy, it's easy to get adequate iodine every day.

Second, *don't starve.* If you've been on a dieting roller coaster, we are so glad our book found you! It's important to know that "starvation diets" (diets with severely restricted caloric intake) are a common cause of an underactive thyroid. Starvation slows the body's metabolism, as the thyroid gland learns to expend energy more efficiently in order to conserve calories for the next "famine." After a starvation diet we have a tendency to gain even more weight than we took off, and we may find it even harder to lose weight the next time we try. A very low-calorie diet can suppress the thyroid function in less than twenty-four hours. After one to three months of such dieting, there is a danger of permanently inhibiting the thyroid function.

Third, *relax*. Many thyroid disorders occur because of excessive stress. Yoga and meditation can help to alleviate stress and anxiety to a great extent. This practice is also useful in maintaining the right balance between the mind and the body. Phase I's stillness and Phase III's solitude also play important roles in keeping stress at bay.

Four, *filter your water*. It's important to drink fresh unfluoridated water (that means no tap water), as fluoride is proven to weaken the thyroid.

Just like obesity and menstrual problems, thyroid disorders are at *epidemic* levels. In the United States, more than 30 million people suffer from thyroid disorder, and that doesn't include the people who have what's known as "subclinical" thyroid issues—meaning their thyroid function doesn't register as lacking according to standard medical tests, but is low enough to have ill effects on the body. Many women go undiagnosed with "borderline" thyroid function, where their thyroid is "okay" according to Western medicine's blood testing system, yet still not working up to par.

You are not alone if your thyroid isn't up to snuff. (Ellen was borderline, and restored her thyroid health *fully* by doing this "all month long" protocol.) We feel that our program can help bring your thyroid into balance, but in addition to our program, we encourage you to read two exciting books: *The Thyroid Solution: A Revolutionary Mind-Body Program for Regaining Your Emotional and Physical Health* by Dr. Ridha Arem, and *Solved: The Riddle of Illness* by Stephen Langer and James Scheer. They are refreshingly holistic and cover the mind, body, and spiritual aspects on everything thyroid.

All Month Long, Part 2—Vitamin E

Vitamin E is an antioxidant that improves circulation by thinning the blood, making it flow more smoothly through our veins. It has been proven successful in increasing ovulation and conception, too. You know when someone has nice levels of vitamin E because her hair tends to be shiny, her skin isn't dry, and her lips aren't cracking.

Food Sources of Vitamin E

Sunflower seeds (1 oz.)	7.4 mg
Almonds (1 oz.)	7.3 mg
Turnip greens (½ cup, cooked)	2.9 mg
Tomato, pureed or sauce (½ cup)	2.5 mg
Pine nuts (1 oz.)	2.6 mg
Wheat germ (2 Tbsp.)	2.3 mg
Avocado (½)	2.1 mg
Spinach (½ cup, cooked)	1.9 mg
Broccoli (½ cup, cooked)	1.2 mg
Olive oil (1 Tbsp.)	1.9 mg

Healthy oils (like wheat germ and olive oil), nuts (like cashews and almonds), and seeds (like sunflower and pumpkin seeds) are all vitamin E all-stars. You can also find vitamin E in broccoli, spinach, and avocado—and who doesn't love avocados?

Vitamin E deficiency is rare for American women. Yet even though we may not be deficient, we may thrive with a bit more. The US Recommended Daily Allowance (RDA) for adult women is 15 mg per day, but that number is contested by many holistic health practitioners, who recommend up to 80 mg per day. Instead of keeping track of numbers, just know that every single one of our recipes contains some vitamin E.

Low-Fat Diets Can Cause Vitamin E Deficiency

Vitamin E is plentiful in oils and other "high-fat" foods. In fact, vitamin E is fat-soluble, so it *needs* fat to be assimilated in the body. Low-fat diets—the kind that steer you away from nutritious sesame seeds and avocados because they are "high in fat"—are dangerous and should be avoided always and forever.

READY, SET, FLOW FOR DAYS 8–21

- All phase long: Be a social butterfly. Unlike Phase I, you do not need extra downtime now. In fact, you will actually thrive with very little.

- All phase long: Work out daily for at least 30 minutes. This could be a walk in the park, a Pilates class, or a competitive tennis match.

- All phase long: Make sure every meal has sufficient protein—10 grams per meal is ideal. Energy Balls (page 142), Ginger Salad with Shrimp (page 145), and Quinoa Stir-Fry (page 149) are excellent protein-rich meal options for the Mother Phase.

- All phase long: Nurture your thyroid with a daily Supported Shoulder Stand (see page 89).

- All phase long: Get plenty of non-exercise activity by physically moving as much as possible, or as we like to say, "hustle." These fourteen days are all about the hustle!

- All cycle long: Support your thyroid by getting plenty of iodine. Our Ginger Salad with Shrimp recipe gets an iodine A+!

The Top Three Habits of the Highly Successful Mother

1. The habit of hustle—be energetic with everything you do during Days 8–21.
2. Make protein-rich meals that have minimal gluten content.
3. Do a daily Supported Shoulder Stand between Days 8–21 (see page 89). Hold for at least 1 minute.

- All cycle long: Support your circulatory system by getting plenty of vitamin E. Our Buff Girl Guacamole recipe on page 139 is packed with it.

Overall, the fourteen days of Mother are extroverted, high-energy, and productive. These energies equate to *doing*, so don't just sit there, *do something!* We are advising you to work hard and play hard. You're feeling frisky this time of the month, too, which may motivate you to be *very* social! Sex is great exercise, plus it creates intimacy—perfect for Phase II.

CHAPTER 7

Phase III: Pre-Menstruation (Days 22–28) VIXEN

Let's get one thing straight: Pre-menstruation is simply the time frame preceding menstruation. There is no rule that it automatically includes the stereotypical symptoms of PMS, such as crankiness, headaches, and foul moods. It does not deserve to have only a negative connotation. It is not a requirement that you experience out-of-control food cravings that lead to eating binges that in turn lead to weight woes.

Here's what's going on in your body during this phase: Estrogen and progesterone levels rapidly increase on or around Day 21, then plateau before strongly decreasing on or around Day 25. By Day 28, we bottom out. This hormone roller coaster is a natural ebb and flow within the body and is not a disease or chronic condition (as Western medicine chooses to label it). The hormonal shifts happening now lead to:

1. A bit more water retention, but not necessarily to the point of discomfort.
2. Lower energy levels, but nothing that an earlier bedtime can't help.
3. A bona fide aversion to social situations, but nothing that solitude can't remedy.

There is *nothing* "wrong" with these three occurrences. Mother Nature is simply ebbing and flowing, like the seasons, the breath, the tide, and the planets. So we repeat: Moderate water retention, low-*ish* energy levels, and introverted tendencies are not bad. They don't need to be "tamed" with drugs of any kind. They are natural . . . and womanly. (And dare we say, beneficial. More on that later!)

Yet today in America the majority of women experience something dreaded, often debilitating. They have premenstrual syndrome (PMS), which may include the following symptoms:

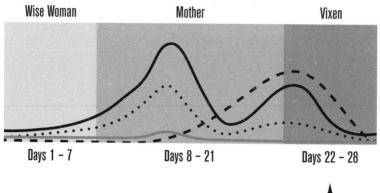

Wise Woman   **Mother**   **Vixen**

Days 1 – 7   Days 8 – 21   Days 22 – 28

↑
**YOU
ARE
HERE**

Estrogen	——————
Progesterone	– – – – – –
Testosterone Produced	· · · · · · · · · · ·
Testosterone Perceived	∼∼∼∼∼∼∼∼∼∼∼

- Breast swelling and tenderness

- Dizziness

- Headaches

- Cramps

- Nausea and vomiting

- Food cravings

- Abdominal bloating

- Noticeable weight gain from water retention

- Stomach upset

- Lower back pain

- Depressed mood

- Crying spells

- Anxiety, irritability, anger

- Trouble falling asleep

If you experience some or all of these symptoms, you're not alone. Too many women (a whopping 80 percent of American female adults, in fact) experience PMS. Studies report that more than 50 percent of women find PMS to be a setback, and 20 percent of American women miss work because of it. It's fair to say that for a few days each month, most American women are less productive, make less-healthy dietary choices, strain their relationships, and are, from dusk to dawn, downright uncomfortable.

We've noticed—and too often—that PMS leads to self-destructive behavior. Overeating, eating junk food, and not exercising are destructive to the body. Days of zoning out with gossip magazines and *Real Housewives* marathons are destructive to the mind. Holding your tongue to such an extent that you lash out at friends and family or go on random crying jags are detrimental to your emotional wellness. Many of us have three weeks of healthful living in body, mind, and spirit, and then PMS sabotages it all. Month after

Could PMS Be a By-Product of Progress?

It's true that women from all over the world say they experience physical changes related to menstruation, but PMS seems to be more common in Western cultures. Several studies concluded that PMS is influenced by cultural factors and the modern demands on women in Western industrialized countries. In fact, women who are married and have children are more likely to suffer from PMS symptoms.

Out-of-Control Eating and PMS: Taryn's Story

I was a serious figure skater as a teen. It's a sport that requires a huge amount of discipline, which I had most of the time. I had no problem adhering to a strict training schedule and diet every day of the month except during PMS. On these four days leading up to my period, I had to have Cheetos and Happy Meals. I'd down a pint of ice cream at ten a.m.! Because of this, I was always playing catch-up the rest of the month, always weighing in seven to ten pounds more than I needed to in order to compete at a high level. I wish I'd known about the 28 Days Lighter Diet then; I would have been much more successful as a figure skater, and I wouldn't have felt so badly about myself during my teen years.

(freaking) month . . . it's enough to ultimately squelch the spirit. In regard to water weight, it gets even more frustrating. Many women retain scary levels of water during Phase III, with certain statistics indicating that for some, it can be as much as three to six pounds of water weight. News flash: This is not normal.

A big bummer for us is the fact that most of our fellow females believe PMS is *normal.* (Ellen did until she was thirty-five!) Why? Because it's so common, of course. But there is another reason, perpetuated at your doctor's office. Get this: Our go-to authority on the woman's reproductive system, our ob/gyn, leads us to believe that PMS is "just the way it goes," and that "there's nothing much you can do about it." Usually, she doesn't take your symptoms all that seriously, and even when she does, she offers a Band-Aid, like a prescription for pain medication or a hormone corral-er, like The Pill. From our holistic point of view, this is a big problem, and explains why the widespread belief that PMS is normal is so gosh-darn widespread.

Our female ancestors didn't seem to suffer from PMS. That's because:

1. They were more in tune with the moon.
2. They were aware of cycles in nature. They shivered in winter and sweated in summer, as there was no AC or central heating. They also went to bed earlier in the winter due to diminished sunlight.
3. They had weekly and seasonal Sabbaths. Today, we live in a 24/7 world, whereas our ancestors "turned off" more often.
4. They ate seasonally. Berries in spring are especially cleansing after a winter of fermented heavy foods. Summer is a time for more raw and water-rich foods, like melon and lettuce.
5. They had limited birth control and thus were pregnant earlier and more often. (Pregnancy has been known to regulate the menstrual cycle.)
6. They didn't have supermarkets filled with crappy, preservative-filled, processed food. Fluoride wasn't in their water systems. High-fructose corn syrup didn't exist. Neither did GMOs.

Yes, you can do something about PMS besides pop a Midol. This is not hearsay. It has been proven that women, through diet, exercise, and lifestyle, can turn their PMS predicament completely around, and quickly—within a few months. So congratulations are in order; just by picking up this book, you're one step closer to smoother pre-menstruation sailing.

Three Deep Thoughts

1. The problem, bigger than this PMS epidemic, is that we live in a society that thinks PMS is just part of being a woman.
2. Pre-menstruation doesn't have to equal PMS.
3. The week before your period can actually be a time of power, charisma, and attraction.

THE BENEFITS OF PRE-MENSTRUATION

Yep, that's right; we said *"benefits* of pre-menstruation." You know how most of us women were brought up to be sweet little peacekeepers? How, if you didn't have anything nice to say, it's better to not say anything at all? That crap just doesn't apply to pre-menstruation.

During this highly intuitive time, your true thoughts are right at the surface. If you acknowledge them and give them a healthy form of expression, you can make important decisions and changes now that would seem impolite or uncool at other times of the month. In fact, we theorize that the stereotype of the premenstrual woman scarfing a bag of chips or pint of ice cream is really an attempt to keep those true thoughts stuffed way down, where we've been taught they ought to be. Pre-menstruation is all about letting it fly, baby. And if you can find a way to talk to your husband about why tripping on the shoes he insists on leaving strewn in the middle of the floor makes you want to throw his remote control out the window *before* you actually hurl it outside, you can make positive changes in your relationship and avoid the need to stuff yourself with empty calories.

Lara Owen said it best in her guide to a balanced menstrual cycle, *Her Blood Is Gold:* "It may be that one of the functions of PMS is that through hostility, women repel those around them, and therefore are able to have a little time to themselves." How's that for a different take on PMS? She goes on: "Before I became conscious of my need to spend time alone during the premenstrual phase, I often experienced a feeling of deep relief when the man in my life took himself out of the house rather than stay around my bad mood . . . I found that when I began to pick up this pattern consciously, I stopped needing to have crazy fights and wild outbursts just before my period; what actually wanted to happen was a clearing up of any relationship difficulties in my life." Let's add another item to the list of functions our menstrual cycle can serve in our life: shrink.

If you find yourself getting incredibly irritable each and every month, use some of the solitude you will now create for yourself during the week as a chance to ask yourself, What am I not saying that needs to be said? What am I not doing that needs to be done? Acting on the answers you get will not only relieve your premenstrual symptoms, but it will also change your relationships and your life for the better.

What's Your Liver Got to Do With Your PMS?

By Laurie Steelsmith, ND

If you want a healthy, happy menstrual cycle, you need a healthy, happy liver. From a Western perspective, the liver is responsible for breaking down hormones (as well as other materials, including alcohol and environmental toxins) into digestible forms so they can be removed by the body. The liver processes estrogen and progesterone, delivers them to the gallbladder, which delivers them to the colon, where they are then—ideally—expelled in the stool. From a Chinese perspective, the uterus, ovaries, and breasts all reside on the liver meridian, or energy pathway. The liver regulates all transformations in the body, and that includes ovulation and menstruation.

Your liver is exquisitely designed to regulate the amount of hormones circulating in your system. The bad news is that pretty much everyone's liver is overworked, and if you drink alcohol regularly, yours is likely *really* overworked. It's hard work to find food that hasn't been encased in plastic, which can leach troublesome chemicals into your dinner. Most personal-care products are chock-full of petroleum by-products. It is the responsibility of the liver to process and eliminate all of these environmental chemicals. Throw regular margaritas or glasses of red wine into the mix, and your liver starts to get bogged down and will fall behind.

You'll get clues your liver is sluggish; gassiness, bloating, slowed digestion, breast tenderness and swelling, breast cysts, and noticeable irritability during the pre-menstruation phase are key indicators. If you recognize yourself in these symptoms, it's important that you embark on the Happy Liver Program outlined on page 174 at least once a year, and incorporate whatever pieces of it work best for you and your lifestyle as you're able the rest of the time. You don't have to do an extreme "cleanse" or "detox" to reap major benefits—namely, a leaner, cleaner body and less irritability, which paves the way for closer relationships, too.

It's What You Do All Month Long, Not Just during Pre-menstruation

Many of you reading this book may only have issues with PMS, so you'll open it up to this chapter and heed the advice given for this phase only. While it will undoubtedly help, it won't do the whole trick. You have to get tuned in with your entire cycle, not just this part of it. It's like patching up a leaky boat in one spot when there are three more holes. You'll sink more slowly, but you'll still sink.

THE PHASE III ARCHETYPE: THE VIXEN

A Vixen is undoubtedly female, *with an edge.* We've labeled Phase III—the "finale" of the cycle—*Vixen* because, ladies, in this phase of our cycle, we're instinctual, going with our guts. The barrier between our wants and our actions is gone. And a woman who knows what she wants and goes after it is *sexy,* dammit.

> *Women complain about PMS, but I think of it as the only time of the month when I can be myself.*
>
> —Roseanne Barr

Vixen (n)
1. A female fox
2. A quarrelsome woman
3. A spitfire
4. A carnivorous female

History is sprinkled with some notable Vixens. French warrior Joan of Arc, descended from a powerless peasant family, claimed divine guidance as she led the French army to several victories in the Hundred Years War. Two key things make her an exemplary Vixen:

1) She had a heightened sense of spiritual connectedness; and 2) she followed her instincts with fervor (even when they may have tipped over the proverbial apple cart). Another great example is pop star Madonna. She is an obvious Vixen, and with her mix of spirituality, sexuality, and ambition, she has conquered the world, pissing off more than a few along the way.

A girl should be two things: who and what she wants.

—Coco Chanel (spoken like a true Vixen)

Like pre-menstruation, the Vixen archetype tends to have a negative connotation. Too little sleep, too much small talk, not enough exercise, and too many Frappuccinos all throw Vixen off her A-game and throw her into *imbalance*. Think bee-yatch instead of red-hot mama. Vixen, just like pre-menstruation, can be horrible or glorious.

Remember: Even though it's just a few days each month, PMS is a disease, just like asthma and arthritis. Truly healing it—not just managing it or suppressing symptoms—involves rebalancing.

So what does a balanced Vixen look like? Well, for starters, she's content, but not too keen on whooping it up. She's confident enough to know that her true self will draw the right people toward her; she doesn't need to go out on the town and scatter her energy. She's conscious of her inner self and wants to commune with it. Her intuitiveness is at a monthlong high. What an opportunity to get clear on what's true for you, and to connect with just the right people who recognize and appreciate what you're really about.

Albert Einstein said, "The intuitive mind is a sacred gift and the rational mind is a faithful servant. We have created a society that honors the servant and has forgotten the gift." This quote really speaks to us in regard to Vixen. We live in a culture that is pointed outward and values logic more than gut feeling. There is, of course, a need for logic, but there is also an incredible need for intuition. When you are intuitive, you know which decisions to make. Your actions are laser-focused—even if they don't make sense to other people, or even your own rational mind. When you are in touch with your intuition, you trust that everything is working out exactly as it needs to, and you know that if something you say or do upsets someone else, that reaction is going to be just what that person needs to learn and grow. When you are in touch with your inner wisdom, you aren't worried about keeping the peace. That's what Phase III is *all about*. We always have access to our intuition, but during the Vixen days, intuition is bubbling to the surface. Feeling slightly bloated, sluggish, and introverted is nature's way of turning your attention toward your literal and metaphorical center: the womb. Don't deny the power that's available to you right now!

We've noticed in ourselves, and in the women we've had the privilege of working with over the years, that when we are really "sold" on our society and all its *yang*-ness, its hustle and bustle, confrontation, and go-go-go, we are at battle with our retreating tendencies. By denying the urge to stay home, nest, to be alone and withdraw from certain social scenes, we exacerbate and perpetuate PMS.

THE VIXEN PLAN: CARDIO, SOLITUDE, AND HYDRATION

The overall theme of the Vixen phase is *abundance.* The question to ask yourself now is, "What can I add?" instead of, "What should I avoid?" It's time to really treat yourself! A walk in the woods is a treat. Staying home and watching a movie in bed instead of going out is downright luxurious. We've noticed that traditional pre-menstruation action steps do the opposite of this, focusing on what we should cut out: Don't drink coffee. Don't eat salty chips. Yada, yada, yada. This does more harm than good to the psyche because we end up walking around the world with a sense of deficiency. It's also incredibly difficult to give up your beloved cup of joe during the few days you are most sensitive. So think abundance with the three Vixen action steps and *add* steady cardio exercise, solitude, and hydration through food and drink. (Yep, still no calorie counting, folks!)

Move—Steady Cardiovascular Exercise

Exercise is your medicine, Vixen. We feel the most important part of the Vixen protocol is, without a doubt, *Move.* Our reasoning is simple: *You gotta keep feeling good,* and exercise is Mother Nature's great antidepressant. Everything else will be much more manageable once you get your move on!

"The inactive body is a residence for depression," says Dr. Maoshing Ni in *Secrets of Self-Healing*. This is especially true when you're a Vixen. Way back in 1998, a publicist said to Ellen, "You sell exercise." Well, if there was ever a moment of truth, it's in this chapter, over fifteen years later. Here, we are selling exercise, *aggressively*. That's because, when it's done right during pre-menstruation, there are soooooo many pros—and zero cons.

The perfect Vixen workout is nothing fancy. There are no bells and whistles, just your basic cardio. Ideally, it's 45 to 60 minutes that's moderate-intensity and low-impact. Go for a hike, take a power walk, or zoom away on your bike . . . these are perfect options for Phase III because they are 1) sustainable for 45 to 60 minutes; 2) solitary (if you want them to be) or socially mellow; 3) low- or non-impact; and 4) they induce sweating.

On a scale of 1 to 10, 10 being very intense, hover around 6 or 7. You don't need to huff and puff to get the job done. In fact, we don't want you to huff and puff at all. You should be able to carry on a conversation at this intensity level, and sustaining 60 minutes should be very doable.

> *The body only profits a little from exercising, but the spirit profits a lot.*
> —Billy Blanks, founder of Tae Bo

When estrogen is low, we are more sensitive to pain. A quick and natural way to remedy premenstrual discomfort is through cardiovascular exercise because it generates two feel-good chemicals in the body, endorphins and serotonin. These "chemicals" literally turn that frown upside down. They help to release tension and soothe our nerves—crucial for the premenstrual grump.

Besides the endorphin and serotonin kick, the second reason for this type of exercise during Vixen is simple: Cardio promotes perspiration. Breaking a sweat is especially advantageous when one is bloated because it releases excess water. Sweating cleanses the body of toxins, as well as helps with overall blood and lymph circulation. Sweating is so good for us!

Favor low-impact activities, like walking and cycling, as opposed to high-impact ones, like jogging and jumping rope, because the uterus is at its heaviest now. Like we mentioned in The Golden Rules (page 46), the added weight—even just a few ounces—could strain the ligaments that hold the uterus in its position. On average for a woman of childbearing age, the uterus is the size of a fist and weighs approximately four to seven ounces. The size and weight will vary depending on how many pregnancies the woman has had, and/or if there are any fibroids or masses present. During pre-menstruation, when the uterine lining is thickest, it can weigh an additional two ounces (or more).

Shifting the uterus out of its current harmonious spot in the lower abdomen causes a "tipped" or "tilted" uterus, which has been known to cause painful periods, infertility, and reproductive problems, because the blood flow to the pelvis can be compromised. This is why we insist on low-impact activities and avoid activities that require both feet off the ground at the same time, like jogging, some forms of dance, tennis, and high-impact aerobics.

Correcting a Tilted Uterus

The Arvigo technique of Maya Abdominal Therapy is a noninvasive massage to the abdomen and pelvis that helps to guide the internal reproductive organs toward their ideal position, relieving tension in the diaphragm. For Kate, getting regular Maya Abdominal Therapy from a professional, and practicing the at-home version on her own for a few months, improved digestion and relieved PMS symptoms. She credits it for being the first step on her path toward drastically reducing her negative experience of the pre-menstruation phase. For more information, and to find a practitioner near you, visit arvigotherapy.com.

Nourish—Hydration

Water is the main component of the human body. The muscles and the brain are about 75 percent water, the blood and the kidneys are about 81 percent, the liver is about 71 percent, the bones are about 22 percent, and adipose tissue (fat) is about 20 percent. Leonardo da Vinci was right when he wrote, "Water is the driving force of all nature."

Dehydration during Phase III is detrimental for three big reasons: First, because the *female body "reacts" to dehydration by clinging to water,* making the should-be-subtle premenstrual bloat not so subtle. Second, *dehydration hinders all of our organs,* causing them to work harder than otherwise necessary. And last but not least, when it comes to weight loss, *water helps the liver remain focused on and capable of burning fat.* When dehydration occurs, the liver goes into "Keep the weight on!" mode.

With the word *hydrate,* we instantly think "drink" or "water," and while drinking water does hydrate (and we want you to hydrate with liberal amounts of fresh, clean drinking water), we also want your meals to have high water content as well. With food, it's not so much about *what* you eat, but rather, what *quality* the foods possess, and much of that has to do with how they are prepared. For Vixen nourishment we're after a deeper hydration strategy, and it's more than just drinking plenty of water; we also want you to *eat* it.

- **Get steamed:** Steaming *adds* moisture, so lightly steam your veggies, your dumplings when you order Chinese takeout, and even poach your eggs.

- **Do soup:** Soups, even with their tendency for high sodium levels, are perfect for Vixen because they are filling, water-rich, and often ultra-nutrient-rich. We have plenty of soup recipes in chapter 8, our diet plan. Try our Leek and Potato Soup (page 156), and our yummy coconut-based soup (page 157) that'll please your sweet tooth. Soup can be a meal, not just an appetizer or a first course. We suggest making a big batch, freezing individual serving sizes, and using your stovetop (not the microwave!) to prepare when you're jonesin' for a bowl. Remember, soup will hydrate and fill you up as it soothes your psyche.

- **Go raw:** Smoothies are a smart breakfast choice for Vixen (see our Blueberry and Walnut Smoothie on page 143) because, usually, most of the ingredients can be raw. Raw food is the most hydrating kind of food. Period. Take a dry roasted cashew and put it next to a raw cashew and you will see a big difference. Sushi is often about 80 percent raw. Snack on raw pieces of fruit, like apples, oranges, and grapes. They are super easy and super hydrating—perfect for Vixen.

- **Add oils to your diet:** We especially love two kinds: olive oil and coconut oil. They can be used externally as an application to skin, and internally in recipes. Oils are moisturizing because they help the body to retain water in the right spots within the body. Oh, and don't think greasy hamburgers and fries—oil can be added in subtle ways. We put a tablespoon of coconut oil in our oatmeal on page 141. Just be aware that heat, light, and air can affect the taste and quality of oils, so store them in a dark, room-temperature cupboard, or in warmer seasons, in the refrigerator. The fats and healthy phytonutrients in oils—as well as the taste—can slowly degrade

Don't Eat Dehydrating Foods

This equates to avoiding processed foods, which have a high sodium content and are often "twice baked." They usually have genetically modified ingredients, food coloring, and preservatives—all of which tax the digestive system and liver. Have you ever noticed how thirsty you get when you eat a handful of Pepperidge Farm Goldfish? Processed foods usually 1) come in a box, bag, or wrapper; 2) have over a dozen ingredients; and 3) many of these ingredients are long, scientific words that we cannot pronounce. They require lots of water for digestion.

The Water Thieves

Things like coffee, sugar, and alcohol are the big baddies of dehydration. Cutting them out, or minimizing their consumption, will probably help your overall health, not just reduce PMS symptoms.

over time, so it's probably best to use them within a year, or within six months once opened.

As for drinking, water isn't the only acceptable beverage. We love herbal teas, like licorice and chamomile, coconut water (best if straight from a young coconut), and kombucha. A hydration rock star, warm vegetarian or chicken broth (see our recipes for both on pages 135 and 137), is a tasty and filling mineral-rich drink, too.

Live—Solitude

Solitude is a state of being alone without being lonely. It's beneficial in that you provide yourself with your own beautiful company. Solitude is a time that can be used for reflection, inner growth, or enjoyment of some sort. All artists know that solitude is necessary for creativity.

Solitude elicits a sense of tranquility, accessing an inner richness from which we draw sustenance. We all need periods of solitude, but in Phase III, Vixen craves it voraciously. In order to remain balanced, she needs an ample supply. Solitude de-stresses, or at least minimizes the stresses of daily life. It allows Vixen to hear the whispers of her soul. The 28 Days Lighter Diet is all about the big picture, and for Vixen, restoring through solitude now, during Days 21 through 28, undoubtedly helps to ward off binge eating and other reactive self-sabotage that leads to subpar women's wellness.

Hormonally, progesterone is making you a homebody, or as the yogis say, you've got an "inward gaze." Have you ever wondered why small talk at a cocktail party can be completely irritating, or how the book club you usually love feels like work during this time of the month? Your tolerance for emitting your energy outward is limited

Sleep Solo

As a wife and mother with a high-energy household, solitude is hard to come by for Ellen, but one thing that she does, for a few nights as a Vixen, is sleep in the guest bedroom.

now, so whatever you call it—alone time, me time, chillin', or (our favorite) solitude—do it. In order to stay balanced, you need a big chunk of it every day during Phase III.

Here's what *not* to do, Vixen: Don't overextend yourself socially by hosting jewelry parties or going out on the town with your beau. (Holiday parties, when they fall in the Vixen phase, tend to be depleting, maybe even weakening the immune system.) Don't invite out-of-town guests to crash at your house, and don't go out to eat (order takeout instead). You have much more social endurance at other times of the month (that's what Phase II is for!), but now other people can get under your skin quickly, so go home, unplug the phone, put on your PJs, and read *Jane Eyre*, in bed.

Exercise can be solitude. Folding laundry can be solitude. Cooking dinner can be solitude. Solitude can be *productive*. Ellen has over an hour of delicious solitude when commuting from NYC to New Haven by train. Solitude is time with your thoughts and feelings in a relaxed manner, and is oh so soothing to Vixen.

"Home Alone" Restorative Yoga Postures

Because restorative yoga can be done alone and at home, it's a perfect opportunity for solitude for Vixen. This three-pose routine takes 15 or 30 minutes, depending on your time allowance. Do the poses in the order shown below, and be sure to close your eyes and/or use an eye pillow for the full effect.

Restorative Yoga Postures
Seated Straddle Forward Fold (Upavistha Konasana)—Hold up to 5 minutes

How to do it: Sitting on the floor, extend both legs out into a wide V shape. (Your legs should form a 90-degree angle, give or take a

How I Know It's Time to Get Out My Yoga Props

Kate: I keep a yoga mat permanently unfurled in my walk-in closet so that I'm inspired to at least do a Downward Dog when I'm getting dressed or undressed. But I know it's time to also get out the bolster, blocks, blankets, and yoga strap when I start getting annoyed by my kids. As I write this book, they are four and two—adorable little creatures with squeezable cheeks and the sweetest propensity to tell me they love me. But sometimes—and it mostly happens during Week 4—when they use their angelic little voices to ask for yet another drink of water at bedtime, or to ask *Why?* ten times in a row, I feel a surge of white-hot rage. It's not pretty, but it's true.

That's when I know that no matter how crowded my calendar may feel, I have to spend twenty minutes alone in my closet, all cuddled up with my yoga props. Every single time, I emerge from that closet a different person: I'm calm, and I've just received some insight on something that's been plaguing me. When I act on that insight, it's like I've added rocket fuel to my productivity level. Then later, when one (or both) of my kids attaches his or herself to my leg while I'm cooking dinner, I can remember to take a deep breath, give them a squeeze, and savor this time when they are so affectionate.

I've been doing yoga on my own at home for close to twenty years, and nearly every time, my rational mind tries to tell me some very good reason why now is not the best time for a session. I have never, not once, *ever* regretted taking a few moments to get my mind and body back on speaking terms. And although I do value the physical relaxation, improved mood, and better sleep and digestion that yoga brings, the reason I keep coming back to it is that it helps me to hear my intuition.

If you're reading this, and it's your Week 4, put down this book and try at least one of the poses that follow. You can amp up the comfort factor by using the bolster under your back in Reclined Bound Angle, and under your torso in Seated Straddle Forward Fold and Wide-Knee Child's Pose. You'll benefit from the extra relaxation a bolster can provide now—when your need for alone time and your intuitive powers are at their peak—more than ever.

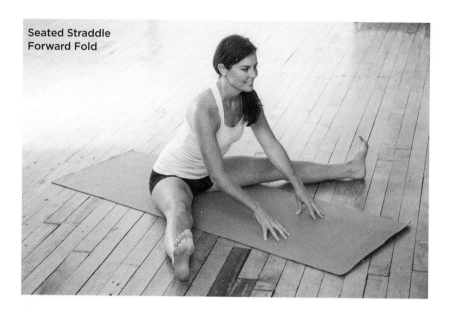

Seated Straddle
Forward Fold

degree.) Inhale and stretch your torso tall, exhale and fold forward, walking your hands away from you along the floor until you feel a stretch in your inner thighs. Keep your back straight (no rounding or hunching), but feel free to bend your knees in order to find a comfortable intensity level.

What it does: This pose releases lower back tension and brings fresh, oxygenated blood into the pelvis.

Reclining Bound Angle Pose (Supta Baddha Konasana)—Hold for 5 to 10 minutes

How to do it: From a seated upright position, bend your knees and bring the soles of your feet together, then inch your feet toward your hips. Allow the knees to drop down toward the floor as you press the soles of your feet together. Always keep the outer edges of your feet on the floor. Exhale and lie back on the floor, resting your hands on your belly or on the floor beside your hips.

What it does: Promotes circulation in and around the reproductive organs and eases tension in the hips.

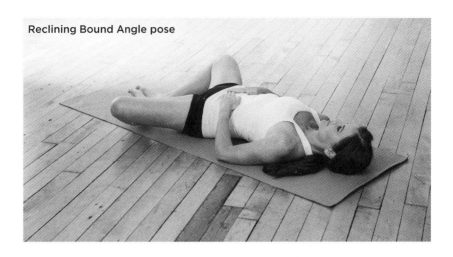

Reclining Bound Angle pose

Legs Up the Wall (Viparita Karani)—Hold for 5 to 10 minutes
How to do it: Find a wall that is clutter-free from the baseboard up, and at least four feet wide. Position your hips as close as possible to the wall and lie back, completely relaxing the head and shoulders on the floor. Bring the legs up the wall, heels resting on the wall, hip distance apart.

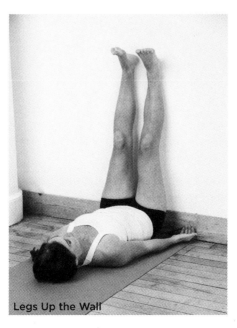

Legs Up the Wall

What it does: This restorative pose brings fresh oxygenated blood to the chest, neck, and head, helping to eradicate mental fatigue. It also promotes the flow of blood and lymph from the feet and legs, which promotes immune function and gives the heart a little rest.

Spine Twist on Back—Hold for 5 to 10 minutes each side

How to do it: Lie on your back with both knees bent 90 degrees, feet off the floor, and shins parallel to the floor. Open your arms out to the sides like airplane wings and rest them on the floor at shoulder height. Exhale and drop both knees to the right and relax there for 5 to 10 minutes. Repeat to the left.

What it does: This pose relieves muscular tension on the lower back. It also gently massages the abdominal organs, promoting digestion and detox.

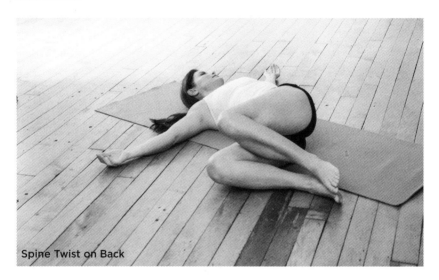

Spine Twist on Back

Wide-Knee Child's Pose, with or without pillow (Salamba Bala-sana)—Hold for 5 to 10 minutes

How to do it: From a kneeling position, bring your big toes to touch behind you as you spread your knees apart. Fold forward, allowing your forehead to rest on the ground. Extend your arms comfortably forward and relax.

What it does: This pose releases lower back tension and helps to calm the nervous system.

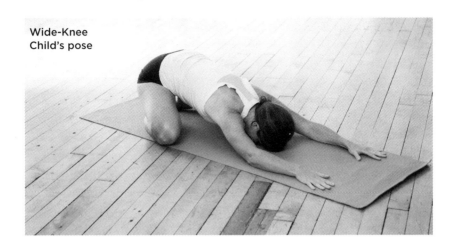

Wide-Knee Child's pose

Kate's Favorite Meditation Pose

How to do it: Lie on your back with your knees bent, feet planted hip-width distance apart on the floor. Futz with the position of your feet until you find the spot where you don't have to use any muscular strength to keep your legs perfectly balanced, like a suspension bridge. Place a thick book or two (telephone books work well) under your head. Place your palms on your belly and feel the inhale and exhale of each breath as you release all muscular effort and allow your body to sink into the floor. Close your eyes and relax.

What it does: Kate finds this pose (adapted from the semi-supine pose taught in the Alexander Technique) much easier to maintain

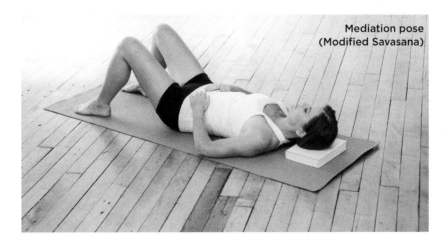

Mediation pose
(Modified Savasana)

for longer periods of time than traditional Savasana. It's great for purging muscular tension out of the whole body, and an ideal way to settle down before bed.

All Month Long—Magnesium, Calcium, and Vitamin D

While it's great to ingest magnesium, calcium, and vitamin D during Phase III, it is essential that you get them all month long. These three Vixen nutrients have been proven to help minimize, and even prevent, PMS symptoms. Let's kick things off with magnesium.

Magnesium is the fourth most abundant mineral in the body. It is critical in over 350 essential biochemical reactions in the body. For women, a magnesium deficiency is linked to hormonal imbalances and PMS. Several studies concluded that PMS symptoms have consistently been found in women with significantly less magnesium in their blood than those with no reported PMS. Without necessary magnesium levels, insulin cannot be produced, and without insulin, glucose conversion is not possible. Failing to receive glucose, the brain detects a lack of sugar and will release signals that trigger sugar cravings. Many women report being obsessed with chocolate (which is rich in magnesium), and such cravings often result in binge eating of sugar-laden junk. Magnesium deficiency has also been discovered as a root cause of dysmenorrhea, or painful cramping during Phase I.

Deficiency in magnesium used to be rare because it is found in abundance in plant and animal foods. Green vegetables (spinach

Food Sources of Magnesium

Buckwheat (1 cup, cooked)	229 mg
Almonds and cashews (½ cup)	135 mg
Garbanzo beans (½ cup, raw)	115 mg
Cocoa powder (¼ cup)	105 mg
Spinach (½ cup, cooked)	80 mg
Oysters (3 ounces)	76 mg
Sesame seeds (1 Tbsp.)	31 mg

Chocolate Has Magnesium and Tryptophan!

Chocolate contains tryptophan, which is a chemical that the brain uses to make serotonin. As we've learned in the Vixen "Move" section, high levels of serotonin can make us feel really good.

is a superstar), cashews and other nuts, beans, seeds, chocolate (!), and whole unrefined grains all contain magnesium, so even with an imbalanced diet, people could still eke out plenty of magnesium. It's different today. Magnesium deficiency is more common now because our overall food supply has been de-mineralized; food isn't supplying what it did in days of yore. You can thank some forms of food processing, overly farmed soil, and genetically modified ingredients for contributing to the decline of quality. For women, a teeny bit of magnesium may be lost each month through menstrual bleeding, especially for those suffering from heavy flows, so we recommend around 400kg/day for women.

Calcium is needed in large quantities and on an ongoing basis. It is well known for its contribution to bone building, but calcium also plays an important role in muscle contractions. Because of this, low calcium levels are linked with painful cramping during pre-menstruation and menstruation. Studies suggest that calcium levels are lower in women who experience PMS, and that increasing the supply of calcium to the body through one's diet (rather than through supplements) may reduce the severity of symptoms. One study looked at 1,057 women with PMS and 1,968 women without PMS. Women with the greatest intake of calcium from food sources had the least PMS symptoms.

Calcium not only helps to relieve cramping but also helps to ease the emotional symptoms associated with PMS, like mood swings and depression. The reason? Too many hormones are released in the body if there is an insufficient supply of calcium. Hormone levels are already elevated during Phase III, so the combined low calcium levels create twice the hormones coursing through our bodies. Yikes! And interestingly, the symptoms of PMS are the same as the symptoms of calcium deficiency.

Another pertinent reason we are obsessed with calcium relates to its important role in weight management. (Most women don't have the slightest clue about this either!) Although you can certainly gain weight if you have a good source of calcium in your diet, if you don't have sufficient calcium in your diet, it is extremely difficult *not* to gain weight. This happens because your body registers a calcium deficiency as starvation, causing the thyroid to release a hormone called parathyroid. This hormone causes your bones to release calcium into the bloodstream. Your kidney then releases a form of vitamin D, called calcitriol, which aids in the absorption of calcium.

The problem with this is that parathyroid and calcitriol also stimulate the production of fat and inhibit the breakdown of fat (a double whammy if you're trying to lose weight). Thus, without enough calcium, fat is being produced and not being broken down, leading to weight gain. If you have good levels of calcium in your diet, these hormones will not be released.

Here are our top four calcium ingredients. We love them, and use them liberally in our recipes in chapter 8:

- **Sesame seeds:** These little white seed wonders are very high in calcium, as well as other important vitamins and minerals. Raw sesame seeds possess almost 1,000 mg of calcium in about ⅔ cup. Tahini, a popular sesame seed–based nut butter, has 426 mg in a little less than ½ cup.

- **Dark green, leafy vegetables:** From greens to spinach to kale, obtaining our calcium from dark green, leafy vegetables is an excellent health choice. Spinach ranks very high in calcium, with 56 mg of calcium per cup. A 100 g serving of collards packs a 145 mg calcium punch. One cup of steamed bok choy has around 158 mg of the mineral. Kale ranks in with 139 mg of calcium, and the spicy mustard green has 103 mg of calcium per 100 g serving.

- **Quinoa:** A light and healthy whole grain, one cup of cooked quinoa offers approximately 60 to 100 mg of calcium, as well as a high amount of potassium, zinc, and protein.

- **Beans:** Many common beans are high in calcium. Cannellini beans are high in calcium—approximately 175 mg of calcium per cup. Black beans are another good source of calcium, with about 120 mg per cup. These beans make an excellent soup base and are featured in several recipes in chapter 8.

There are three "asides" with calcium:

1. Supplements in pill form don't seem to do the trick. It's best if calcium is ingested in meals rather than supplemented in pill form. Many studies suggest that calcium tablets aren't easily absorbed by the body.
2. People think calcium and they think milk, but actually green leafy vegetables are the richest sources of calcium.
3. Calcium is dependent on our third Vixen nutrient: vitamin D.

Vitamin D is calcium's BFF. In order for your body to absorb calcium, it needs vitamin D. Without enough vitamin D, the body leeches calcium from its stores in the skeleton, which weakens our bones. You can get vitamin D in three ways: through the skin (with the sun's help), from the diet, and from supplements (which we don't recommend). We think the best vitamin D–rich foods include egg yolks and saltwater fish, like tuna and cod.

Ellen is convinced that the best way to get vitamin D is from exposure to the sun. Many of us are lathered in high SPF creams every day of the year, creating a faux fortress where the sunlight can't penetrate. While we don't want you to get sunburned, we do

Food Sources of Vitamin D

Cod liver oil (1 Tbsp.)	1,360 IUs
Salmon, cooked (3 oz.)	447 IUs
Tuna fish, canned (3 oz.)	154 IUs
Egg yolk (1)	41 IUs

A sample menu for Vixen is water-rich and light:
Breakfast: Blueberry and Walnut Smoothie (page 143)
Lunch: Escarole and Bean Soup (page 154)
Dinner: Easy-Peasy Arugula Salad (page 147)

want you to catch some rays. Twenty minutes of morning sun is ideal, and unless you live in a tropical environment, you will probably go months without sun. This is where food comes in. Mother Nature gives us options here—do a bit of both!

READY, SET, FLOW FOR DAYS 22–28

- All phase long: Do 60 minutes of low-impact cardio at least every other day, preferably every day.

- All phase long: Get a daily dose of solitude. Heed your urges to stay in. Find a quiet spot in your house to hide, and do some delicious restorative yoga poses. Meditate in your car for 10 minutes before you come into the house after work.

- All phase long: Prioritize hydration. Drink plenty of water and tea (mix in plenty of herbal blends so you don't over-caffeinate); eat soups, smoothies, and steamed, boiled, or raw foods whenever possible; and avoid the great dehydrators—caffeine, alcohol, and processed foods.

The Top Three Habits of the Highly Successful Vixen

1. See exercise as a form of "mood medicine."
2. Drink water and herbal teas instead of coffee and soda.
3. Seek out solitude. The Vixen knows that alone time is crucial for good health and happiness.

- All cycle long: Magnesium and calcium (which depends on vitamin D for absorption) are anti-cramping minerals, so add more magnesium-, calcium-, and vitamin D–rich foods to your diet, and allow yourself small chunks (no more than 20 minutes) of unprotected time in the sun to boost your levels of vitamin D.

Because of pain sensitivity and feelings of discomfort, it's easy to fall off the wagon in Phase III, convincing yourself to put on sweatpants and lounge in bed instead of doing your steady cardio. We know—we've been there. Just knowing that we are making ourselves more susceptible to mood swings and food binges helps us to stay on course. Keep your eye on the prize, ladies, and that's a stress-free, pain-free, frump-free (!) pre-menstruation phase.

CHAPTER 8

The 28 Days Lighter Diet

The food you eat can be either the safest and most powerful form of medicine or the slowest form of poison.

—Ann Wigmore, renowned health educator

You can trace every sickness, every disease, and every ailment to a mineral deficiency.

—Dr. Linus Pauling, winner of two Nobel Prizes

These two quotes rock our world! They completely sum up the 28 Days Lighter Diet. Our food plan follows their lead by being *nutrient-rich*. Like everything else we preach, it's not about taking things away; it's about adding things in. As such, it's not vegan, gluten-free, raw, or low-carb. The 28 Days Lighter Diet is chock-full of good-for-women, body-building minerals and vitamins that get and keep the female body humming along perfectly. Food will be our *feminine* medicine as we eradicate deficiency bite by bite.

We could fill the pages of many books on the subject, but let it be known that women and men have different dietary needs. Women need more iron than men because we lose iron with each menstrual period. Women need more iodine than men because iodine inhabits the breast tissue and the ovaries, which are nonissues for men. Women need more calcium to ward off osteoporosis. Because men tend to be bigger, they need more calories and protein than we do. We may be made out of the same building materials as men, but our materials are used in different proportions than men's building materials. (This is why there are women-specific multivitamins.)

The guiding principle for the 28 Days Lighter Diet is Five and Five: Five minerals and five vitamins that women need to prime their feminine pumps. The big five minerals for menstruating women are calcium, iodine, iron, magnesium, and zinc. The big five vitamins are vitamins A, B6, B12, D, and E. The goal of the 28 Days Lighter Diet is to ensure that you're getting ample amounts of these precious commodities into your body.

You've already read up a bit on the five minerals and five vitamins in the Wise Woman, Mother, and Vixen action plans, but here is a collective rundown:

- Calcium is the most abundant mineral in your body. It is essential for the development and maintenance of strong bones and teeth, and that's where about 99 percent of the body's calcium is found. Calcium also helps the heart, nerves, muscles, and other body systems work properly. Calcium deficiency is linked to heightened PMS symptoms. Aim for 1,000 mg per day. Calcium all-stars: spinach, milk and milk products, dried herbs, walnuts, and almonds.

- Iodine is necessary for the proper functioning of the thyroid. With inadequate thyroid activity, women are more likely to experience excessive fatigue, excess weight that won't budge no matter how much you eat or exercise, and infertility. The ovaries require ample amounts of iodine as well in order to function fully. Aim for 150 micrograms per day. Iodine all-stars: shrimp, eggs, and blueberries.

- Iron is essential for everyone, but especially vital for menstruating women. We lose an average of 30 to 40 mg of iron during each period. Even a slight iron deficiency can result in lethargy and fatigue. Aim for 18 mg per day. Iron all-stars: chicken, lentils, black and cannellini beans, spinach, walnuts, quinoa, almonds, blueberries, and broccoli.

- Magnesium helps to maintain normal muscle and nerve function and is known for its abilities to combat stress and promote relaxation. Deficiency is linked to menstrual cramps and many symptoms of PMS. Aim for 320 mg per day. Magnesium all-stars: oats, coconut milk, almonds, and pine nuts.

- Zinc is involved in more body functions than any other mineral. Zinc affects menstrual regularity and female sexual organs. Without zinc, the carbon dioxide exchange that happens at the cellular level could not occur at a rate fast enough to keep humans alive. Research shows that zinc levels are low in women with PMS, and there is a high correlation between zinc deficiency and depression in women. Aim for 8 mg per day. Zinc all-stars: shrimp, coconut milk, garlic, and spinach.

- Vitamin A allows for the proper development of reproductive organs, including the uterus, cervix, and vagina. Since vitamin A is an antioxidant, it helps to maintain the strength of the reproductive tissues. Aim for 700 mg per day. Vitamin A all-stars: parsley, eggs, carrots, apples, and broccoli.

- Vitamin B6 allows the brain to produce serotonin, in turn helping women to feel relaxed rather than depressed. When the body doesn't get enough vitamin B6, it will have a harder time getting rid of excess estrogen. Vitamin B6 also helps to reduce bloating during Phase III. Aim for 1.7 mg per day. Vitamin B6 all-stars: poultry, eggs, fish, potatoes, brown rice, quinoa, and cooked spinach.

- Vitamin B12 deficiency can lead to a type of anemia called pernicious anemia, which causes extreme fatigue. Vitamin B12 can also help to decrease depressive symptoms that are sometimes associated with PMS. Aim for 2.4 mcg per day. Vitamin B12 all-stars: chicken, fish, milk, and eggs.

- Vitamin D is necessary for the absorption of calcium, making it as important as calcium to the female body. It's important to note: We can ingest vitamin D through foods and beverages, or the body can manufacture it by itself through exposure to sunlight. Aim for a minimum of 600 mg per day. Vitamin D all-stars: fish, milk, and egg yolks.

- Vitamin E protects our cell membranes and keeps the skin, heart, nerves, muscles, and red blood cells healthy. It can help to alleviate some of the symptoms associated with PMS. Aim for 15 milligrams per day. Vitamin E all-stars: pine nuts, avocados, coconut oil, and olive oil.

We know what you might be thinking: "I eat plenty, and I'm actually kinda overweight, so how could I be nutrient-deficient?" Well, you can be and most likely are. We are living in strange times. Your nutrient deficiency is probably contributing to your weight woes to boot! Research reports that 20 percent of American women are iron-deficient. At least 70 percent of American women are iodine-deficient. As much as 71 percent of American women aren't getting enough calcium. And three-quarters of US adults are deficient in vitamin D. The list goes on! What we *are* getting is plenty of calories that provide us with nada. Zilch. Zippo. They are empty. They are like a gift box with no present inside. This is why it is very possible to be obese and malnourished at the same time! (Excuse the exclamation mark—we're getting fired up now!)

JUST SAY NO TO EMPTY CALORIES

Lasting weight loss begins with just saying no to empty calories. We don't count calories in the 28 Days Lighter Diet, but we don't *waste* calories by eating crappy food either. A genuine enemy to women's wellness—and to lasting weight loss—is food with no nutrients. Our modern society is loaded with them. Soda. Wonder Bread. Swedish Fish. These are the obvious examples. Most of us know before eating a handful of Skittles that they are not nutritious. However, today, things have become tricky. Our food has been de-mineralized through its soil, genetically modified through science, overly processed, and ultra-pasteurized. That chicken cordon bleu may seem like it's "feeding" you, but its nutrition level could be close to nil, thanks to factory farming and the fact that it was nuked in the microwave moments before it arrived on your plate.

We can no longer think of foods as having a fixed value; for such value varies according to the soil content.

—Dr. Henry Bailey Stevens, University of New Hampshire

Gertrude Stein famously said, "A rose is a rose is a rose." Well, we say the opposite about ingredients—*A potato isn't a potato isn't a potato.*

A potato grown organically in high-quality soil and prepared with love can have 70 percent or more nutrients than a potato grown in mineral-deficient land. This is a fact. Ellen has chickens in her (urban) backyard for this reason. She resorted to this because free-range, organic eggs are costing up to $8/dozen. She can now get the best eggs possible for her family and her neighbors in a cost-effective way.

> *I am against calorie counting. Measure food by hunger. Only eat when you are hungry.*
>
> —Anne Marie Bennstrom, legendary weight-loss guru and founder of The Ashram

Steering clear of evil empty calories requires some vigilance and effort. First, pay special attention to the quality of the original ingredients. Are they organic? Are they in season? Are they fresh, canned, or frozen? *These things matter.* An organic apple in season from a well-loved orchard is different from a pesticide-sprayed apple shipped in from far away in February. The well-loved apple will most likely be higher in vitamins A and C, will include fewer toxins, and will simply taste better. There are several books on this subject we recommend, especially *In Defense of Food* and *The Omnivore's Dilemma*, both by Michael Pollan.

The second step to avoiding empty calories is to pay special attention to food preparation. Is it microwaved? Is it twice-baked? Is it overly processed to the point of nonrecognition? This is what ultimately forced Ellen into her kitchen. She wanted quality control, since even her local gourmet deli nuked their soups (gasp!). The bottom line: The best way to eliminate empty calories in your diet is to shop for yourself and cook for yourself.

FOOD SHOPPING

There's no doubt about it—the grocery store can be a scary place. And that doesn't even broach the question of how to find the time to get there. Trust us, at one time, we were each grocery store- and cooking-averse. We remember aimlessly walking the aisles,

We Highly Recommend Avoiding Microwaves

Research has concluded that foods cooked in a microwave, even for as little as 30 seconds, lose some or all of their nutrients. Worse yet, microwaving certain food, like meat, can turn its molecules into carcinogens. It's also important to know that being near the microwave itself is dangerous, as it emits radiation and high levels of EM (electromagnetic) emissions that are unhealthy for every living thing.

overwhelmed with choices, underwhelmed with the produce quality, and daunted by cost, asking the age-old question, "What am I going to do about dinner?" Feeding yourself is hard enough. Add a family into the mix and whoa, it's a big responsibility. We aim to take away the torture by breaking it all down for you in two steps: 1) The pantry staples; and 2) the weekly basics.

The Staples

The staples are things that have a pretty long shelf life and make up the base ingredients for many of your meals. Ellen buys most of her staples at Whole Foods, her local food co-op, and/or gets them direct from various online distributors. We know Whole Foods has the bad rep of being pricey. The good news about pantry staples is that they have a long shelf life—meaning, you can stock up when they're on sale and be done for a while (check out their coupons at www.wholefoodsmarket.com/coupons). Kate gets a lot of staples at Trader Joe's and her new favorite store, Ocean State Job Lot. Check out Costco, Sam's, and even Wal-Mart—you can find great staples in unlikely places if you keep your eyes open for them. Even Amazon carries a lot of this stuff, and you can set it up to automatically ship to you every month. Here's a list of our top pantry staples:

- Coconut oil (organic, extra virgin, and cold-pressed)

- Maple syrup (organic, grade A or B)

- Olive oil (organic, extra virgin, and cold-pressed)

Storage Is Important

Store all staples in a cool, dark place, such as a pantry closet. Maple syrup, once it's opened, needs to be refrigerated. Nuts should also be refrigerated or even frozen, especially in summer months, as they can easily go rancid from the slightest amount of heat. Oils are light-sensitive, so tuck them away in a cupboard, away from sunlight.

- Sea salt (Himalayan or Celtic)

- Spices (our favorite spots for spices are online at worldspice .com or mountainroseherbs.com)

- Rolled oats (old-fashioned, quick, or steel-cut)

- Brown rice (organic)

- Pasta (organic)

- Quinoa (organic)

- Beans (dried or canned, organic), preferably from Eden Organics, which doesn't use industrial chemical Bisphenol A (BPA) in its can liners

- Nuts and seeds (raw, unsalted, including walnuts, almonds, pecans, flax seeds, pumpkin seeds, sunflower seeds)

- Honey (raw, local)

- Frozen seafood, wild-caught when possible (Note: A frozen bag of shrimp or salmon fillets in the freezer and a lone red pepper in the vegetable drawer makes a fabulous and respectable dinner when you're overdue for a grocery run. Frozen seafood is often cheaper than fresh, too.)

The Weekly Basics

The weekly basics are things that don't last long, so we need to replenish them weekly, or even twice weekly. If you are like us, you may go to a few places in order to find the best of the best. Ellen "makes the rounds," hitting up Whole Foods and Trader Joe's, and she recently started growing her own produce. Kate can't handle the thought of going to multiple stores, so she shops primarily at Whole Foods, and figures the extra money she spends she gets back in time and energy that she doesn't have to spend driving around to multiple places (she also makes one trip to Trader Joe's—a bit of a schlep for her—every six weeks or so to stock up on nuts, quinoa, and frozen seafood).

It's a personal choice; find what routine works best for you. Farmer's markets can be great (but are seasonal in many parts of the world), and you may have a corner deli that works in a pinch. Ellen has a few Italian markets in her neighborhood and often finds the best produce there, and definitely the freshest bread.

Produce, dairy products, meats, and breads are your weekly necessities (for the most part). When you have the ingredients on hand, you can prepare your own meals, which is a big part of the 28 Days Lighter Diet plan, putting you in control of your nutrition, your wellness, and your weight.

MEAL PREPARATION

If you are at all like Ellen, the kitchen could be the most daunting place (second only to the grocery store). Ellen did not grow up with Martha Stewart and was not exposed to the art of cooking until her mid-twenties, but even then, she just ate the food and applauded the chef. Now, she's a solid short-order cook (and an aspiring Julia Child). It didn't happen overnight, but rather one recipe at a time, starting with a couple of basic recipes and wholesome breakfasts. Be gentle with yourself—just one homemade meal per day is a good start! Let your motivation come from wellness. Remember, the best way to keep the doctor, extra pounds, and PMS away is with good nutrition.

As you read through these recipes, notice that we never microwave and never use hard-to-find/exotic ingredients. We use the stovetop, the oven, and for dressings, soups, and smoothies, a blender. There is nothing extraordinary about our ideal kitchen. We recommend splurging on a good cast-iron skillet if you don't

How to Maintain a Cast-Iron Skillet

A trusty iron skillet is a kitchen's best friend—it's cheap, conducts heat well, and even lends the food that's cooked in it an extra smidge of iron. But they do require a little bit of care to ensure that they don't rust and that food doesn't stick to them. You want your cast-iron skillet to be seasoned—that means it has developed a lovely, all-natural, nonstick coating of cooking oils.

When you first get a skillet, coat the pan with a good layer of olive oil, put it upside down in the oven, and turn it up to 500 degrees. The high-heat bath will seal the pan and give it a nice, healthy start. To keep that sheen going and to foster it over the long term, never use soap on your skillet. To clean, get a stiff scrub brush and use only hot water on it.

Kate's husband Scott has a trademark technique of putting water in the pan, setting it to boil, then turning the pan off and letting the hot water soak in the pan while doing the other dishes. Then he does a quick scrub and swish with clean water in the sink. Finally, he puts the still-wet pan back on the burner and puts it on low, encouraging the pan to dry quickly, so rust never gets a chance to set in. (The only caveat: You have to remember to turn off the burner! A few times, Kate has come down from putting the kids to bed and found their empty skillet sizzling away on the stove.)

The end result is a pan that's worthy of being an heirloom, with visual evidence of all the amazing and wholesome meals made in it.

already have one, as it can help to boost your iron levels. Also be sure to acquire a wooden cutting board and a serrated knife. With these tools, your kitchen is complete. Even a little kitchenette can be adequate. Now it's recipe time, with five categories: foundations, breakfasts, soups, salads, and one-pot meals.

RECIPES

Foundations

Foundations are nice to have on hand and especially great to make yourself, so as to guarantee their nutrient-richness. If you are "kitchen-shy," we recommend starting with the foundations. Master them, and you'll soon gain confidence in your cooking abilities. Plus, you'll have the base ingredients for many of the "bigger" recipes that follow in this chapter. (Note: We've indicated the phases for which these recipes are most conducive after the recipe title.)

Vegetable Stock (Phases I, II, and III)

The nutrients in vegetable stock are bountiful, as the vitamins and minerals in the veggies themselves seep into the water as they cook. You can use vegetable stock instead of water when you make rice or quinoa, and instantly transform these staple grains into nutrient-delivery systems. You can drink a warm cup of vegetable stock all by itself in lieu of tea or coffee, and, of course, you can use it for all soups. Our ancestors used it like medicine for healing livestock, sick babies, and nursing mothers.

NUMBER OF SERVINGS: 6

Ingredients

2 tablespoons olive oil

1 large onion

2 celery stalks, including leaves

3 large carrots

The stems of any greens you've cooked up in the last week (store them in the crisper drawer until you have time to make stock)

3 scallions, chopped

3 cloves garlic, minced

3 sprigs fresh parsley

3 sprigs fresh thyme

2 bay leaves

1 teaspoon sea or Himalayan salt

2 quarts water

Directions

1. Scrub vegetables and then chop into 1-inch chunks. Keep in mind: The greater the surface area, the more quickly the vegetables will yield their flavor.

2. Heat oil in a large soup pot. Add onion, celery, carrots, stems of greens (if using), scallions, garlic, parsley, thyme, and bay leaves. Sauté over high heat for 5 to 10 minutes, stirring frequently.

3. Add salt and water and bring to a boil. Lower heat and simmer, uncovered, for 30 minutes. Strain. Discard vegetables.

Chicken Broth (Phases I, II, and III)

Much like vegetable broth, chicken broth is abundant in nutrients. When you've had chicken (or turkey), don't throw out the bones until you've used them for broth. In fact, immediately following your chicken dinner, make the broth and freeze it (or freeze the bones until a more opportune time). That way, you'll have it on hand for future recipes. And if you or anyone in your household starts to get a tickle in their throat or ache in the bones, you'll have an age-old immune system booster on hand and ready to go.

NUMBER OF SERVINGS: 6

Ingredients

2 to 3 pounds bony chicken pieces, or carcass of a roasted
   chicken that you've already eaten the meat off of
2 celery stalks with leaves, cut into chunks
2 medium carrots, cut into chunks
2 medium onions, quartered
2 bay leaves
½ teaspoon dried rosemary
½ teaspoon dried thyme
8 to 10 whole peppercorns (optional)
2 quarts water

Directions

1. Place all ingredients in a soup pot. Slowly bring to a boil, then reduce heat and skim foam off the top. Cover and let simmer for 2 hours.

2. Strain broth and discard vegetables, seasonings, and chicken bones. (Any excess chicken meat can be saved, pulled off the bone, and added to the stock.)

3. Refrigerate overnight, then skim the fat that collects at the surface.

Tart Cherry Granola (Phases I and II)

There tends to be too much added sugar and also many unwanted preservatives in store-bought, prepackaged granola. Making it yourself ensures its quality, but honestly, it's cheaper and tastes better, too. Win, win, win!

NUMBER OF SERVINGS: APPROXIMATELY 10

Ingredients

4 cups rolled oats

2 cups walnuts

2 cups sliced almonds

1 cup coconut flakes

1 cup coconut oil

1 cup maple syrup

2 cups dried cherries (preferably with no added sugar)

Directions

1. In a large bowl, combine oats, walnuts, almonds, and coconut flakes and mix.

2. In a saucepan, warm the coconut oil until it becomes liquid and then stir in the maple syrup.

3. Take the coconut oil and maple syrup mixture and pour it into the oat mixture. Stir well so as to coat everything. Keep the cherries on the side.

4. Spread the mixture about ¼-inch thick onto ungreased cookie sheets (you'll need about four standard cooking sheets) and bake at 325°F for 40 minutes, or until the oats turn golden brown.

5. Cool for 2 hours and then pour back into the big bowl. Add the cherries and toss. Store in an airtight container.

Buff Girl Guacamole (Phases I, II, and III)

Ellen lives by this simple rule: Don't leave the grocery store without a couple of avocados! Avocados are a super food, with twenty essential nutrients, including loads of women-friendly vitamin E and B-vitamins. This guacamole makes a great dip or a topping for Almost Eggs Florentine (page 140), and goes well with all of our quinoa dishes.

NUMBER OF SERVINGS: 3

Ingredients

3 ripe avocados
1 lime (for its juice)
½ teaspoon sea or Himalayan salt
¼ cup red onion, minced
½ cup cilantro, chopped
1 jalapeño, seeds removed and then diced

Directions

1. Prepare the avocado by scoring the inner meat with a small knife and scooping the diced avocado into a large bowl.

2. Pour lime juice and salt on top. Mash and stir with a fork until desired consistency.

3. Stir in the red onion, cilantro, and jalapeño. Transfer the guacamole to a smaller bowl and serve immediately.

Breakfast Recipes

Over the years, we've been quietly appalled by some of our clients' breakfast choices. They either don't eat breakfast at all, or they eat bagels, muffins, and croissants on the run. While we love a good croissant, it is not a nutrient-rich breakfast. After all, breakfast is the most important meal of the day, and we have worlds to conquer. Here, we make nutrient-rich breakfasts that contain a solid amount of protein.

Almost Eggs Florentine (Phases I and II)

We think of this recipe as a "winner's breakfast." All of our five vitamins and five minerals are represented here—a total home run. We recommend using fresh spinach, but frozen spinach is an okay option, too.

NUMBER OF SERVINGS: 4

Ingredients

    2 tablespoons olive oil, divided
    4 cups raw spinach, chopped
    8 eggs, poached
    ¼ teaspoon sea or Himalayan salt
    ½ teaspoon pepper
    ½ cup grated Parmesan cheese
    ½ cup shredded Cheddar cheese

Directions

1. In a skillet, use half of the allotted olive oil and sauté the spinach for approximately 5 to 10 minutes, mixing periodically.

2. Grease a shallow baking dish with the other half of the olive oil. Using tongs, place sautéed spinach into this greased baking dish, lining the bottom. Arrange the cooked and drained poached eggs over the top of the spinach. Sprinkle with salt and pepper and then, lastly, the two types of cheese.

3. Bake eggs at 400° F for 3 minutes, or until cheese is melted and lightly browned. Remove from oven and then cut into squares around each egg and serve immediately.

Good Morning Oatmeal (Phases I and III)

After you see how simple (and quick) it is to make our oatmeal, you will never use instant oatmeal packets again. Ours takes about 3 more minutes than the microwave crap version, but is years apart in taste and nutrition.

NUMBER OF SERVINGS: APPROXIMATELY 4

Ingredients

2 cups quick oats

4 cups water

2 tablespoons coconut oil

2 tablespoons maple syrup

Directions

1. In a medium-size saucepan, combine oats and water over medium heat on the stovetop. Cook for approximately 5 minutes, stirring occasionally.

2. Turn off heat and add the coconut oil and maple syrup.

3. Pour into bowls, top it off with our Tart Cherry Granola, and serve immediately.

Energy Balls (Phases II and III)

When we snoop around our clients' kitchens and pantries, we often come across "power bars"—brands like Luna, Kind, thinkThin, and Slim-Fast are stowed away for an on-the-go boost or a pre-workout snack. These energy balls serve the same purpose as those bars but are cleaner. They don't have any unrecognizable ingredients and much less sugar. Make Energy Balls the day before (or days before!), and you can literally grab and go, just as easy as a pricey bar.

NUMBER OF SERVINGS: 4 (2 PER SERVING)

Ingredients

2 cups almond butter

½ cup honey

½ cup coconut oil

2 cups coconut flakes

Directions

1. In a blender, combine the almond butter, honey, and coconut oil and puree until well mixed and the consistency is smooth and buttery.

2. Put coconut flakes in a wide-mouthed bowl.

3. Using a spoon, scoop out tablespoons of the mixture, roll into a ball with your hands, and then roll it in the coconut flakes, coating each ball thoroughly. Store in an airtight container.

Blueberry and Walnut Smoothie (Phases II and III)

Smoothies can go either way—good for you or not so good for you. Here, we make the good-for-you kind with nutrient-rich ingredients that hydrate but don't overdo dairy or sugar. If you don't have blueberries, feel free to swap in other berries. We especially love raspberries, strawberries, and mulberries. Again, fresh is best, but frozen works well, too.

NUMBER OF SERVINGS: 2

Ingredients

1 apple, sliced and cored

2 cups frozen or fresh blueberries

1 tablespoon coconut oil

½ cup walnuts

4 to 6 ice cubes or ½ cup coconut milk or almond milk (optional)

Directions

Add all ingredients to the blender and blend on high until smooth.

Salads

Salads are a girl's best friend. Hydrating, nutrient-rich, and low in sugar, salads are a great choice, especially for Phases II and III. (They are great for Phase I as well, as long as you don't eat them straight out of the fridge.)

Spinach Salad with Warm Vinaigrette (Phases I, II, and III)

The warm dressing in this recipe makes it a favorite winter salad, and if you don't have pecans on hand, use walnuts, pumpkin or sunflower seeds, or sliced almonds.

NUMBER OF SERVINGS: APPROXIMATELY 6

Ingredients

1 cup pecans, whole or chopped
1 tablespoon olive oil
1 medium shallot, minced
½ cup red wine vinegar
1 teaspoon honey
¾ teaspoon Dijon mustard
Pinch of sea or Himalayan salt
Ground black pepper, to taste
2 pounds spinach, washed, stemmed, torn into bite-size pieces, and thoroughly dried

Directions

1. Place the pecans on an ungreased cookie sheet and bake for 10 minutes at 325° F. Remove from oven and set aside.

2. In a saucepan on the stovetop, heat the olive oil and add the shallot. Cook until fragrant, about 30 seconds. Whisk in the vinegar, honey, and Dijon mustard for another 2 minutes (approximately). Remove from heat and season with salt and pepper.

3. Combine the spinach and pecans in a large bowl. Add the vinaigrette and toss to coat. Season with additional salt and pepper and serve immediately.

Ginger Salad with Shrimp (Phases I, II, and III)

Our Ginger Salad with Shrimp is a crowd-pleaser, packed with flavor and aroma. You can take the marinated shrimp to the outdoor grill—weather permitting—making it a festive barbecue option.

NUMBER OF SERVINGS: 6

Ingredients

1 cup olive oil (for marinade; a bit of it will be discarded)

1 lemon, juiced

3 cloves garlic, minced

2 pounds large shrimp, peeled and deveined with tails attached

½ cup fresh ginger root

½ cup Dijon or hot mustard

1 tablespoon honey

1 tablespoon water

1 head of iceberg lettuce or Napa cabbage, washed and chopped

Directions

1. There are three steps to this recipe. The first step is the shrimp. In a mixing bowl, mix together olive oil, lemon juice, and garlic. This is a marinade. Pour it into a large resealable plastic bag and add the shrimp. Seal and shake and allow the shrimp to marinate in the refrigerator for 2 hours.

2. After 2 hours, pour mixture into skillet and sauté, cooking shrimp for 5 minutes per side, or until opaque. Once thoroughly cooked, discard the remaining marinade.

3. The second step is the ginger dressing. Place the small chunks of ginger root, mustard, honey, and water into a blender and puree until smooth, approximately 3 minutes.

4. The third step is to put it all together. In a large salad bowl, combine the chopped lettuce (or cabbage) and toss with the ginger dressing. Take the shrimp and lightly toss the shrimp into the salad as well. Serve with a scoop of Buff Girl Guacamole (page 139) as a yummy addition!

Senora Salad (Phases I and III)

The Senora Salad has it all—protein, fiber, healthy fats, flavor, and ample amounts of our 5:5 nutrients. Be sure you don't skimp on the lime juice—it's the ingredient that pulls this salad together—so squeeze it fresh from an actual lime (not from a bottle).

NUMBER OF SERVINGS: 4

Ingredients

1 head of romaine lettuce, chopped
1 can black beans, rinsed and well drained
1 cup tomato, seeded and chopped
¾ cup radishes, thinly sliced
1 red bell pepper, chopped
1 ripe avocado, diced
½ cup crumbly feta cheese
¼ cup fresh lime juice
¼ cup olive oil
2 tablespoons honey
2 tablespoons fresh cilantro, finely chopped
1 garlic clove, peeled and minced
1 teaspoon jalapeño pepper, finely chopped

Directions

1. Toss all salad ingredients in a large bowl—the lettuce, beans, tomato, radish, pepper, avocado, and feta.

2. In separate bowl, mix the lime juice, olive oil, honey, cilantro, garlic, and jalapeño.

3. Pour dressing over salad and toss.

Easy-Peasy Arugula Salad (Phases I and III)

If you're leery of the kitchen, this is the salad for you! It will build your culinary confidence for sure. One thing—try to use unpasteurized Parmesan cheese (Ellen finds it at her local Italian deli). Parmesan cheese is the recipe's standout ingredient, and tastes better and is more nutritious when it is raw.

NUMBER OF SERVINGS: 4

Ingredients

   2 bunches arugula, washed, dried, and torn
   ¼ cup olive oil
   ½ lemon, juiced
   Pinch of sea or Himalayan salt
   Pinch of pepper
   ½ cup walnuts
   1 block of Parmesan cheese (you'll use only about ½ cup of cheese)

Directions

1. In a serving bowl, drizzle the arugula with the oil, squeeze in the lemon juice, and sprinkle with salt and pepper.

2. Toss to coat, then add in the walnuts and toss again.

3. Use a vegetable peeler to shave thin pieces of Parmesan over the top.

Tasty Tahini Dressing

This scrumptious salad dressing is high in calcium, protein, and probiotics—friendly bacteria that aid digestion found in the fermented miso. Savory and satisfying, it's also great drizzled over steamed vegetables or as a dip for raw vegetables. It's also forgiving—if you don't have miso, use tamari or shoyu. If you want more of a kick, throw everything in the blender with a clove of raw garlic. If you want a dressing to throw over cooked and chilled soba noodles, substitute toasted sesame oil for the olive oil (and toss in a couple cups of chopped cucumber, carrots, celery—whatever crunchy veggie you have on hand—with a sprinkling of chopped cilantro).

NUMBER OF SERVINGS: 4

Ingredients

   3 tablespoons tahini
   2 tablespoons miso (may substitute tamari or soy sauce to taste)
   ½ lemon, juiced
   1 tablespoon extra virgin olive oil
   Water, as desired

Directions

Combine all ingredients in a bowl and whisk in water until it reaches desired consistency.

One-Pot Meals

As the following one-pot recipes can attest, cooking can be quick and tasty and doesn't have to be laborious. In just one pot, you get terrific amounts of protein, fiber, nutrients . . . everything you need! No need for side dishes, simplifying dinnertime.

Quinoa Stir-Fry (Phases I, II, and III)

Quinoa is an ancient grain, dating back over three thousand years. The Incans called it the "Mother Grain"—apropos for Phase II. It has a nutty flavor that mixes well with other strong flavors, like the ginger in this recipe. It is also a good source of iron, magnesium, folate, and protein.

NUMBER OF SERVINGS: 4

Ingredients

¾ cup quinoa, rinsed until the water runs clear

½ teaspoon sea or Himalayan salt, finely ground, divided

1 tablespoon olive oil

1 carrot, thinly sliced

1 red bell pepper, cored, seeded, and chopped

2 teaspoons grated ginger

1 clove garlic, sliced

1 small red chile, chopped (optional)

2 cups snow peas, trimmed

¼ teaspoon black pepper

1 egg, beaten

4 ounces grilled chicken breast, cut into 1-inch chunks

2 scallions, chopped

½ cup cilantro, chopped

Directions

1. Place quinoa in a small saucepan with ¾ cup water and ¼ teaspoon salt. Bring to a boil, then reduce heat to low. Cover and cook, undisturbed, until quinoa absorbs water, about 15 minutes. (FYI: Quinoa is cooked like rice, not pasta.) Remove from heat, fluff with a fork, and leave uncovered.

2. Heat olive oil in a large skillet over medium-high heat. Sauté the carrot, stirring occasionally for about 1 minute. Add bell pepper, ginger, garlic, and chile. Cook, stirring frequently, for about 2 minutes. Add peas, sprinkle with remaining ¼ teaspoon salt, and pepper, and cook, stirring frequently, for another minute.

3. Remove vegetables and place them in a large bowl.

4. Pour the quinoa into the skillet (no need to clean it, as we'll use the juices from the vegetable sauté) and pour the egg into it. Cook, stirring constantly, until egg is evenly distributed, about 2 minutes, or until you see the egg turning pale yellow within the mixture.

5. Add vegetables, chicken, fresh scallions, and cilantro, and cook 1 minute more. Serve warm.

Quinoa and Black Beans (Phases I, II, and III)

Quinoa is not only high in protein but also low in calories. This dish is a low-cost meal that takes less than 30 minutes to make. We think it's a perfect dinner in general, but especially if you are aiming to lose weight.

NUMBER OF SERVINGS: 4

Ingredients

1 teaspoon olive oil
1 onion, chopped
2 cloves garlic, peeled and chopped
¾ cup uncooked quinoa
1½ cups vegetable or chicken broth
1 teaspoon ground cumin
¼ teaspoon cayenne pepper
Salt and pepper to taste
1 cup corn kernels (can be frozen or fresh)
2 cans black beans, rinsed and drained
½ cup cilantro, chopped

Directions

1. Heat the olive oil in a medium-size saucepan over medium heat. Stir in the onion and garlic, and sauté until lightly browned. Mix quinoa into the saucepan and cover with vegetable/chicken broth. Season with cumin, cayenne pepper, salt, and pepper. Bring the mixture to a boil. Cover, reduce heat, and simmer 20 minutes.

2. Stir corn and black beans into the saucepan, and continue to simmer about 5 more minutes.

3. Turn off heat and add the cilantro. Serve warm. Add a scoop of Buff Girl Guacamole (page 139) for more deliciousness.

Chicken and Broccoli over Almond Rice (Phases I, II, and III)

This recipe demands chopsticks—the rice will be sticky enough, and the broccoli very "grab-able." Chopsticks tend to slow down fast eaters and make us more aware of our food. We like to keep the broccoli crispy, so try not to overcook it.

NUMBER OF SERVINGS: 6

Ingredients

4 cups chicken or vegetable stock
2 cups brown rice
2 cups sliced almonds
1 tablespoon olive oil
1 bunch fresh broccoli (about 3 cups)
1 celery stalk, chopped
1 onion, chopped
4 skinned and boned, grilled chicken breasts, cut into bite-size pieces
¼ cup parsley, chopped (as a garnish)

Directions

1. Combine the chicken/vegetable stock and rice. Bring to a boil, then cover and simmer for approximately 30 minutes, or until rice is fluffy.

2. Turn off heat and stir in the almonds. Set aside.

3. In a skillet, using the olive oil, sauté broccoli, celery, and onion for about 3 to 5 minutes; then stir in the already-grilled chicken.

4. Split the rice between six bowls and spoon the chicken and broccoli mixture on top. Garnish with parsley and serve immediately.

Pine Nut Pesto Pasta (Phase II)

Pine nuts can be pricey (up to $19.99/pound at Whole Foods—yikes!), but they are fiber- and nutrient-rich—high in iron, magnesium, zinc, and vitamin E—and thus worth every cent. Plus, the other ingredients in this recipe are relatively inexpensive, so the overall meal will still be reasonable. As in our Easy-Peasy Arugula Salad, try to score some unpasteurized Parmesan cheese.

NUMBER OF SERVINGS: APPROXIMATELY 8

Ingredients

1 pound bow-tie pasta

4 cups Parmesan cheese, shredded, divided

3 cups pine nuts, divided

2 cups fresh basil, chopped

2 tablespoons garlic, minced

½ cup olive oil

Directions

1. Boil the pasta according to instructions (al dente works the best for this recipe).

2. In a blender, combine 2 cups of the Parmesan cheese, 1½ cups of the pine nuts, all of the basil, all of the garlic, and all of the olive oil. Puree on low until mixture is well blended. (It doesn't take long!) Set aside.

3. Place the remaining pine nuts on an ungreased cookie sheet and toast in the oven for approximately 10 minutes at 350° F, or until golden brown. Set aside.

4. Rinse pasta. Stir in pesto mixture. Blend in the remaining 2 cups Parmesan cheese and the toasted pine nuts. Serve warm or cool.

Soups

Soups, with their warmth and iron-rich ingredients, are especially awesome for Phase I. Their amazing ability to hydrate makes them great for Phase III, too. Please note: All of these recipes provide six servings. If you don't have six people for dinner, make a big batch anyway—just freeze the remaining soup and reheat at a later time; then your future nutrient-rich meal will be faster than takeout.

Escarole and Bean Soup (Phases I and III)

When Ellen moved to the Italian-centric city of New Haven, Connecticut, she fell in love with Escarole and Bean Soup. In fact, her 50 percent Italian husband is the king of "E and B," and says the key is lots and lots of fresh garlic.

NUMBER OF SERVINGS: 6

Ingredients

2 tablespoons olive oil
1 white onion, chopped
6 cloves garlic, minced
6 cups chicken (or vegetable) broth, divided
4 cups chopped escarole
2 cans cannellini beans

Directions

1. Using the olive oil, sauté the onion and garlic in a large pot with a few tablespoons of the chicken/vegetable stock. Do not brown.

2. Add the escarole. After approximately 5 minutes on a medium heat, the escarole should be tender but still a little crispy.

3. Now add the rest of the stock, and the beans. Simmer for 20 minutes on low. Serve warm.

Lentil Soup (Phases I and III)

Lentils are high in protein and fiber, low-cost, and easy to prepare. We recommend them especially for Phase I, as they are also high in iron.

NUMBER OF SERVINGS: 6

Ingredients

¼ cup olive oil

1 onion, chopped

2 carrots, diced

2 celery stalks, chopped

2 cloves garlic, minced

1 bay leaf

1 teaspoon dried oregano

1 teaspoon dried basil

2 cups dry lentils

6 cups vegetable stock

1 cup spinach, rinsed and thinly sliced

2 tablespoons balsamic vinegar

1 pinch of sea or Himalayan salt

1 pinch of ground black pepper

Directions

1. In a large soup pot, heat olive oil over medium heat. Add onions, carrots, and celery. Cook and stir until onion is tender.

2. Stir in garlic, bay leaf, oregano, and basil. Then cook for 2 additional minutes.

3. Stir in lentils and add stock. Bring to a boil. Reduce heat, and simmer for at least 1 hour, or until lentils are soft.

4. When ready to serve, stir in spinach, and cook until it wilts (approximately 3 to 5 minutes). Stir in vinegar, and season to taste with salt and pepper, or more vinegar if desired.

Leek and Potato Soup (Phases I and III)

During Phase III, when you are craving comfort food, choose this creamy and warm soup instead of fattening mac and cheese or salty potato chips.

NUMBER OF SERVINGS: 6

Ingredients

2 tablespoons olive oil

1 large or 2 small leeks (about 1 pound), chopped

5 cups chicken stock

1 pound russet potatoes, diced

1 teaspoon sea or Himalayan salt

¾ teaspoon pepper

1 cup cream

2 tablespoons snipped chives

Directions

1. In a large soup pot over medium heat, use the olive oil and sauté the chopped leeks and cook until wilted, about 5 minutes.

2. Add chicken stock, potatoes, salt, and pepper, and bring to a boil. Reduce the heat to a simmer and cook for 30 minutes, or until the potatoes are falling apart.

3. Turn off heat, let cool for a few minutes, and pour mixture into blender and puree, stirring in all of the cream. Serve immediately, with some of the snipped chives sprinkled over the top of each bowl of soup.

Coconut Chicken Soup (Phases I and III)

The chicken in this soup is chicken broth, not actual chicken meat, and the coconut isn't coconut oil or flakes, it's coconut milk. You'll feel like you are dining in Thailand with this recipe. Get ready for big flavor and a warm belly!

NUMBER OF SERVINGS: 6

Ingredients

4 cups chicken stock

2 cups coconut milk

1 lemon, juiced

¼ teaspoon dried chili flakes

1 teaspoon ginger, finely grated

½ teaspoon sea or Himalayan salt

¼ cup parsley, chopped (optional)

Directions

1. Bring stock to a boil, skim off the foam that collects on top, then stir in the coconut milk, lemon juice, chili flakes, and ginger. Simmer for about 15 minutes.

2. Add salt and garnish with parsley. Serve warm.

Kate's #1 Secret for Eating Healthy When You're Busy

Kate cooks five dinners and four breakfasts for her family of four each week, plus she cooks her own lunch five days a week, since she works at home. (They eat out once a week and have a communal pizza night with friends once a week, and she and her husband alternate cooking breakfast each day). That's twenty-five meals a week, which equals a lot of time in the kitchen.

Her best tip for making meal prep easy and darn near stress-free is devoting an hour or two to cooking on Sunday afternoons. Each weekend, she makes a few things to have on hand for the week, like chicken stock and a pot of quinoa; chili and granola; a big batch of oatmeal and a huge pot of kale soup; beans and a roasted chicken. These elements serve as the basis for several upcoming weekday meals; for example, the chicken stock becomes risotto one night and soup for another couple of lunches. Chili makes one dinner for four, a couple of lunches for her, and adds spice to cheese quesadillas for another dinner. The roast chicken makes one dinner, with the leftovers used for a couple of chicken-salad lunches. The carcass (stored in a Ziploc bag in the freezer until an opportune time) will fuel a further Sunday cooking session.

Best of all, that time in the kitchen—when there's no pressure to feed hungry bellies—is a highlight of Kate's week. It's just her, her cooking tools, and her thoughts (and sometimes a little Nina Simone on the stereo). It's multitasking at its best—cooking and mind-body practice combined into one.

THE DEVIL IS IN THE DETAILS

There are some loose ends we want to tie up when it comes to how we eat, because some seemingly small things can be game-changers. These aren't so much about what to eat, but more pieces of food philosophy that we've discovered to be helpful guideposts on the quest toward eating healthfully. May they help usher you through those moments when you're feeling confused by all the dieting lore that's circulating out there in the public consciousness and wondering how it all pertains to you.

To Snack or Not to Snack?

We believe in three meals a day and that's it, really. We've all heard about the "five small meals/day" scenario, and to be honest, it may be necessary for certain medical conditions, for kids, and pregnant women, but in general, not so much, especially if your goal is to lose weight. If you must snack, think "whole," like a piece of fruit or a handful of nuts.

Should We Drink Water with Meals?

We suggest drinking before eating, not during. If you must, take little sips during the meal. We don't want to dilute digestive juices, because when diluted, they are hindered and food isn't processed as readily.

What about Alcohol?

Alcohol is okay in moderation because it can be social and de-stressing for some. However, we must admit, unless it's a glass of red wine (which is chock-full of antioxidants), it's ultimately a big glass of empty calories. We do not recommend getting into the habit of drinking a glass of wine every night, as it could get in the way of a good night's sleep, on top of adding up to 200 "wasted" calories into your diet. Make drinking a Friday-night treat or a once-a-month splurge . . . or, if you're really serious about losing weight, only on special occasions, like Thanksgiving.

How Late Is Too Late for Eating at Night?

This may surprise you, but if you are in the processes of losing weight, Ellen suggests nothing after six p.m.! She wants you to wake up craving breakfast. (There is a direct correlation between late-night eaters and breakfast skippers!) If you are simply maintaining, seven or eight p.m. is okay. Again, life gets in the way and this isn't always possible, so be flexible and just do your best.

Is Gluten Really Bad?

Gluten, which is found in wheat, isn't necessarily awful. The problem with it is twofold. First, Americans eat too much of it, and in excess it can create mucus, clog the digestive system, and cause inflammation. Second, wheat has been extensively hybridized (genetically engineered) to the point where the body has trouble recognizing it as food, and therefore struggles to digest the gluten within it. We suggest minimal gluten intake by making two out of three meals wheat- and flour-free when possible.

What Are Your Thoughts on Juicing?

We are big fans of fresh green juice. It's packed with vitamins and minerals and is a great way to get your veggies. Many people go on juice fasts, which we think is fine, too, but only when you are under the guidance of an experienced health counselor.

Do You Do Desserts?

Of course; we're human! Just be picky. Eat only the best, and make it worthwhile. Desserts aren't necessarily "empty calories." Pastries made with fresh, whole ingredients do have protein, fiber, and vitamins. Ellen's go-to dessert is dark chocolate–covered raisins, which are high in iron. One of Kate's favorites is a de-pitted date with a little schmear of peanut or almond butter, which offers potassium, magnesium, selenium, and calcium.

INSPIRED EATING

Now that we've gone over the "what" and the "how," we want to cover more of "why" to change your diet. When you take control of what goes in your belly, you take control of your destiny, because, as the adage goes, *you are what you eat*. In fact, the state of your body right now, weight-wise and reproductively, is in large part due to what you've been eating *and not eating* in recent months and years.

If you desire a smoother menstrual period, greater hormonal balance, and lasting weight loss, the way you eat needs to shift. Namely, shop and cook for yourself as often as possible. Make it your way of life.

Start making homemade meals that include high-quality *building* ingredients, and the weight loss will follow. By building your metabolism, strengthening your endocrine system, and increasing your mineral reserve, you will grow leaner. Plus, your energy levels will soar and you will be a highly functioning female when your menstrual cycle flows without a hitch. Let the vision of your abundant vitality motivate you to choose your food with wisdom, confidence, and inspiration.

On the flip side, diets that deprive your body weaken it, making it more susceptible to weight *gain*. How ironic! In your heart and from personal experience, you already know this is the truth, so from this point forward, say it with us: I will stop depriving and start building.

Total wellness, here we come!

PUTTING IT ALL TOGETHER

Here is a general plan that you can follow for each week of the month. For a more detailed food and exercise plan, see Appendix B: The 28-Day Plan.

All Month Long			
Days	**Theme**	**Nourishment**	**Movement**
1–7	Restoration	Eat warming, iron-rich foods. **Foods we love right now:** broths and beans	Part 1: Be still. Part 2: Gentle seated yoga.
8–21	Circulation	Eat protein-rich, circulation-enhancing foods. **Foods we love right now:** shrimp, ginger, and avocado	30 minutes daily—anything goes: cardio, stretch, or strength. You've got the energy to move!
22–28	Contempla-tion	Eat calcium-rich, hydrating foods. **Foods we love right now:** salads, soups, and smoothies	45-60 minutes daily—steady, low-impact cardio. Remember, exercise will help eradicate bloating and moodiness.

Signature Yoga Pose	Healthy Living Tips	Phase Motto
Kate's Favorite Meditation Pose	Part 1: Use a hot water bottle. Part 2: Sleep 30 to 60 minutes more each day.	The Wise Woman knows you can "accomplish more by doing less."
Supported Shoulder Stand	Part 1: Socialize as much as possible. Part 2: Physically move as much as possible.	The Mother says, "Don't put off for tomorrow what you can get done today. Live each day to its fullest."
Wide-Knee Child's Pose	Seek a daily dose of solitude.	The Vixen under-stands that "Soli-tude stimulates the creative mind."

IT'S NOT "ALL OR NOTHING"

The 28 Days Lighter Diet program is meant to inspire you, not enslave you. Take what works for you and leave the rest behind. It is *not* all or nothing. We've been our own guinea pigs, testing the program in this book on our own bodies and in our own lives. Do we do it all perfectly all the time? Nope. But we obey the Golden Rules and try our best after that!

Many of the women we've worked with over the years have used parts of our program for weight loss and for eradicating PMS or other menstrual discomforts. We feel as though we've had a 100 percent success rate in that our program in its entirety, and also with its individualized tips, has *helped*. Some women have experienced lasting weight loss. Some women have smoother and more regular cycles. The most frequent feedback we receive, however, is, "I don't feel at war with my body anymore." Hip hip hooray! Moving toward wellness is always a reason to celebrate!

Here are some examples of how the 28 Days Lighter Diet program has helped.

Marilyn: "Consulting with My Cycle"

As a type-A New Yorker, I was a robot with my workouts. I set the alarm for six a.m. and did the same thing Monday through Friday every single day of the month for years—an hour of high-impact, intense Tae Bo. It never occurred to me to "consult" with my cycle. So at age forty-three, I don't think it was a coincidence that I had what is called a prolapsed uterus, and needed surgery to repair my uterine ligaments.

After surgery Tae Bo didn't feel good, so I started power-walking and taking Pilates class instead. I also began to use Days 1 and 2 as chill-out days, where I would give myself permission to sleep in. Shockingly, I dropped five pounds, and I feel like I lost it without trying! Emotionally, I have much less anxiety, and feel more in tune with myself and the rhythms of the universe.

Tori: "The Powers of Red Raspberry Leaf Tea"

When I was about ten years old, my grandmother told me about red raspberry leaf tea for women's health, and she actually grew and prepared the leaves herself. I remember her steeping the leaves in the summertime. She'd add real plump raspberries into the pitcher of tea, along with ice cubes for a refreshing, fruity beverage that was beautiful to look at as well. My whole family loved it. I had forgotten about this family "heirloom"; thanks for reminding me. It's an easy habit to embrace. For about three months, I've been brewing a big batch of the tea on Day 22 and sipping it all throughout Phase III. By doing this, I've virtually eliminated my PMS symptoms. No more headache. No more breast tenderness.

Taylor: "Eating Rice and Quinoa More Often than Pasta"

In college, my roommates and I lived on pasta. It was cheap and easy to make, and it filled us up. However, I was unhappy about my weight, so I sought out Ellen for assistance. She told me to go a week without pasta, and opt for rice and quinoa instead, just as a test. She said, "Let's see how it feels," which was really interesting, as I never paid attention to how food "felt."

Well, it felt great—like I was digesting food faster—and my energy level skyrocketed, too. Without counting calories or being obsessive about exercise, I lost four inches around my waist, and I was sold. Now, I may have pasta once a month, but it's not a staple in my diet. Rice and quinoa are just as cheap and easy to make, and I'm amazed at how a simple switch can have such a dramatic effect.

Ellen: "Be True to Nature"

I've revealed a lot about myself in the pages of this book, but there's one more thing I want to share with you, and that's my understanding of nature. I've done a complete 180. I once ate Power Bars, used tampons, worked out to Jane Fonda at midnight, and ate watermelon in December. I used to drive through a rural area and believe I was entering nature, but was somehow removed from it. My cycle has shown me that I don't *visit* nature, I *am* nature. It's not something I can be separated from. This deep understanding alone—orienting my life from this perspective—has made me reproductively sound, and, I feel, is the ultimate take-away from this book.

Kate: "Awareness Is the First Step"

I was doing a lot of the pieces we suggest in this book before writing it. But our research led me to start keeping track of my cycles using the Energy Wheel. And I am astounded at how much information and insight it's given me. I've learned that my appetite spikes around ovulation, that my energy plummets 6–12 hours before my period starts, and that I tend to get sick during Phase III. Using the Energy Wheel has really made me see that we women are always on our cycle—to ignore it is to ignore who we are. Also, by adding a few quick notes of what I was doing each day, my collection of Energy Wheels has become a fabulous record of what it felt like to be me at any given time.

Since our cycle simply starts again as soon as it ends, looking at my past Energy Wheels helps me make the most of each trip through the phases, and helps me trust the signals my body is constantly sending me. And, let me tell you, that feels really good.

Study nature, love nature, stay close to nature. It will never fail you.
—Frank Lloyd Wright

CHAPTER 9

Off-Track Cycles:
Common Problems and Their Solutions

So you want to follow along with our plan, but your cycle is erratic or your period has gone missing. What's a girl to do? Well, first, know that you are not alone. Most women in the United States, at some point during their menstruating lives, hit a bump in the road due to stress, pregnancy, or lifestyle changes. We've guided many women toward a beautifully balanced cycle by implementing other holistic modalities, like herbal remedies, moon gazing (yes, we are going there!), yoga, and alternative medicine. If your menstrual cycle isn't even close to 28 days long, or when your version of Phase I and/or Phase III wreaks a little (or a lot of) havoc in your life, have no fear, help is here. Once you have even a glimpse of menstrual predictability, the rest of the book with its three-phase action plan will promote cyclical balance, too.

HEAVY PERIODS

The average woman sheds 1 to 1.4 ounces of blood each period—about as much as will fit in a shot glass. But some women shed much more. This may or may not be problematic. If the blood is bright red and clear of clots (small clumps of uterine lining), and you aren't debilitated by fatigue or cramps, you're just on the heavier end of the spectrum. If you bleed so much that you feel totally wiped out, or the bleeding is accompanied by intense cramps, then that's a clue your cycle is out of balance. You may suffer from menorrhagia, which is defined as losing 5.5 tablespoons (2.75 ounces) or more of blood during your menstrual cycle.

Key symptoms include:

- A menstrual cycle that lasts more than seven days

- The need to change a sanitary pad or tampon every hour for days

- Soaking through even the thickest pads

- Large blood clots

In their awesome book, *The Woman's Book of Yoga & Health* (a book we believe should be on every woman's bookshelf), Linda Sparrowe and Patricia Walden write that recurring heavy bleeding can cause you to lose too much iron, making you susceptible to iron deficiency and anemia. It can also be a symptom of something more serious, such as endometriosis or fibroids (both of which we'll cover in just a bit).

If you bleed so much that you feel totally wiped out, or the bleeding is accompanied by intense cramps, then that's a clue your cycle is out of balance.

If you regularly, as Kate's friend Veronica used to say, "hemorrhage as if from a massive head wound," your goal is to truly rest as much as possible until the flow comes down. If you do any sort of formal movement, do Cobbler's Pose and Seated Straddle Pose—both of which tone and nourish the uterus—followed by a nice long Corpse Pose or Kate's Favorite Meditation Pose. Once your period stops completely, do Seated Straddle Pose (see page 114 for instructions) daily—as it tones and nourishes the uterus—and follow it up with a nice long Corpse Pose.

Stress absolutely affects the heaviness of bleeding, so meditation is another key action step for you. Lie in Kate's Favorite Meditation Pose (illustrated on page 119), close your eyes, and relax there for at least 10 minutes every day.

Traditional Chinese medicine (TCM) has a great track record when it comes to curing heavy bleeding. Ellen recommends seeking out a TCM practitioner in your area for as little as one session. They can give you a specific herbal formula, often custom-made precisely for you. The Chinese herbs alone just may do the trick!

Ready, Set, Flow! Heavy Bleeding Healing Steps:
1. Rest as much as possible while bleeding is occurring.
2. Do Seated Straddle Pose every day of the month you are not bleeding, followed up with Final Relaxation Pose.
3. Do 10 minutes of meditation daily.

4. Seek out a TCM practitioner and have them create an herbal formula that meets your specific needs.

ENDOMETRIOSIS

Endometriosis occurs when cells that respond to the hormonal call to swell and bleed—the very types of cells that line the inside of the uterus—are found outside the uterus. They either start out as cells attached to the interior uterine wall and lose their way as they migrate out of the uterus during the period, coming to rest in other spots within the abdominal cavity (such as the walls of the pelvis, the bowel, or the pelvic organs); or they begin life outside the uterus as a non-hormonally triggered cell, and at some point evolve into cells that respond to surges in estrogen the same way that uterine cells do.

In either case, if your doctor suspects you have endometriosis (a conclusive diagnosis requires laparoscopic surgery), rest is your priority during the first day or two of your period. Health-care providers of all stripes believe endometriosis is linked to stress, so sticking with the 28 Days Lighter Diet throughout the month will help you to build more reflection, quiet, and stress-reducing exercise into your life.

You know we're all about taking a stand for *all* women to minimize their use of tampons, but if you have endometriosis, it's even more important, as you don't want to encourage any more endometrial tissue to find its way outside the uterus. Exposure to dioxin—a carcinogenic by-product of the bleaching process used in making tampons and paper—has been linked in animal studies to a much higher incidence of endometriosis. A 1990s study by S. E. Rier and colleagues found that a whopping 79 percent of rhesus monkeys who were exposed to dioxin for a study ten years earlier developed endometriosis. That's 79 percent. We ingest dioxin in all kinds of ways—it is pervasive in our modern environment—but you certainly don't need to also stick it in your vagina. Buy unbleached, organic tampons if you must, but just say no to your standard, bleached-within-an-inch-of-its-life tampon.

To further help your body to remove any environmental toxins it may be harboring, follow our Happy Liver Program outlined in the section on fibroids, on page 174. The information on severe cramps will also help.

Ready, Set, Flow! Endometriosis Healing Steps:

1. Stop using tampons immediately.
2. Follow the Happy Liver Program on page 174.
3. Exercise daily (except when menstruating) to promote circulation and detoxification, and to take advantage of the days you feel good.

SEVERE CRAMPS

There are two different types of heavy-duty cramps: primary and secondary. Primary dysmenorrhea (the scientific name for cramps) is caused simply by your straight-up menstrual cycle, while secondary is caused by something else, such as endometriosis or pelvic inflammatory disease. Secondary dysmenorrhea doesn't typically respond to the types of lifestyle, diet, and activity changes we cover in the 28 Days Lighter Diet, but the good news is, simple yoga poses can help to lessen the intensity of your cramps, and the stress relief they provide can also make your perception of the cramps less intense. (Also see the sidebar, on the next page.)

Other changes to consider are really focusing on increasing your magnesium and omega-3 fatty-acid intake through food (and supplements, if dietary changes don't produce noticeable effects), and getting acupuncture—all of which have numerous studies that support their effectiveness.

Herbal teas can help to relieve the pain of cramps, too—specifically, red raspberry leaf, chamomile, and ginger. You can buy bagged tea at most supermarkets. We especially love Yogi Tea and Traditional Medicines brands for their high-quality, organic ingredients. (See our Ginger Tea recipe on page 91.) Red raspberry leaf is a tonic for a healthy uterus and has been used for centuries and across cultures for its therapeutic qualities. Chamomile induces muscle relaxation. Ginger promotes circulation in and around the womb. (Ginger can be an acquired taste—Kate hated it until she was well into her thirties. Now, she loves the way it warms her up from the inside out.)

Exercise Helps to Ease Cramps— True or False?

By Katy Bowman, MS

Studies investigating the effect exercise has on dysmenorrhea have led to two potential reasons that exercise can help. The earliest research (from the 1940s) concluded that problematic periods were the result of alignment (body-placement) issues. Treatments from this research led to the teaching of corrective exercise and postural adjustments. Better body positioning meant less strain to abdominal tissues and decreases in the pressures to the spinal nerves.

More-recent studies into exercise and dysmenorrhea have looked into biochemical causes of heavy or painful periods. Fluctuating protein compounds as well as stress can be risk factors for problematic periods. Either way, exercise, in general, can be beneficial for stress reduction and, if used specifically, to aid in creating a more suitable position for the working uterus.

On the other end of the spectrum, heavy exercise has been shown to disrupt the natural cycle of ovulation. So which is it? Is exercise beneficial or not?

As a biomechanist studying the strength systems of the pelvis, I have found that many women have habits that alter the pelvis's natural internal environment. And as an exercise scientist, it is also clear that many women don't move at all. While your best remedy for severe cramps will be tailored to your unique body and lifestyle, the following recommendations will help your personal uterus function, and thus, help you to feel better.

- Mobilize the pelvic and hip areas, especially the groin, through targeted stretches and massage techniques. The muscles connecting the pelvis to the legs and torso are chronically tight in a sedentary population. If you sit (at work or in a car) more than a few hours a day, it's possible that the angle of your pelvis (and, therefore, uterus) is altered from its optimal positioning.

- Walk more: The functions of the body—especially circulation—require upright movement. While many modes of exercise are great for stress relief (who doesn't love a great spinning class or a rowing session), walking creates loads of circulation to the uterus that can't be found in other movement activities.

- Book a session with an alignment professional: Learning a few ways of adjusting your body to decrease extreme loads to your abdomen or pelvic area can be used for the rest of your life. What a bargain!

- Gradually work squatting into your life: No need to hoist a lot of weight or do 200 reps. A daily gentle yoga squat (with a rolled-up mat under your heels to improve balance, if necessary) or even lying on your back with your legs up in a squat position can do wonders for your hips and pelvis.

Ready, Set, Flow! Severe Cramps Healing Steps:
1. Do yoga during Phases II and III.
2. Increase your magnesium and calcium intake.
3. Drink woman-friendly herbal teas, like red raspberry leaf, ginger, and especially chamomile to hydrate, warm, and relax your body.

FIBROIDS

Fibroids are benign tumors that grow on the uterine walls. They contain estrogen and grow as a response to excess estrogen in your system. If you have fibroids, you are in good (and large) company. The Department of Health and Human Services Office of Women's Health's website estimates that as many as 80 percent of women will develop fibroids before they turn fifty. You may have them and not even know it. Unless you're having trouble getting pregnant, or experiencing problematic symptoms—such as pain, heavy bleeding, or cramps—you don't need to worry about them (although of

Acquire an Herbal Tea Habit

Many women are totally turned off just thinking of herbal tea. They think they are drinking "flowers" or something that tastes a little like dirt. Many women reach for a caffeinated tea or another cup of coffee just because they want something warm. It's too bad, because herbal teas are your friend! You can add lemon, honey, or agave to make them more appealing. Give them a second try, as they are such a great way to ingest healing herbs on a daily basis. (Honestly, we've never met a woman who couldn't deal with red raspberry leaf tea—it's downright yummy!)

Ginger helps to regulate digestion—which can get all wacky in those days leading up to your period—and is a powerful anti-inflammatory; hence, its effectiveness on cramps. It's like nature's Motrin. Also, making your own tea can be a lovely little ritual for yourself. Put it to boil before you cook dinner or do the dishes, and when you're done with your household labor, you'll have a lovely little pick-me-up.

course your doctor or other health-care provider will be better able to advise you).

If you are experiencing troublesome symptoms, there are things you can do. The same yoga poses for severe cramping will also help if you have fibroids, as traditional Chinese medicine believes they arise as a result of sluggish circulation in the pelvic area. These poses really get things flowing all throughout your lady parts. Acupuncture is really great for improving the circulation of blood, lymph, and qi; seek out a licensed acupuncturist if you'd like to use TCM to treat your fibroids.

There are a few ways you can reduce the amount of estrogen circulating in your system. First, decrease the amount of estrogen you take in. We get outside estrogen through eating meat that's been pumped full of hormones and pesticides that mimic hormones in the body, so opt for organic meat, dairy, and eggs. Second, increase

The Happy Liver Program

By Laurie Steelsmith, ND

Your liver plays an important role in maintaining hormonal balance in your body. But if it isn't functioning well—and many of our livers are overburdened by alcohol consumption, environmental toxins, and prescription drugs (including The Pill)—it won't be able to process estrogen efficiently, meaning there will be an excess of estrogen floating around in your bloodstream.

There are simple ways to keep your liver happy. Incorporate as many of these suggestions as you can into your daily life, and dedicate yourself to doing as many of them as possible for a period of at least two weeks at least once a year.

- Sip lemon water. Lemon is an astringent and helps the liver do its detoxification work. Squeeze a whole lemon into forty-eight ounces of water and grate a little bit of peel into the water as well; then drink it throughout the day.

- Eat organic and avoid meat. You want to give your liver a break from pesticides, chemicals, and antibiotics, so eat the cleanest food you can muster and minimize your meat consumption, as most farm animals are given hormones and antibiotics regularly.

your body's ability to neutralize excess estrogen by supporting the liver, which is responsible for processing excess estrogen. (See the Happy Liver Program sidebar, above.) Third, you can talk to an ND or other health-care provider about supplementing with natural progesterone, which will help to neutralize excess estrogen. Often applied in cream form during the last 14 days of your cycle (from ovulation until your period begins), this is a remedy suggested by Laurie Steelsmith, ND, in her must-have book, *Natural Choices for Women's Health*.

On an emotional level, traditional Chinese medicine posits that fibroids are a side effect of unexpressed creativity. If you have

- Drink dandelion root tea. Drink one cup twice a day of this liver-supportive herb.

- Eat more artichokes, beans, beets, and cruciferous vegetables. These foods contain compounds that help the liver work more efficiently. Cruciferous vegetables include broccoli, cauliflower, kale, cabbage, Brussels sprouts, and bok choy.

- Sweat more. Following the exercise prescription in this book will help you to release toxins through the skin via sweat, but spending time in a low-heat sauna (at least three times a week for at least 45 minutes) or attending Bikram yoga classes will help to clear out some of the backlog of toxins. Just be sure to shower after and scrub your skin with a loofah so you don't reabsorb anything icky that your body has just released.

- Dry-brush your skin. Use a natural bristled skin brush to remove dead skin cells and increase circulation before you shower each morning. Always sweep the brush toward your heart to encourage the flow of lymph (the waste-removal medium of the immune system).

a blog idea, neglected painting habit, or crafting desire, consider your fibroids a kick in the pants to devote time to scratching your particular creative itch. If you need more inspiration, we love this quote from renowned acting teacher Stella Adler: "Life beats down and crushes the soul, and art reminds you that you have one." That stifled feeling might also be the result of being in a relationship or a job that feels like it's going nowhere. If that sounds like you, your fibroids are here to show you how your outer circumstances affect your internal environment.

If you have fibroids that are causing you trouble each month, whether it's emotional and/or physical, your doctor may suggest the ultimate solution: removal of the uterus. In fact, fibroids are the most common reason for hysterectomies. An important thing to keep in mind if this is an option you're considering is that fibroids often resolve themselves after menopause. As Tracy Gaudet, MD, writes in her fabulous guide to women's wellness, *Consciously Female,* "I'd guess nine out of ten women with fibroids have no problems after menopause, because fibroids are estrogen-dependent. After menopause, estrogen falls and the fibroids shrink. So if you are close to that point in life and can endure your present symptoms a little longer, know that the symptoms will soon pass."

Ready, Set, Flow! Fibroids Healing Steps:
1. Be proactive with your doctor and find out exactly where your fibroids are located and if they should be surgically removed.
2. Seek out a traditional Chinese medicine (TCM) practitioner. TCM has a proven track record when it comes to fibroids!
3. Start expressing yourself and your creativity, through art, decor, fashion, or even by simply keeping a journal.
4. Do yoga during Phases II and III.
5. Decrease estrogen in your body by eliminating estrogen sources in your diet, like meat, dairy, and soy.

POLYCYSTIC OVARY SYNDROME (PCOS)

Polycystic ovary syndrome is caused by a hormonal imbalance—specifically, too much of a "male" hormone called androgen. This can cause acne, infertility, extra facial and body hair growth, and ovarian cysts. Studies are showing that PCOS affects about one out of every fifteen women. The million-dollar question is, "Where is the androgen coming from, and why?" The answer is unclear, and each case varies. The good news is that one thing does minimize hormone imbalance overall: regular exercise.

Regular exercise has been proven to lessen the symptoms of PCOS, so following our 28 Days Lighter Diet plan of exercising every day of the month, except for the days of your period, is perfect advice here. "When it comes to PCOS, the best prescription I could give is a pair of running shoes," says Susan Lark, MD, in *Dr. Susan Lark's Hormone Revolution.* We couldn't agree more!

And yet, PCOS is mysterious, so we recommend naturopathic doctors (NDs) that specialize in women's wellness. A qualified ND can help you to navigate lifestyle strategies that can remedy or manage PCOS.

Ready, Set, Flow! PCOS Healing Steps:

1. Exercise every day, except for Day 1 (and possibly Days 2 and 3, depending on how you feel).
2. Read *Dr. Susan Lark's Hormone Revolution.*
3. Find a naturopathic doctor (get a referral from a friend, or from naturopathic.org) who specializes in women's wellness.

IRREGULAR CYCLES OR A MISSING PERIOD

Many women go off The Pill and it takes years for their periods to regulate. Other women get off track during times of high stress: Ellen's client, Lucinda, moved from New Zealand to the USA and seemingly left her period behind!

Lots of factors influence irregularity; diet, stress, insufficient sleep, and pharmaceuticals can easily throw off a menstrual cycle, causing it to be too long, too short, or AWOL. If you have a period that comes randomly or doesn't come at all, here is our most New Age advice yet—moon gazing.

The Light of the Moon Is No Joke

By Laurie Steelsmith, ND

Our connection to the moon is incredibly powerful. After all, we are mammals—our uterus waxes and wanes in regular cycles, the same as the moon. That gorgeous orb is a reminder and a means for us to get in touch with our own feminine nature. In our culture, we're conditioned to look at life as some sort of nonstop boot camp. But the moon shows us that we have cycles of growth and cycles of contraction. Spending more time in the moonlight will encourage you to honor your own rhythms (and can work on your biology to make those rhythms more harmonious, too).

Shannon: Moon-Gazing Testimonial

I grew up in a town with one stop sign and had a very consistent 29-day menstrual cycle until the age of eighteen, when I left to live in the "big city" of Chicago. Immediately, my period changed. During my entire freshman year, I had a total of two periods! In the summer, when I'd be back at home on our 300-acre farm, my periods would fall back into their 29-day pattern again. I realize now that the city lights tricked my hormones into submission. Growing up in the country, I was acutely aware of the moon, yet in the city, I was intellectually and physically unaware and disconnected. This was the difference, I'm certain of it.

New Haven midwife Joni Stone avers that the easiest thing a woman can do for restoring (and maintaining) cyclical balance is to pay attention to the moon and all of its phases. Don't worry; you don't have to journey into the wilderness. All you have to do is go outside at night and stare up into the sky—or as Ellen dramatically puts it, be drenched in moonlight—for at least five minutes a night. Notice what phase the moon is in. Is it waxing or waning? Is it a new moon or a full moon? Stand out there and take in the moonlight through your senses. Doing this every night might be tough, but do it as often as possible. That's all there is to it!

The theory at work here is simple: Before electricity and artificial light, the moon was the main influence on the menstrual cycle, and women tended to ovulate and give birth on the full moon and bleed on the new moon. Research has concluded that the moon governs the flow of ocean tides as well as human body fluids.

Ready, Set, Flow! Irregular Menstruation Healing Steps:

1. Pay more attention to the moon and to artificial light in and around your environment. Either start sleeping with an eye mask to block out streetlights and night lights, or invest in blinds that block out 100 percent of the outdoor light. On nights when there is a full moon, open the shades.

INFERTILITY

Being unable to conceive a child can be one of the most heartbreaking and frustrating experiences in a woman's life. According to the Centers for Disease Control and Prevention, one in six couples is infertile, and fertility problems strike one in three women over the age of thirty-five. While there are many causes of infertility, one cause in particular, hormone imbalance, is something this book aims to rectify. You know that hormone imbalance can lead to many physical challenges; it can also lead to ovulation problems, the most common cause of infertility in women.

Before getting pregnant with her son, Luca, Ellen struggled for years to conceive a child. At the time, she owned a fitness studio and was exercising excessively, seven days a week, and was exhausted. According to her ob/gyn, everything regarding her reproductive system was A-okay, but according to her acupuncturist, she had too much stress in her life. His advice was very simple: "You need lazy days."

Ellen's lazy days arrived when she sold her studio, and for the first time in her adult life, didn't have to roll out of bed and work out. Three months into her "retirement," she was pregnant naturally.

We share this story with you for two reasons: One, excessive exercise, too much stress, and a workaholic lifestyle are all detrimental to fertility. Two, traditional Chinese medicine (TCM) looks at the subtler workings of the female body—things that Western medicine doesn't have a test for. If you are struggling with conception, getting a TCM assessment could provide a doable lifestyle change that could lead to pregnancy!

Ready, Set, Flow! Infertility Healing Steps:

1. Chin up, girl! Infertility can often turn into *fertility* through balancing hormones, and if you are following the guidelines in this book, you are already working on that.

2. Make managing your stress a top priority. Take relaxing baths (but not during Phase I), meditate, do yoga, sleep in, and seek out other activities that help to reduce anxiety and fear.

3. Get a TCM assessment of your energy levels and reproductive health.

Remedy Matrix for Common Cycle Problems

Ailment	Defining Symptom	Physical Component
PMDD	Mood swings, depression, anxiety, bloating, insomnia, constipation, fatigue to the extent that it's interrupting your normal life for a few days each month.	Too little pregnenolone—the precursor to all reproductive hormones—and/or an imbalance in the ratio of estrogen (too much) and progesterone (too little).
Severe cramps	Either sharp, contraction-like pains, or a dull, congested ache.	More often experienced by young women, often changes after pregnancy—either goes away or can get worse.
Endometriosis	Heavy bleeding and severe cramping that doesn't go away after Day 1.	Often seen in tandem with immune disorders, including asthma, allergies, fibromyalgia, chronic fatigue syndrome, and endocrine diseases.
Irregular cycles	Cycles are longer or shorter than 28 days, and are generally unpredictable.	Perimenopause
Fibroids	Maybe none, maybe heavy cramping, bleeding, or abdominal pain.	Caused by excess estrogen in the system.
PCOS	Irregular cycles, acne, excess facial hair, ovarian cysts, and high insulin levels.	Pituitary gland doesn't produce enough FSH and luteinizing hormone, which affects ovulation and menstruation, and can lead to an excess of testosterone.
Infertility	Difficulty getting pregnant.	Numerous physical causes, including hormone imbalances that lead to problems with ovulation.

Emotional Component	Remedies	Mantra
Anger, unexpressed emotions. Progesterone is a feel-good hormone; when the level is too low, it plays a role in promoting anxiety, irritability, and depression.	Solitude, journaling, heart-to-hearts, steady low-impact cardio, hydrating foods.	"Tell it like it is."
A uterus that works much harder than it needs to, to shed its lining, suggests a woman who works much harder than she needs to in order to prove her worth. Ask yourself: What is my perfectionism and/or my desire to "wow" people costing me?	Yoga poses that soothe the uterus; a diet of warm foods (plenty of soups, stews, oatmeal, etc.); an extra 60 minutes-plus of rest per day while the cramps last; saying no to things that don't light you up, particularly during the first few days of your period; keeping the pelvis and hips open and working well via stretching, walking, and squatting.	"Easy does it."
Is triggered and made worse by stress.	Curtail tampon use, exercise daily (except during first day or so of period) to improve circulation and detox, follow the Happy Liver Program on page 174 to boost body's ability to purge toxins and excess hormones.	"Let it go."
Feeling cut off with nature and own internal wisdom.	Remove sources of ambient light from your bedroom or use an eye mask for sleeping. Get in touch with the cycles of the moon. Sleep with your shades open when the moon is full.	"Let there be darkness as well as light."
Associated with stifled creativity, whether that's a blog idea you've never gotten around to pursuing, or a dead-end job or unfulfilling relationship.	Reduce exposure to environmental estrogens, boost your liver's ability to function (and clear out excess estrogen), get your creative ya-yas out or find other outlets for your talents, do circulation-boosting exercise, prioritize cruciferous veggies.	"Go for it."
Emotional eating can be a cause. Consider getting support from a therapist, coach, or trusted friend on getting your emotional needs met in other ways.	Increase exercise and eat a diet low in inflammation-producing foods, such as gluten and sugar—both of these help you lose a few pounds, which also helps.	"I ask for what I want."
Frustration, feeling out of control, feeling out of touch or angry with your body.	Consider lifestyle changes that will help you downsize your stress levels. Seek out a licensed acupuncturist or Doctor of Oriental Medicine with a track record in treating infertility (ask for referrals).	"I nurture myself."

CHAPTER 10

Lifestyles of the Cyclically Balanced

By this point, you've been exposed to all the information we currently have on how to get more in sync with your cycle—the how and the why. We've poured everything we have into these pages with the intention of helping you wake up to the pleasures and powers of your feminine cycle, so you can feel at home in your body and give a cease-and-desist order to your monthly physical, emotional, and spiritual dysfunctions.

Here's the kicker: We know that information doesn't necessarily lead to transformation. If it did, the self-help industry would have put itself out of business long ago. You can't just read about something and expect it to change your life. It won't. (Bummer! We know; we've tried!) Change requires action. And to make sure the actions you take will a) work, and b) stick, you have to do two important things first:

1. Acknowledge the pain your current way of being is costing you.
2. Inspire yourself with a compelling vision of how you'll feel and what your life will be like when you are no longer in the grips of that habit.

FIRST, LET'S GET REAL—REALLY REAL

This chapter is all about helping you to do both of those things. Let's get the tough part over with and look at what it's costing you to push yourself consistently throughout the month, stuff your emotions back down when they're naturally rising to the surface, ignore your inner wisdom, and use the impending arrival of your period to eat crap. Take a few minutes to jot down a quick list of the current ailments and weight gain you're experiencing that encouraged you to pick up this book in the first place.

Now take a good look at your list. For each ailment you listed, write down the negative impact it's having on your life. If, for example, you wrote down ten days of painful, swollen boobs, write down, "Don't want anyone to touch them, so I shut down on the sex front for those ten days. Need to have two sets of bras. Feel self-conscious of my extra-large chest. Feel kind of freaked out that my body changes so much on a monthly basis—like it dictates what I do and how I feel." You can see how this can quickly and easily add up to quite a list of downsides!

Here's Ellen's list from 1992, her junior year in college, when her menstrual woes were at their worst:

- Two days of PMS that included raging cravings for salt and carbs, and thus two days of overeating salt and carbs, two days of feeling bad about my out-of-control eating, and two days of feeling frumpy as a co-ed.

- One day (Day 1 of period) of debilitating menstrual cramps, barely able to walk down the hallway of my dormitory. I skipped classes, missed work, and basically took a sick day. I was always hoping Day 1 fell on a Sunday, so I'd be AWOL less. (One sick day per month adds up to twelve days/year, which is more than two work weeks.) God forbid if I had a tennis match on Day 1, as I would lose.

- Twenty-six days of dreading the next time!

We know this is not a fun process, and yet it's crucial for your lasting happiness; if you aren't fully aware of how your current habits are affecting you, you won't be committed to changing them. You'll think, "Oh, so what if I eat a whole bag of chips when I'm PMS-ing, or run a race on the first day of my cycle, or never get around to meditating—it's not *that* important." Making this list is all about showing you that consistently making positive, informed choices *is* that important, thank you very much.

The good news about this taking-a-hard-look-at-the-costs exercise is that it actually makes change a whole lot easier. When you know, down deep in your bones, why you personally want and need to change, you no longer feel like you're denying yourself by making new choices. We've said it before and we'll say it again: This plan is not about depriving yourself. It's not even about fixing problems. It's about adding foods and activities to your normal routines that will result in a smoother ride all month long. Acknowledging the pains of the spot you're currently in will help you to see that you're not sacrificing anything; rather, you're empowering yourself to make better choices in a way that feels exciting (not depressing).

> When you know, down deep in your bones, why you personally want and need to change, you no longer feel like you're denying yourself by making new choices.

When you clearly see the angst and drama of your current state of being, you lose the "I just have to buckle down, work hard, and be a good little girl" mind-set that loses its power to inspire change more quickly than a five-year-old laptop battery. While it doesn't mean that what you do from here on out will be effortless, it will help you find the ease in the process. Being present to your current pain is a great motivator, and it allows you to get into that space where you're in the flow. Ahhh, what a great feeling that is!

AND NOW FOR THE FUN PART

This is where you start to see—*really* see—where you're headed, which is crucial. That vision of what's possible when you're no longer bogged down by the list of woes you just created will be like a tractor beam, calling you to take the right actions that will get you where you want to go instead of reverting back into old habits that only keep you stuck in the list you just created.

To get you thinking about how your life could be when you start implementing the changes we outline in this book, we want to share a little story with you about what life is like when you're in sync with your cycle. And like all stories, this one starts at the beginning. Day 1, to be exact.

You're in the bathroom and see the first spots of your period. Phew, you think, here's my cue to take it easy the rest of the day. You knew it was imminent, of course, so you have your fem-care product of choice at the ready. (Kate says: "I invested in not one but two DivaCups, and keep one in the upstairs bathroom and one in the downstairs bathroom, so no matter where I am, it's within arm's reach, and I don't have to do an awkward panties-not-quite-pulled-up-to-avoid-getting-blood-on-them shuffle to retrieve my protection. I also work on the couch instead of at my desk on at least Day 1, and sometimes into Day 2, too.")

You come out of the bathroom and start heating the water for your hot-water bottle (if you're at home), or throw a shawl over your abdomen and make yourself a cup of tea if you're at work. If you're at the office, your work BFF notices the shift in your energy and gives you a wink. If you're at home, your pet seemingly magically shows up to snuggle at your feet. You finish up what you're absolutely obligated to do, bow out of anything strenuous—whether it's physically, emotionally, or mentally rigorous—and then spend the evening quietly, letting the dishes sit in the sink or the laundry go unfolded.

Your husband notices the hot-water bottle and suggests getting takeout. (You order warm soup.) Either before you go to bed (as much as an hour earlier than usual, because you know your body is working hard to shed that lining and you want to help make its job as easy as possible) or right after you wake up the next morning, you spend ten minutes or so in Goddess Pose, enjoying the space it creates in your abdomen and upper chest, and the deep breaths that happen naturally as a result of that extra breathing room (literally).

Day 2, you still allow yourself to move pretty slowly. You make arrangements with your husband to wake up with the kids so you can sleep in, and/or your boss to come in a little late. When you notice your stress levels beginning to rise at work or from being with the kids, you opt to find a quiet place—a sunny window, or a spot outside—and just sit and breathe. After a few minutes there, you're thinking clearly enough to return and do what needs to be done with minimal drama. You make it a point to do a little journaling about some decision or problem that's vexing you, and are surprised at how quickly you get an aha moment about what to do next. And you go to bed at least thirty minutes earlier than your normal bedtime or let yourself doze on the couch in the afternoon while your child naps.

Over the next couple of days, you gradually ramp back up to a normal activity level, adding in some more active yoga poses. If you still use tampons, you switch to pads or panty liners after the first couple days of heavy bleeding. If you're a pad or DivaCup devotee, you get out the panty liners—whether they're disposable or cloth— around this time. Even though you're still technically menstrual, you're noticing that your energy is building. So you spontaneously add some things into your schedule that you had purposefully planned to be light, knowing that you'd be on your period and your energy levels would be dependent on how that particular period transpired. If your period is particularly crampy, heavy, or debilitating, you continue to take it pretty easy during this time, and make a note to dial down the stressful activities as much as you can throughout the month and stick to the more-restorative yoga poses until your period ends.

Once you have completely finished bleeding, around Days 5–7, you're feeling back in the swing of things. The memory of your period quickly recedes and you ramp up to feeling your most kick-ass—you can pull together big presentations with ease, your clothes are fitting their best, and you have a certain sparkle in the photos your husband snaps of you.

You're ready to get out there and socialize, and look forward to reconnecting with your friends after being pretty quiet for the last week or so. Your body is craving more movement after the stillness as well, and you're drawn to higher-intensity workouts, like spin class, power yoga, strenuous hikes, singles tennis, or skiing. But you don't feel like you have to kill yourself, because now you want to be able to exercise formally for at least thirty minutes a day for the next two weeks. You know that fitness should feel good—not like punishment. You trust that whatever you can do on a daily basis will add up to plenty. On days you don't make it out on a walk or to the gym, you do several rounds of Sun Salutations (see page 83) at home. You may also decide to bike to work a couple days a week, or do your errands on foot. Your energy levels are at their peak now, and you want to take full advantage of them. Heck, maybe you even hang your laundry out to dry, just for the excuse to be outside, using your body.

On the diet front, you're eating plenty of protein: eggs or yogurt for breakfast, leftover Quinoa Stir-Fry (see recipe on page 149) for lunch, and a roast chicken with salad for dinner. If you truly need a snack, you reach for a handful of almonds and wash them down with a cup of Ginger Tea (see recipe on page 91). You have a real sense that the food you're eating is fueling the dynamism you're feeling now.

At work, you're happy to roll up your sleeves and crank out the good stuff. Right around ovulation time, the great ideas are flowing and you have a few occasions where it feels like you get several days' worth of work done in just a few hours. If you have something big planned, like a vacation or a move, you've been careful to schedule it for this Mega Phase so you have your highest energy levels happening just when you need them most.

Because your intuition is coming up close to the surface right around Day 14, you're carving out a little room in your schedule for reflection, whether that's through meditating, journaling, or just brainstorming with a piece of paper and a pen. The ideas that surface when you do this help you to express yourself more clearly to your partner, friends, and kids. And by putting in the effort to tune into those insights and put them to good use, you know you're laying the groundwork for a less emotional (read: bitchy) premenstrual time.

All along, you're jotting down how you feel mentally, emotionally, and physically on your Energy Wheel, which helps you to remember where you are in your cycle and become more aware of when ovulation is actually happening. If you're open to getting pregnant, or actively trying to have a baby, you know exactly when to dim the lights and surprise your husband with your nakedness. And if you're not, you know when to be extremely conscientious about either abstaining or using condoms or your diaphragm. You're also noticing which days in your cycle tend to be most intuitive for you and when your energy dips tend to occur, so you can plan your schedule during future cycles accordingly.

Around Day 21—although it can be as early as Day 18—you begin to notice the first signs that your premenstrual time has arrived. Maybe it's the first blush of breast tenderness, or your pants are just a hair tighter. As soon as you catch wind that your body's shifting into its next phase, you start to prioritize your alone time. If you go to the gym, you opt to ride a machine and go into the zone with your favorite play list instead of taking a class. You combine your exercise with your stress relief and head out for a long walk over lunch instead of eating with friends, or opt out of one weekday dinner/bed/bath routine with the kids to lace up your shoes and go on a walkabout. (Because you knew it was coming, you've had a chance to ask your sister, friend, husband, or mother to cover for you.)

Food-wise, you're having more smoothies for breakfast, or oatmeal cooked in plenty of water. You make it a point to whip up a big pot of soup, so you always have an easy lunch on hand that'll help you stay hydrated and get plenty of mineral-rich greens without a lot of prep. The Easy-Peasy Arugula Salad (page 147) is perfect right now. Ideally, you cook up an extra meal or two in preparation for the first day of your period, when you're really not going to feel up to cooking. And you do it at some point when the house is quiet, so you can really absorb yourself in the creative process and turn your time in the kitchen into an opportunity to decompress and reflect.

When you start to notice your irritation levels going from 0 to 60 in 3.2 seconds (you trip on a kid's toy and immediately start bellowing, for instance, or you pick a fight with your husband because something your mom said upset you, but you didn't let yourself tell her what you really thought about it and you need an outlet for your frustration), you either head out the door to get a sweat going with some low-impact cardio, or find some way to create solitude for yourself. Maybe you even set up a PMS babysitting co-op, so you can send your kids to your friend's house when you're having a tough Day 25, and she can do the same. (Sound crazy? Share this book with a friend and turn down the corner on this page. Of course, it helps if you're not in the same phase at the same time.) Maybe you opt to sleep in the guest bed a couple nights so you can be pleasant to the people you love during waking hours.

You also get a ton done on your creative projects, because the solitude they require that can feel so hard to come by when you're in Mega mode is so appealing right now. In fact, you start looking forward to your premenstrual time as an opportunity to really make major progress on those projects that call to your heart but don't ever seem to make it to the top of your to-do list. You still get a little bloated and a little moody, but you're no longer debilitated by your symptoms. (If you are, you know it's time to recalibrate.)

By being in better touch with your cycle, you know much earlier when something seems to be "off" with your health, and you get to your doctor, naturopath, acupuncturist, chiropractor, shrink, coach, or any combination of these, *before* you veer off into total emergency land. You also become present to how much your body truly does fluctuate each month, which helps you to appreciate your dynamic and resilient body more. And that appreciation helps you treat your body better; it's the equivalent of closely tending a garden and enjoying the bounty it provides even more because of the awareness you bring to the growing process, versus sticking some plants in the ground, watering them occasionally, and being shocked when you get something edible and only mildly disappointed when the plants whither in the sun. There's a scientific principle that says the very act of observing something affects the outcome. The simple act of paying closer attention to your own personal fluidity helps the tide flow with you rather than against you.

And perhaps most important, when you deepen your appreciation of the menstrual cycle, you pass your point of view on to your daughters, sisters, and friends. You become an important piece of helping womankind heal from the concept of "the Curse" and help us all to feel more connected to our true biological and spiritual nature. We know it sounds woo-woo to say so, but it's absolutely true. As renowned anthropologist Margaret Mead said, "Never doubt that a small group of thoughtful, committed citizens can change the world. Indeed, it is the only thing that ever has." Here's your opportunity to be the change, and to help all current and future females and society at large make peace with and respect the true nature of being a woman. Amen to that.

And for ongoing support and resources to keep your cyclically balanced lifestyle going, visit us at 28dayslighterdiet.com. We've created lots of other goodies to keep you going, and look forward to connecting with you there!

Acknowledgments

We'd like to thank our agent, Stephanie Kip Rostan, for enthusiastically climbing on board our train from the moment she first opened our e-mail, and for using her considerable savvy on our behalf.

We'd like to thank Lara Asher, our editor at skirt!, who kicks butt in the very nicest way. (I, Kate, consider myself truly blessed to be able to work with you twice!) And our heartfelt thanks to everyone at Globe Pequot Press / skirt! for launching our concept into the world.

We'd like to thank our contributors, Laurie Steelsmith, Linda Sparrowe, and Katy Bowman, for lending their considerable expertise with grace (and for being fun to work with to boot), and the women who provided testimonials, for their openness.

We'd like to thank Joni Stone, CPM, and traditional Chinese medicine expert extraordinaire, Dr. J Yan, for sharing their vast knowledge, especially regarding the mind/body/spirit connection. Huge thanks also to Ellen's big brother, Dr. John Barrett, for helping us to navigate the medical research world and encouraging us to write our book.

We'd like to thank Mitch Blank and Arthur Cohen for translating our vision into clear and beautiful charts and photographs.

And finally, we'd like to thank our children's preschool teachers and our husbands for watching our kids while we kicked out the jams on this book.

Appendix A: The Energy Wheel

Energy Wheel

Go to 28dayslighterdiet.com for downloadable PDFs that you can print and fill out each month.

Appendix B: The 28-Day Plan

Day	General Mood	Food Focus
1	Very low energy, at times even "weak"	Breakfast: Good Morning Oatmeal (page 141) Lunch: Stir-fried veggies and rice Dinner: Any warming soup Snack: A mug of herbal tea with honey
2	Low energy	Breakfast: Almost Eggs Florentine (page 140) Lunch: Grass-fed burger Dinner: Quinoa Stir-Fry (page 149) Snack: Handful of dried apricots
3	Low energy	Breakfast: Scrambled eggs and toast Lunch: Leftover Quinoa Stir-Fry Dinner: Chicken and Broccoli over Almond Rice (page 152) Snack: Couple squares of dark chocolate
4	Mellow	Breakfast: Warm toast with almond butter Lunch: Leftover Chicken and Broccoli over Almond Rice Dinner: Easy-Peasy Arugula Salad (page 147) Snack: Raisins and almonds
5	Mellow	Breakfast: Good Morning Oatmeal (page 141) Lunch: Ginger Salad with Shrimp (page 145) Dinner: Lentil Soup (page 155) Snack: Dark chocolate–covered raisins
6	Feeling light but low stamina	Breakfast: Almost Eggs Florentine (page 140) Lunch: Chicken Broth (page 137) that you've spiced up with miso, a dash of tamari, a handful of chopped greens, and leftover rice Dinner: Senora Salad (page 146) Snack: Date with a smear of almond butter
7	Feeling light	Breakfast: Warm toast with almond butter Lunch: Vegetarian chili or bean-based soup from the take-out joint on the corner Dinner: Soba noodles with Tasty Tahini Dressing (page 148) and chopped raw veggies (whatever you have in the fridge) Snack: Roasted pumpkin seeds
8	Feeling light	Breakfast: 1 cup of Greek yogurt with ½ cup of Tart Cherry Granola (page 138) Lunch: Leftover soba noodles Dinner: Quinoa and Black Beans (page 151) Snack: Roasted seaweed
9	Good energy	Breakfast: Whole-wheat or gluten-free toast with smashed avocado Lunch: Leftover Quinoa and Black Beans Dinner: Take-out sushi (order the seaweed salad to start) Snack: Dried apricots

Exercise Option	Lifestyle Tips
Do the Reclining Bound Angle Pose, with long exhales (page 116).	Use a hot-water bottle on your lower abdomen; sleep in; or go to bed 30 minutes early.
Practice Loving-Kindness Meditation while lying in Kate's Favorite Meditation Pose (page 119).	Take a shower instead of a bath; prioritize downtime.
Do the Wise Woman Yoga sequence (page 63).	Go to bed early; try the Dreamy Trick to Help You Get More Zzz's on page 71.
Do the Wise Woman Yoga sequence (page 63), or maybe take a low-intensity walk.	Take a quick nap.
Do the Wise Woman Yoga sequence (page 63), and/or take a low-intensity walk.	Linger in bed in the morning; make a list of things you want to tackle when your energy is totally back in a day or two.
Do the Wise Woman Yoga sequence (page 63), and/or take a low-intensity walk.	Start working a notch harder—gradually amping up intensity instead of diving in headfirst.
Do the Wise Woman Yoga sequence (page 63), and/or take a low-intensity walk.	Find a simple way to honor the end of the menstrual phase: Tuck your period panties in the back of the drawer, put your sweatpants away, or some other simple ritual that's meaningful to you.
Go to a Zumba class; do a Supported Shoulder Stand before bed (page 89).	Walk to work.
Take a long walk with a friend.	Chase your kids around the park before dinner.

Day	General Mood	Food Focus
10	Good energy	Breakfast: Tart Cherry Granola (page 138) and almond milk Lunch: Leek and Potato Soup (page 156) Dinner: Pine Nut Pesto Pasta (page 153) and simple green salad Snack: Hard-boiled egg
11	High energy	Breakfast: Good Morning Oatmeal (page 141) Lunch: Leftover Pine Nut Pesto Pasta Dinner: Quinoa and Black Beans (page 151) Snack: Ginger Tea (page 91) with honey
12	Very high energy	Breakfast: Blueberry and Walnut Smoothie (page 143) Lunch: Leftover Quinoa and Black Beans Dinner: Lamb burger with roasted or steamed broccoli Snack: Roasted sunflower seeds
13	Very high energy	Breakfast: Energy Balls (page 142) Lunch: Half of a turkey sandwich and cup of soup Dinner: Ginger Salad with Shrimp (page 145) Snack: Pumpkin seeds
14	Very high energy	Breakfast: Scrambled eggs with leftover Pine Nut Pesto and toast Lunch: Leftover Ginger Salad with Shrimp (page 145) Dinner: Spinach Salad with Warm Vinaigrette (page 144) Snack: Handful of almonds
15	High energy	Breakfast: Avocado on toast Lunch: Take-out sautéed veggies and rice (Indian, Chinese, or Thai) Dinner: Coconut Chicken Soup (page 157) Snack: Small Blueberry and Walnut Smoothie (page 143)
16	High energy	Breakfast: Energy Balls (page 142) Lunch: Turkey sandwich with extra lettuce and tomatoes Dinner: Pine Nut Pesto Pasta (page 153)
17	High energy	Breakfast: Good Morning Oatmeal (page 141) Lunch: Leftover Pine Nut Pesto Pasta Dinner: Senora Salad (page 146) Snack: Hard-boiled egg
18	Good energy	Breakfast: Whole-wheat or gluten-free toast with almond butter Lunch: Hummus and veggie wrap Dinner: Chicken and Broccoli over Almond Rice (page 152)

Exercise Option	Lifestyle Tips
Do 20 minutes of Sun Salutations (page 83) in the morning, ending with a Supported Shoulder Stand (page 89).	Take the stairs wherever you go; stay late at work to get a jump on that big project.
Hit the gym for weights and cardio.	Make calls and set up fun outings for next week.
Take a yoga class.	Listen to music while making dinner and dance along.
Run or hike with a friend.	Instead of e-mailing your colleagues, walk over to their desks to relay your message.
Do 30 minutes of Sun Salutations (page 83), ending with a Supported Shoulder Stand (page 89).	Get out and circulate in the evening—a party, a dance class, a networking event. Go!
Socialize and energize; grab your racket for a couple sets of tennis.	Have that important meeting.
Do 30 minutes of Sun Salutations (page 83), ending with a Supported Shoulder Stand (page 89).	Go out dancing with your girlfriends.
Take a 90-minute yoga class.	Garden for 30 minutes if it's spring or summer, rake if it's fall, shovel snow if it's winter.
Do 30 minutes of Sun Salutations (page 83), ending with a Supported Shoulder Stand (page 89).	Get outside after the kids go to bed and bask in the moonlight.

Day	General Mood	Food Focus	
19	Good energy	Breakfast: Huevos rancheros with extra guacamole Lunch: Quinoa and Black Beans (page 151) Dinner: Shrimp cocktail and a Caesar salad Snack: Celery sticks with almond butter	
20	Good energy	Breakfast: Energy Balls (page 142) Lunch: Bean burger on a gluten-free bun Dinner: Spinach Salad with Warm Vinaigrette (page 144) Snack: Dark chocolate–covered raisins	
21	Good energy	Breakfast: Banana and almond milk smoothie Lunch: Grilled salmon with rice and string beans Dinner: Two slices of arugula pizza Snack: Cashews	
22	Good energy but irritable	Breakfast: Energy Balls (page 142) Lunch: Spinach Salad with Warm Vinaigrette (page 144) Dinner: Coconut Chicken Soup (page 157) Snack: Raw veggies dipped in Tasty Tahini Dressing (page 148)	
23	Good energy but irritable	Breakfast: Green juice (try Ellen's fave: kale, celery and carrot) Lunch: Escarole and Bean Soup (page 154) Dinner: Ginger Salad with Shrimp (page 145) Snack: Energy Balls	
24	Introverted and sensitive to discomfort	Breakfast: Good Morning Oatmeal (page 141) Lunch: Leek and Potato Soup (page 156) Dinner: Quinoa Stir-Fry (page 149) Snack: Herbal tea with honey	
25	Introverted and sensitive	Breakfast: 1 cup of Greek yogurt with 1 cup of strawberries Lunch: One sushi roll and a cup of miso soup Dinner: Senora Salad (page 146) Snack: Piece of fruit	
26	Low energy	Breakfast: Energy Balls (page 142) Lunch: Turkey sandwich with extra lettuce and tomatoes Dinner: Escarole and Bean Soup (page 154) Snack: Roasted seaweed	
27	Low energy	Breakfast: Good Morning Oatmeal (page 141) Lunch: Leftover Escarole and Bean Soup Dinner: Quinoa and Black Beans (page 151) Snack: Hummus with cucumbers	
28	Very introverted and low energy	Breakfast: Good Morning Oatmeal (page 141) Lunch: Coconut Chicken Soup (page 157) Dinner: Easy-Peasy Arugula Salad (page 147) Snack: Apple	

Exercise Option	Lifestyle Tips
Do a 20-minute run on the treadmill and follow it up with a Pilates mat class.	Have a "date night" with your partner or spouse
Run on the treadmill for 15 minutes, then do another 15 minutes on the seated rower.	Get out and about in the evening; you're about to go into quiet mode, so make the most of it.
Do a 45-minute low-impact exercise DVD at home by yourself.	Dim the lights and lie in Kate's Favorite Meditation Pose for 20 minutes.
Go for a 30-minute power walk and follow it up with the Vixen Restorative Yoga series (page 114).	Stock up on herbal teas—chamomile, red raspberry leaf, nettle, or dandelion root.
Go on a soulful sunrise hike.	Do the Vixen Restorative Yoga series (page 114) before or after work.
Do 20 minutes of walking on the treadmill, 20 minutes on the elliptical, and 20 minutes on the stair-climber for 60 minutes of steady cardio.	Set your cell phone on "mute."
Map out a 20-mile cycling ride, fill your water bottle, and go!	Have a cup of red raspberry leaf tea for dessert.
Take your dog (or your friend's dog) for a walk in the woods.	Soak in the tub by candlelight.
Charge up your iPod and go for a solo power walk.	Turn in early with a good book.
Instead of lunching with coworkers, take a midday stroll and then eat at your desk.	Go straight home from work for a full evening of alone time.

Bibliography

Buckley, Thomas, and Alma Gottlieb (eds.). *Blood Magic: The Anthropology of Menstruation*. Berkeley: University of California Press, 1988.

Colbin, Annemarie. *Food and Healing: How What You Eat Determines Your Health, Your Well-Being, and the Quality of Your Life*. New York: Ballantine Books, 1986.

Delaney, Janice, Mary Jane Lupton, and Emily Toth. *The Curse: A Cultural History of Menstruation, Revised Edition*. Urbana: University of Illinois Press, 1988.

Ehrenreich, Barbara, and Deirdre English. *Witches, Midwives, and Nurses: A History of Women Healers*. New York: The Feminist Press, 1973.

Gray, Miranda. *Red Moon: Understanding and Using the Creative, Sexual, and Spiritual Gifts of the Menstrual Cycle, Revised Edition*. Dancing Eve, 2009.

Groover, Rachael Jayne. *Powerful and Feminine: How to Increase Your Magnetic Presence and Attract the Attention You Want*. Fort Collins, CO: Deep Pacific Press, 2011.

Iyengar, Geeta. *Yoga: A Gem for Women*. Spokane, WA: Timeless Books, 2005.

Kent, Tami Lynn. *Wild Feminine: Finding Power, Spirit & Joy in the Female Body*. New York: Atria Books, 2011.

Ni, Maoshing, MD. *Secrets of Self-Healing: Harness Nature's Power to Heal Common Ailments, Boot Your Vitality and Achieve Optimum Wellness*. New York: Avery, 2008.

Owen, Lara. *Her Blood Is Gold: Awakening to the Wisdom of Menstruation, Revised Edition*. Wimborne, UK: Archive Publishing, 2008.

Rier, S. E., et al. "Endometriosis in Rhesus Monkeys *(Macaca mulatta)* Following Chronic Exposure to 2, 3, 7, 8-tetrachlorodibenzo-p-dioxin," *Fundamental and Applied Toxicology*, Vol. 21 (1993), pp. 433–41.

Rier, S. E., et al. "Serum Levels of TCDD and Dioxin-like Chemicals in Rhesus Monkeys Chronically Exposed to Dioxin: Correlation of Increased Serum PCB Levels with Endometriosis," *Toxicological Sciences*, Vol. 59, No. 1 (2001), pp. 147–59.

Sparrowe, Linda, and Patricia Walden. *The Woman's Book of Yoga & Health: A Lifelong Guide to Wellness.* Boston: Shambhala, 2002.

———. *Yoga for a Healthy Menstrual Cycle.* Boston: Shambhala, 2004.

Steelsmith, Laurie, ND. *Natural Choices for Women's Health: How the Secrets of Natural and Chinese Medicine Can Create a Lifetime of Wellness.* New York: Three Rivers Press, 2005.

Stein, Elissa, and Susan Kim. *Flow: The Cultural Story of Menstruation.* New York: St. Martin's Griffin, 2009.

Weschler, Toni, MPH. *Taking Charge of Your Fertility: The Definitive Guide to Natural Birth Control, Pregnancy Achievement, and Reproductive Health, Revised Edition.* New York: Collins, 2006.

Resources

TAMPON REPLACEMENTS
DivaCup (good for years of use)
divacup.com

Lunapads Washable Cloth Pads and the DivaCup
lunapads.com

Party In My Pants Cloth Pads
partypantspads.com

Softcup (two versions—one is reusable for one cycle, the other is disposable and designed for one use)
softcup.com

USEFUL WEBSITES
American Association of Naturopathic Physicians
naturopathic.org

The Arvigo Techniques of Maya Abdominal Therapy
https://arvigotherapy.com

Ellen Barrett Fusion Fitness (Ellen's website)
ellenbarrett.com

LocalHarvest: Find Food Co-ops and Farmer's Markets near You
localharvest.org

Lunaception—A Feminine Odyssey into Fertility and Contraception
lunaception.net

Mountain Rose Herbs
mountainroseherbs.com

Ms. Mindbody (Kate's website)
msmindbody.com

Museum of Menstruation and Women's Health
mum.org

National Certification Commission for Acupuncture and Oriental Medicine
nccaom.org

The 28 Days Lighter Diet
28dayslighterdiet.com

COOKBOOKS

Feeding the Whole Family (3rd ed.) by Cynthia Lair (Sasquatch Books, 2008)

How to Cook Everything (2nd ed.) by Mark Bittman (Houghton Mifflin Harcourt, 2008)

Nourishing Traditions by Sally Fallon (New Trends Publishing, 1999)

RECOMMENDED READING

Consciously Female by Tracey W. Gaudet, MD (Bantam, 2004)

Dr. Susan Lark's Hormone Revolution by Susan M. Lark, MD (Portola Press, 2007)

An End to All Disease by Lt. Lawrence F. Frego (Authorhouse, 2006)

The Fourfold Path to Healing by Thomas S. Cowan, MD (New Trends Publishing, 2004)

French Women Don't Get Fat by Mireille Guiliano (Vintage, 2007)

How to Be a Woman by Caitlin Moran (Harper Perennial, 2011)

Moon Time by Johanna Paungger and Thomas Poppe (Rider, 2005)

Spiritual Nutrition by Dr. Gabriel Cousens (North Atlantic Books, 2005)

Index

About the Authors

A coach, writer, and yoga teacher, **Kate Hanley** teaches busy, frazzled women how to slow down, breathe deep, and trust their gut, even when life is moving a million miles an hour. She's the author of *The Anywhere, Anytime Chill Guide*, a regular contributor to national magazines—including *Parents, Yoga Journal, Whole Living,* and *Real Simple*—and a frequent speaker at everything from corporate events to moms' group meetings. Kate has also appeared on *The Today Show* and been a recurring guest on *Martha Stewart Living Radio* on Sirius/XM.

Kate lives in an ever-evolving fixer-upper in Providence, Rhode Island, with her husband and two kids. Visit her at msmindbody .com.

Women's wellness expert **Ellen Barrett, MA,** is known worldwide for her innovative workout videos, including *Prevention* magazine's best-selling *Flat Belly Diet* series, and also, for her long-running Fit TV show, *All-Star Workouts*. As a 2010 graduate of The Institute for Integrative Nutrition (IIN), she has emerged as a go-to expert for women and weight loss. Ellen lives in New Haven, Connecticut, with her husband and son. For further information regarding Ellen's workshops and retreats, visit www.ellenbarrett.com.

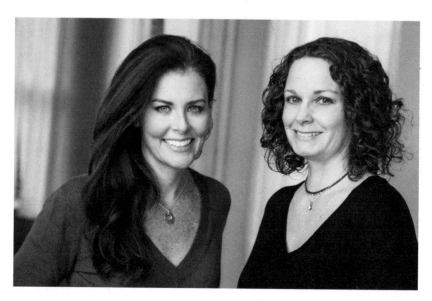

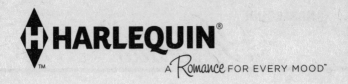

Love the Harlequin book you just read?

Your opinion matters.

Review this book on your favorite
book site, review site, blog or your own
social media properties and share
your opinion with other readers!

"Gawdamn dumb-assed lawmen," someone close to Longarm swore. "Bastards think they can just come into a town and do whatever they want because someone pinned a piece of tin on their chest."

"I think you need to leave our town immediately," the store owner said.

"No," Longarm told them. "Someone here stole this mare in Vulture's Nest early this morning. There is a horse thief in this town who I mean to apprehend and arrest before I leave."

"We don't even know if that mare belongs to you," a man said, looking around for support. "Boys, this jasper might have found or stole the badge."

Edwards drew himself up. "Let's see your bill of sale on that bay mare, Marshal. Also, I'd like to see more proof as to your identity."

"I don't have a bill of sale on that mare," Longarm said, feeling his position eroding as surely as if he stood on a sandy riverbank.

"Well, in that case, we have a problem," Jim said. "You come barging into the store, pistol-whip me and you don't have proof you even are a lawman, much less that you own that mare. Boys, I think we need to teach this uppity stranger a hard lesson!"

The crowd started to advance on Longarm . . .

DON'T MISS THESE
ALL-ACTION WESTERN SERIES
FROM THE BERKLEY PUBLISHING GROUP

THE GUNSMITH by J. R. Roberts
Clint Adams was a legend among lawmen, outlaws, and ladies. They called him . . . the Gunsmith.

LONGARM by Tabor Evans
The popular long-running series about U.S. Deputy Marshal Long—his life, his loves, his fight for justice.

SLOCUM by Jake Logan
Today's longest-running action Western. John Slocum rides a deadly trail of hot blood and cold steel.

BUSHWHACKERS by B. J. Lanagan
An action-packed series by the creators of Longarm! The rousing adventures of the most brutal gang of cutthroats ever assembled—Quantrill's Raiders.

DIAMONDBACK by Guy Brewer
Dex Yancey is Diamondback, a southern gentleman turned con man when his brother cheats him out of the family fortune. Ladies love him. Gamblers hate him. But nobody pulls one over on Dex . . .

WILDGUN by Jack Hanson
Will Barlow's continuing search for his daughter, kidnapped by the Blackfeet Indians who slaughtered the rest of his family.

— TABOR EVANS —

LONGARM

AND THE
BLACK WIDOW

J

JOVE BOOKS, NEW YORK

This is a work of fiction. Names, characters, places, and incidents are
either the product of the author's imagination or are used fictitiously,
and any resemblance to actual persons, living or dead, business
establishments, events, or locales is entirely coincidental.

LONGARM AND THE BLACK WIDOW

A Jove Book / published by arrangement with
the author

PRINTING HISTORY
Jove edition / June 2000

All rights reserved.
Copyright © 2000 by Penguin Putnam Inc.
This book may not be reproduced in whole or in part,
by mimeograph or any other means, without permission.
For information address: The Berkley Publishing Group,
a division of Penguin Putnam Inc.,
375 Hudson Street, New York, New York 10014.

The Penguin Putnam Inc. World Wide Web site address is
http://www.penguinputnam.com

ISBN: 0-515-12839-2

A JOVE BOOK®
Jove Books are published by The Berkley Publishing Group,
a division of Penguin Putnam Inc.,
375 Hudson Street, New York, New York 10014.
JOVE and the "J" design
are trademarks belonging to Penguin Putnam Inc.

PRINTED IN THE UNITED STATES OF AMERICA

10 9 8 7 6 5 4 3 2 1

Chapter 1

"Custis, come on in and close the door behind you," Billy Vail said, urgently motioning his tall United States deputy marshal inside his office. "I've got a job that only you can handle."

Longarm shook his head. "Billy, you know that flattery won't work with me. In fact, I become suspicious when you start giving me compliments."

"Lock the door."

Longarm stopped. "We're in the United States Federal Building. What—"

"For once, will you just do as I say?"

Longarm studied Billy's face and decided the man really did want his office door locked. So he turned the bolt and asked, "What's got you so spooked?"

"Sit down, Custis. I've got a very difficult problem and I'm not sure how to handle it."

"Sounds serious."

"It's *damned* serious," Billy said, looking grim.

Custis Long eased down in the chair. "You look like your wife just died."

"No, but someone else did. And I'm afraid it's someone

1

very important who died in a very bad way."

Longarm steepled his fingers and leaned back in his chair. "Why don't you start at the beginning," he suggested. "And make sure you don't forget to tell me why someone else can't handle the problem because I'm long overdue for a vacation. Remember?"

"Of course. But it might have to wait."

"Billy, I—"

"United States Senator John Hawk has just been murdered along with a federal employee who was delivering a special piece of legislation that needed to be reviewed and signed by the senator."

"Regarding?"

"Regarding the sale and transfer of thirty thousand acres of extremely valuable Ute Reservation lands." Billy frowned. "You've probably read about the Ute land and all the controversy that its pending sale has caused. The Indians will be reimbursed, but it won't amount to nearly as much as Colorado will receive when it sells the land at a public auction to the highest bidder."

"From what I've read, the Ute people are justified in being upset because that land was promised to them in a treaty," Longarm said. "I know quite a few Ute Indians and I also know how much land our government has already cheated them out of."

"I agree. We both know that the treaties our government has made with the Indians aren't worth the paper they are written on." Billy held up his hand when Longarm started to object. "Listen, I'm as sympathetic to the Indians as you are and agree that it's unfair. However, we don't make the law, we *enforce* it, and there seems to be little doubt that the murder of Senator Hawk and the federal dispatcher was committed by a Ute."

"Who says?"

"Our boss. He called me in to see him not more than

2

twenty minutes ago and laid out the circumstances. It seems that Senator Hawk had employed several Utes on his cattle ranch. He treated one of them, a fella named Liberty, like a second son. But Liberty must have been plotting to steal those land transfer documents they are missing."

"Did anyone actually see Liberty kill Senator Hawk or that federal dispatcher?" Longarm asked.

"No but, given the circumstances and evidence of the Indian's sudden disappearance, there is little doubt he committed both murders."

"That's not enough for a murder conviction."

"I know that," Billy agreed. "But the senator was very popular in his part of the country and I expect a lot of citizens will be up in arms. They're probably hunting Liberty right now. At any rate, whoever finds that Ute undoubtedly will also find the land transfer documents."

Longarm shook his head. "Billy, I sure don't want to get into this mess. I have friends among those people."

"Don't you think I know that? You're the only one in this department that has any real contacts among the Ute. They probably trust you. Right?"

"Some do," Longarm said cautiously.

"So they'll help you find Liberty and see that justice is done."

"Not necessarily."

"Listen to me," Billy said, his voice revealing his inner strain. "Our federal director . . . my boss and *your* boss . . . is very aware of the sensitive nature of this case. When the newspapers learn about the murders, our toes are going to be put over the coals."

"The news hasn't gotten out?"

"It has in Pagosa Springs. Pagosa is the town nearest to where the Senator lived and ranched when he wasn't in Washington, D.C. Have you ever seen Hawk Ranch?"

"No, but I've heard it's impressive."

"It is," Billy agreed. "I was there about eight years ago. I had tracked another Ute, a fellow named Charlie Four-Fingers into that country and, I'm sorry to say, had to kill him in a shoot-out that was just a mile south of Hawk Ranch. When Senator Hawk learned I was winged, he insisted that I recuperate at his cattle ranch. I've never been treated so royally in my life. The place is a mansion and sits overlooking an immense alpine valley. It's the most beautiful setup I've ever seen and one of the largest in southwestern Colorado."

"Nice people, huh?"

"Most of them," Billy said, looking away.

"What is that supposed to mean?"

"The senator's wife was born and raised in that country and her family had a terrible reputation. Her maiden name was . . . let me see . . . yes, Kilbane. And they literally wiped out the Utes who used to own that ranch land. Senator Hawk married Nettie Kilbane and, since she was an only child, the ranch passed on to Nettie and John."

"What about Nettie's mother?"

"She died of unknown causes about two months previous to Mr. Kilbane's death."

"Unknown causes?" Longarm asked, eyebrows raising in question.

"That's right. She suddenly took sick and died."

"No coroner's inquest or autopsy?"

"There is no doctor in Pagosa Springs. No coroner. Old Grandma Kibane just died one night and was buried the next day."

"And the reason for her husband's death?"

"The same . . . cause unknown."

Longarm blinked. "I don't like the sound of that."

"Neither did a lot of other people. But the Kilbanes were a very private family with few friends and no shortage of enemies. From what I learned just in the several weeks that

4

I was recovering on their ranch, the family had been pretty ruthless in grabbing land from both the Utes and whites. They'd become land barons and they had some gunmen on their payroll who could . . . shall we say . . . discourage settlers from taking up whatever public lands remained open to homesteading."

"So," Longarm interrupted, "we have a family with a murderous reputation and then two sudden and unexplained deaths within a very short period of time resulting in Nettie inheriting a cattle empire."

"That's right." Billy frowned. "And I should probably tell you that Nettie has a nickname that is less than flattering."

"What is it?"

"The Black Widow."

Longarm blinked. "Why?"

"There are a lot of people who believe she not only *poisoned* her own mother and father to gain control of Hawk Ranch, but that she also poisoned her first husband."

"Do you think she might also have had Senator Hawk murdered?" Longarm asked.

"To tell you the truth, I wouldn't put it past the old gal. When you see Nettie Hawk, the first thing you'll notice is her eyes. They lack even a shred of warmth or humanity. Mrs. Hawk had coal-black hair and dark skin. She might be part Indian. I don't know or care. I have heard that her daughter, Della, is her spitting image. As is their only son."

"What is his name?"

"Jake. He's in his mid-twenties."

"How old is Della?"

"A year or two older than her brother. She's addled in the head, though."

"Crazy?"

"That's right. Criminally insane might be a more apt de-

scription, although she has never been allowed to leave the ranch."

"Then how can you say—"

"Della was about fifteen when I was recuperating at Hawk Ranch," Billy explained. "I remember looking out my window to see her holding a small bird that had fallen out of its nest. Della was playing with the baby bird, unaware that she was being watched."

"What did she do?"

Billy looked quickly away.

"What?" Longarm insisted.

"The bird was almost ready to fly," Billy reluctantly continued. "It actually could fly . . . but not well or far. There were a few barnyard cats, and it soon became apparent to me that Della was playing a sick game. She'd hold the bird up and let it fly, then the cats would pounce on it when it landed. Della would rescue the bird, then turn it loose again. Over and over to be attacked by the cats."

"So what finally happened?" Longarm asked.

"The cats killed and ate the bird. And you know what Della did?"

"No."

"She broke into hysterical laughter. I tell you, Custis, it made the hair on the back of my neck stand up on end!"

"I'll agree it's sick, but that doesn't mean the girl is addled."

"No," Billy agreed, "it probably doesn't. Most likely, Della is just cruel and sick in the head. And I guess it wouldn't have upset me so if she'd been older or even a boy. But she was a beautiful child. She's a Kilbane to the core and the spitting image of her evil mother."

"Sounds like a wonderful family," Longarm remarked cryptically.

"Be careful," Billy pleaded. "Don't trust *any* of them. I can't tell you how glad I was to leave that ranch as soon

6

as I was fit to travel. There is a darkness there that I can't begin to describe."

Longarm waited for more, and when it didn't come he grew impatient. "There are things about the Hawk family you aren't telling me. If I'm going to take on this case, I have to know *everything*."

"I'm afraid that I've already told you about all I know."

Longarm smoked for a few minutes, then said, "Even if Liberty did murder Senator Hawk and the other fella, I doubt that the Utes would help me in a capture and arrest. They've been cheated so many times by the white man that they'd most likely stand in my way."

"I was afraid that you'd say that." Billy stood up and marched around his desk, heading for the door.

"Where are you going?" Longarm asked.

"I'll tell the director that I talked you out of this one. I'll tell him that I insist on taking the case myself."

"Whoa!" Longarm shouted, also jumping up from his chair. "Hold on a minute here. You can't do that."

"Watch me."

Longarm was a big man, standing well over six feet, and he grabbed Billy by the coat and pushed him back down in his chair. "Don't be a complete fool. You got a wife and kids to support."

"I'm not going to send you into a situation where you haven't any chance of coming out alive."

"Sit down and let's talk some more before you get us both fired. I want to know whatever else you can tell me about the late Senator Hawk and his evil family."

Billy's shoulder's sagged. "Whiskey?" he offered.

"Sure."

Longarm clucked his tongue. "Man, this must *really* be bad if you're offering me some of that private hooch you keep hidden in your drawer."

"It is bad," Billy said looking upset. "You must under-

7

stand that Nettie was once one of the most beautiful women in Colorado and her daughter is now every bit as striking."

"But evil," Longarm added.

"That's right. I also remember that Della could be extremely charming when she wanted something . . . a ploy she must have learned from her mother."

"So?"

"So be very careful when you are around Della Hawk. And watch out for Jake, too. I wouldn't trust either one as far as I could throw them. And the same goes for their mother."

Longarm shook his head. "What a nest of vipers!"

"Vipers?" Billy asked. "More like a nest of black widow spiders, all filled with deadly poison. And do you know what?"

"What?" Longarm asked, almost afraid to ask.

"Della Hawk might just be sane enough to kill them all and become the next Black Widow."

Despite himself, Longarm shuddered.

Chapter 2

Longarm stood up and said, "When do you want me to head for Pagosa Springs?"

"The next train south leaves tomorrow at eight."

"I'd hoped to stay around for at least a day or two."

"I'm sorry," Billy said, sounding as though he really meant it. "I've heard rumors that you and Miss Lacy had plans to take your vacations together starting tomorrow. Where were you going?"

Longarm shrugged. "We thought we might go down to Santa Fe and soak up some sunshine and eat more than our share of that good Mexican food."

"It'll still be there for you both after this Senator Hawk assignment."

"I expect so," Longarm replied, "unless Karen finds someone else to spend her vacation time with. There aren't many as pretty or fun as Karen Lacy. She could have her pick of any bachelor in the building."

"I know," Billy said with a thin smile. "And, if I were fifteen years younger and still single . . . well, I'd probably hand in my badge rather than miss a chance to go traveling with that woman."

"No you wouldn't have," Longarm countered. "And anyway, there are always more fish to fry."

"Not as pretty as Miss Lacy. What are you going to tell her?"

"The truth."

"That wouldn't be a good idea, Custis. What I've told you about Senator Hawk and his family is confidential and much of it was just my own personal observations and opinions."

"Do they really call Mrs. Hawk the Black Widow?"

"Only in private." Billy went over to his friend. "Curtis, could I give you a little more friendly advice?"

"Would it make any difference if I said no?"

"I suppose not."

"Then let's hear it quick," Longarm answered. "Because I've got a train to catch in the morning and a lot of loose ends to tie up first."

"My advice is simply to avoid the Hawk family as much as possible once you arrive in Pagosa Springs. If the Black Widow murdered her husband . . . for whatever reason she may have had . . . and then pinned the death on that poor Ute Indian, you're going to have to avoid those people and try to save Liberty's hide. There will be a lot of anger about the death of Senator Hawk and you know how many people up there hate the Utes."

"People usually hate those that they most unjustly wrong. It's a way of handling their guilty consciences."

"You may have that right," Billy said. "But don't get tangled up in that web. Nettie or her daughter, Della, are capable of anything."

"And Jake?"

"I don't know about him. He was away much of the time I was there recuperating and I didn't have a chance to watch him like I did the girl. But I expect he's as rotten as the rest of his family."

"I'll keep that in mind," Longarm said on his way out the door. He exited the U.S. Marshal's Building and walked next door to the Denver Mint where Karen Lacy was employed. There was an armed security guard at the entrance to the building, but when he recognized Longarm, he waved him past.

"I'd like to see Miss Lacy," Longarm told a clerk who was in charge of directing people to the proper offices.

"So would I," the man said with a chuckle. "You lucky dog, you."

"Cut the crap," Longarm told him. "I'm in a hurry."

"All right. You know where to find her."

Longarm marched down the long marble-floored hallway and entered room six where Karen worked as a payroll supervisor. He caught her eye and she smiled.

This isn't going to be easy, Longarm thought, watching Karen hurry over to greet him. *Damn Billy and this miserable timing!*

"Custis, what a nice surprise! I didn't expect to see you until after five o'clock." Karen was a short, brown-eyed girl with the figure of a Greek goddess and a sweet, happy temperament to match her exceptional looks. "Get off early?"

"Yeah. Listen, can we step out into the hallway and talk for a moment?"

"Of course. Have you changed your mind about wanting to go to Santa Fe?"

He tried to avoid a direct answer. "Sort of."

"That's all right," Karen said cheerfully. "It's never as important where you go as who you go with. Right?"

"Right," he agreed, taking Karen's arm and leading her outside. When they were alone in the hallway, Longarm said, "I'm afraid that we're going to have to postpone our vacation for a little while."

11

"Oh no!" Karen wailed loud enough to be heard up and down the hallway. "What happened?"

"Senator John Hawk and a federal dispatcher carrying some important land documents were murdered at the senator's ranch in Pagosa Springs. The documents would have made it possible for the state of Colorado to purchase Ute Reservation land for a fraction of its true value, then resell the land to mining and timber logging companies."

"Oh, Custis! What—"

"It'll all be in tomorrow's newspaper. I didn't know about the land deal but I'm sure that it was hushed up by the senator's office for political reasons. It's an outrageous means of taking away even more of the Ute's land. I'm sure that there was a lot of money that stood to be gained by the mining and timbering companies."

"What has that to do with the murders?"

"That's what they want me to go and find out," Longarm told her. "I've been chosen to handle this because I speak a little Ute and am on friendly terms with several of their leaders."

"Who do they believe killed Senator Hawk and the dispatcher?"

"Some poor Ute that Senator Hawk apparently treated like a second son. His name is Liberty. He is missing, of course, as are the documents that the senator was supposed to sign."

Karen sighed. "I almost sympathize with Liberty. I mean, it certainly wasn't right for him to commit murder but . . . well, I guess there is a point when a person or a people simply can take no more raw injustice. Do you think that Senator Hawk stood to profit from this reservation land grab?"

"I'd be willing to bet on it. Billy didn't say that but it stands to reason. Senator Hawk was known as a man who

always took care of himself first . . . and the people of Colorado second."

"I'm ashamed to admit that I voted for the man."

"Don't feel so guilty. Senator Hawk was the slickest politician I've ever seen," Longarm explained. "He was great for backslapping and making public pronouncements that led people to believe he was always fighting in their best interests. But the truth was quite the opposite."

Karen took his hand. "When do you have to leave for Pagosa Springs?"

"I'll be taking the Denver and Rio Grande south to Trinidad tomorrow. It leaves at eight o'clock in the morning."

"In that case," Karen said, "we really don't have much time, do we?"

"No."

"What if I decided I'd like to visit Pagosa Springs and traveled south with you tomorrow morning?"

"Uh-uh," Longarm grunted, shaking his head. "This is going to be a messy case that involves some very evil and clever people. People that would murder anyone to achieve their aims. Karen, I couldn't let you have any part of this trouble."

"But I could just—"

"No," Longarm said emphatically. "It wouldn't work."

Karen looked away. Longarm knew that he'd both disappointed and injured the beautiful young woman's feelings.

"I'll be back in less than a month," he whispered, gently turning her head so that he could see tears in her lovely eyes. "Will you wait for me?"

"What if there are other 'cases' waiting that Mr. Vail and your director decide only you can handle?" She sniffled. "What if this happens all over again with some other terrible crime?"

13

"I'll tell them they can have my badge before I will ever bring tears to your eyes again."

Karen found a handkerchief and dabbed away her tears. "You'd really say that?"

"You have my solemn word on it."

Karen raised up on her toes and kissed his mouth. "You wait out here and I'll go back to my desk and grab some things. We'll leave right now and go do something fun together."

"Like?"

"Like a nice dinner or a show or . . . well, use your imagination, Marshal Long!"

Curtis chuckled and watched her hurry back into her office. He had wined and dined many women but this one really was special.

It was too early for supper or a show so they walked arm in arm to Longarm's apartment so that he could get his packing out of the way. "This won't take but a minute," he said, grabbing some clean shirts, underclothes, socks and pants and stuffing them all into a battered old suitcase.

Karen watched him with obvious amusement. "I can't believe the way you pack! Your shirts will look as if you slept in them for a week."

"Then I'll just wear a coat over them until the wrinkles go away," he reasoned aloud. "And anyway, I'm going to Pagosa Springs. It's a rough little mountain town filled with miners, loggers, and cowboys."

"All the same," Karen replied, "when we finally go on vacation together, I insist on packing for you. Okay?"

"Suit yourself."

Longarm grabbed his straight razor and a few miscellaneous items and shoved them into the suitcase. When he turned around to ask Karen if she would hand him a pair of sturdy walking shoes, he was surprised to see that the woman had quickly removed her blouse and chemise and

14

appeared to be in the process of disrobing completely.

"What's this?" he asked.

"I thought we should go to bed and work up an appetite for supper," she answered, unable to hide a mischievous grin. "But if you are already hungry, maybe it was a bad idea."

"It is a *great* idea," Longarm told her, unbuttoning his own shirt. "So good that I'm surprised that I didn't think of it first."

"Yes, I'm surprised at that myself." Karen finished undressing and Longarm clucked his tongue with admiration as he fumbled at removing his boots. "Damn but you are beautiful!"

"Even better to touch."

"Yeah, I remember," he said, kicking off one boot and nearly tripping over the pants that had fallen to his ankles.

"Having a little trouble, big boy?" She pulled back the bedspread.

"Nothing I can't handle."

Longarm sat down in a chair, tore off his remaining boot and then his pants and stockings. He crossed the hardwood floor of his apartment in three strides and lay down beside the eager young woman. Karen immediately drew him to her bare bosom and began kissing his mouth.

"Let's make this something that neither of us will soon forget," she whispered, voice already hoarse with desire.

"Yeah," he panted, lowering his face to her lush breasts and then sucking on her pink nipples. "A night to remember!"

Karen loved for him to work his tongue around over her nipples and he was more than happy to give her that special pleasure. She moaned and arched her back, hands stroking the hard muscles of his bare buttocks and then searching for his manhood until he turned slightly and her hand closed on his stiffness.

"Oh, Custis, I'm really going to miss this!"

"Me too," he replied, pushing her legs apart and slowly easing his throbbing rod into her warm wetness.

Karen moaned as he began to thrust in and out. "Custis, please, please take your time. We have all evening and all night. Do it to me slow and easy, Custis. Don't come soon even if I ask for it!"

"I'll make you *beg* for it."

"Oh," she breathed, her legs wrapping around his hips and her womanhood hungrily massaging his slick rod. "This is what I really love most about you. Isn't that shameful and wanton?"

"No, it's just honest."

Longarm increased the tempo of his thrusting. He slipped his finger into her honeypot and found the source of Karen's most intense pleasure. When she began to thrash under his expert lovemaking, he slowed things down a little until she really did beg for him to return her to a plane of exquisite ecstasy.

"Come now, big boy! I can't stand this another second!"

"Yes you can," Longarm grunted, lips drawn back from his teeth and eyes glazing with his own pleasure.

In response, Karen began to thrash and strain under his hard, demanding body. Her short but perfect little legs trembled and tugged forcing him even deeper inside. When her mouth flew open, Longarm felt her entire body stiffen then shudder. That's when he finally released his own torrent of hot seed, muffling her cries with his tongue and his mouth.

They had a fine steak dinner with wine, flirting shamelessly in their favorite restaurant. Later, they returned to Longarm's bed and continued their vigorous lovemaking until they fell asleep locked in each other's arms.

When they awakened, it was nearly seven o'clock and

no real time for a good-bye. Karen dressed quickly and gave Longarm a hug. "Please be careful and come back to me soon."

"I will," he promised as she hurried away.

Chapter 3

Longarm's train ticket was in second-class coach, only a little removed from the riffraff that packed into third class. Second class bought you a well-cushioned seat instead of a wooden bench but it was a big step down from the luxury of first class where men like Senator Hawk reigned supreme.

"Ah, Marshal Long!" the short, florid-faced conductor exclaimed. "It's good to see you again so soon."

"Good to see you, Mike. How are the wife and kids?"

"Me boy Sean has just gotten hired on this railroad. Maybe he'll be an engineer someday." O'Connor tore Longarm's ticket in half. "So, Marshal, will you be travelin' far this trip?"

Longarm stifled a yawn. "I plan to sleep all the way down to Trinidad."

"And I don't suppose that your trip has anything to do with the murder of Senator Hawk? Would it, now?"

"So you've heard?"

"Sure. That bloody news was in the paper this morning. Ah, such a terrible thing. And will you be going after that scalawag Indian when you arrive in Pagosa Springs?"

"He might be innocent."

The conductor scoffed at the suggestion. "His name is Liberty. But I wouldn't give him any liberties. No sir! I'd shoot that Indian full of holes. Those savages can't really be taught our civilized ways. One minute they'll be sayin' the rosary, the next shooting an arrow into your back."

"They don't use bows and arrows anymore."

"No matter! The only good Indian is a dead Indian. Eh, marshal?"

Longarm didn't bother to answer. He liked O'Connor but the man was much too free with bigoted opinions that had no basis in fact.

"I knew Senator Hawk well," the conductor continued. "He was a fine gentleman. And to think that he actually befriended the savage who took his life!"

"What was the senator's family like?"

O'Connor clasp his hands together, rolled his blue eyes to the ceiling, and pursed his lips thoughtfully. "The Hawk women were the most beautiful creatures this side of heaven."

"Did you ever talk to the senator's daughter, Della?"

"I'm afraid that I never had that pleasure. You see, they always traveled first class as befit so rich and famous a family."

"Isn't there a son named Jake?"

"And a tall, broad-shouldered fella he is . . . like you, Marshal Long. Black hair and eyes. Handsome man, that young Jake Hawk."

"Did you ever see Liberty?"

"No sir!" O'Connor's expression turned sour. "Marshal, my employer don't allow heathen in first class or second class. But who is to say if the murderin' hostile might have traveled a time or two in third class, though that seems unlikely. If you catch up with that one, my advice would be to shoot first and ask questions later."

Longarm stretched out in his seat. "I'm going to catch up on my sleep now and I don't want to be disturbed."

"I'll see that you are left alone." O'Connor winked and whispered, "And I'll not be forgetting that no one else on the train needs to know that you are a marshal, eh?"

"That's right." Longarm closed his eyes.

Longarm had put in a lot of miles on trains. He liked them, and their rocking motion suited his need for sleep. But he'd only slept for a couple of hours when the conductor roused him into wakefulness. "Marshal, we've got awful trouble in third class! Would you mind helping us out a little?"

"What's wrong?"

"There's a terrible donnybrook going on! I heard passengers screamin' and shoutin' like wild animals."

Longarm knuckled sleep from his eyes. "Why didn't the fella in charge of that coach handle the trouble?"

"Poor old Mr. Riley has been knocked out colder than a cod!"

"I'll see what I can do," Longarm promised.

"I knew that you'd not let us down."

The Irishman looked so distraught that Longarm placed a comforting hand on his shoulder. "You just stay here and calm down. It's bad for your heart to get so excited."

"Yeah, but they're tearing up third class something awful! And poor Mr. Riley—"

"I'll handle it," Longarm assured the man who seemed to be having difficulty breathing. "Sit and calm down. You've a wife and children to consider and it wouldn't do for you to have your heart quit, would it?"

"Me missus needs me wages."

"Then take it easy."

Longarm forcibly pushed O'Connor into his seat. He removed his brown Stetson, checked his .44 Colt revolver, which he wore on his left hip, butt forward. Besides the

Colt, he carried a twin-barreled derringer attached to his watch fob.

"Marshal, be careful and don't let them kill poor old Mr. Riley, who will retire in just six more months."

Longarm hurried down the aisle and exited the rear of his second-class coach. He sucked in a blast of cool Colorado air, drew his Colt, and threw open the door, yelling, "United States Marshal, everyone freeze!"

He needn't have bothered with such a dramatic entrance because the fight was over and battered combatants lay sprawled everywhere. It must have been quite a battle because almost every man in the coach had been bloodied.

"Kindly don't shoot us, Marshal," a big-shouldered bruiser with a handlebar mustache said, spitting out a tooth. "We were just having a little fun. And, as you can see, everyone is now behaving."

Longarm spied Conductor Riley laid out unconscious. Riley had to have been in his seventies, and, from the looks of him, he'd put up a pretty good scrap before someone had knocked him senseless.

"Did you cork the conductor?"

"Naw, I was trying to help him when someone . . . I forgot exactly which fella . . . caught him with a roundhouse right."

Longarm holstered his sidearm and eased Riley onto a bench. "This old man shouldn't have to put up with this kind of thing at his age."

"That's true. He ought to retire."

"Who started the fight?" Longarm asked.

The big man pointed to a groggy miner who had blood trickling out both his ears. "He did."

"Why?"

"He started giving that city Indian over there a bad time. Wouldn't leave him alone and finally went after him with a hunting knife. Cut him on the arm and the Indian pistol-

21

whipped him for his trouble. That's when the fight started."

Longarm hadn't noticed the Indian until now. He was well dressed and wore expensive boots and a cream-colored Stetson hat that would have set him back at least twenty dollars. Longarm judged the Indian to be in his late fifties or early sixties because there were strands of silver in his long, black hair. The Indian seemed not to notice that blood was dripping from his coat sleeve.

"What do you have to say about this?" Longarm asked.

The Indian had been in a trancelike state, but now he raised his head and looked directly at Longarm. "This fight is over. There is no reason why you can't go back to wherever you came from, Marshal."

"I'd better have a good look at that knife wound."

"I don't need . . . or want . . . your help. Besides, it's only a flesh wound."

"It's bleeding heavily and needs to be bandaged. Maybe we can find a doctor in one of the other coaches."

"Don't bother."

Longarm removed his handkerchief. "Use this as a bandage."

The Indian stood up. He was about five-feet-ten-inches tall, barrel-chested with thick shoulders. "Thanks," he said, taking the handkerchief, then removing his coat and rolling up his sleeve.

"That's pretty nasty," Longarm observed. "It ought to be looked at by a doctor and stitched."

"I'll go right on living."

Longarm frowned because the Indian wasn't being the least bit cooperative. Not that this should be surprising. The man had probably been taunted and tormented right up to the breaking point. The fact that he'd been able to defend himself so ably without killing his attacker was impressive. Longarm asked, "What is your name?"

"Jerome Ochoa."

"Mine is Custis Long, and I think it would be a good idea if you joined me in the second-class coach."

"Don't you know that Indians aren't allowed in first or second class?"

"That's a rule that needs to be broken."

"Don't bother. I can take care of myself, Marshal."

"I'm sure you can, but join me anyway. That's an order . . . not a request."

Jerome headed up the aisle. When they entered the second-class coach, they ran smack into Conductor O'Connor who bristled, "Marshal, you know better than to bring him up here with the respectable folks."

"Mr. Ochoa isn't welcome back there in third class."

"Well he ain't welcome here either!"

"The seat next to mine is empty. I'll take full responsibility."

"Marshal, company rules say no savages are allowed in second class!"

"Get out of my way, O'Connor," Longarm bristled. "Or better yet, go see if you can help your friend Mr. Riley."

"The company says I can't leave my coach."

"Move or I'll knock you aside!"

O'Connor muttered his displeasure but did as he was told. Longarm escorted Ochoa up the aisle to his seat. "Stay put."

Longarm hurried back to the third-class coach, and bursting inside, shouted, "If there is any more trouble, I'll have you *all* thrown off this train!"

"What'd you do with that dirty damn Injun'," the troublemaker who had pulled his hunting knife demanded. "I ain't even halfways finished with him yet!"

Longarm grabbed the miner and propelled him up the aisle. When they exited the coach, he noted that the train was laboring up a steep grade. "This is where you get off, Buster!"

Longarm tossed him into the air then watched with satisfaction as the man rolled end over end until he smacked up against a boulder. Satisfied, Longarm returned to his seat. "Well, that miner one won't be causing us any more trouble."

A faint smile raised the corners of the Indian's mouth. "You heap tough federal marshal."

"Tough enough," Longarm answered. "Now, do you want to tell me who you *really* are?"

"Just another ignorant savage."

"Bullshit!" Longarm snapped. "You handled that miner like a professional, although you did allow him to cut you pretty good."

"I'm not as young and as quick as I once was."

"Are you a lawman?"

"Not anymore."

"Don't speak with forked tongue," Longarm warned.

"I'm a Navajo," Ochoa confessed, dropping his mockery. "I was a scout for the army and later, I was the chief of police on the Navajo Reservation."

"So what are you doing on this train?"

"I was in Denver on business. I heard about the murder of Senator Hawk and the federal dispatcher as I was boarding this train."

"And now you are heading back to Arizona?"

"I might hold over awhile in Pagosa Springs."

"Why?"

"Why not?" Ochoa answered. "From what I have heard and read, Liberty has already been tried and found guilty in the public's opinion. If he isn't dead, the kid might need a friendly Indian in his corner."

"You could step into something way over your head."

"I've got nothing better to do than to try and save some poor Indian kid's life." Ochoa frowned. "So what is your

24

role to be in this investigation? Or have you already decided that Liberty is guilty?"

"Don't insult me," Longarm growled. "If the kid is guilty, he'll probably hang. If he's not guilty, I'll find that out too."

"And if he's already been lynched?"

"Then I'll find out who lynched him and they'll be arrested and brought to trial for murder."

"You make it sound pretty cut and dried."

"It isn't," Longarm said. "If you wore a badge then you know that much."

"I still have my badge and the capacity given to me by the Navajo people to arrest the guilty and bring them to face justice."

To prove his words, Jerome reached inside his coat and extracted his badge. Longarm studied it for a second noting with wry amusement that Jerome's title was "BIG CHIEF."

"Nice badge, but this isn't the Navajo Reservation, and that piece of metal doesn't get you anything in the great state of Colorado."

Ochoa slipped the badge back into his pocket. "Before you pitched that sonofabitch off the train, did you happen to relieve him of his wallet and valuables?"

"No."

"You should have because he cost me the price of a good suit coat and doctor's visit."

"I'll pay those expenses."

"Do that and you'll be beholden to me."

Longarm glanced sideways at him. "How do you figure?"

"Old Navajo rule says that when a man does a favor for another man, he is in his debt."

"Seems like it ought to be the other way around."

"Yeah, but the rule is the rule."

"Are you going to be a thorn in my side when we get to Pagosa Springs?"

"Probably. But I might save your hide if someone takes a dislike to you asking questions."

"Look. I can handle this."

"I don't know that for sure and . . . even if I did, I'd still insist on investigating. The white man has screwed the red man too many times to take anything for granted. That's why I'm going to Pagosa."

"Yeah, Chief, but there's a big difference between us."

"I know. You're younger and taller, but I'm much handsomer."

Longarm cracked up. "Be serious."

"Okay. You're also a white man and I'm just an Injun."

Longarm's smile faded. "I'm a *federal* marshal. You're a tribal officer of the law with no authority off the Navajo Reservation."

"You already said that."

"Yeah, but I don't have the feeling you got it the first time around."

"I'll behave," Ochoa promised.

Longarm looked straight into the man's dark eyes. "I think that you'll do whatever you please and the consequences be damned."

Ochoa frowned. "For a man who only met me five minutes ago, you seem to be making a lot of assumptions about what I will or will not do. I'm curious, Marshal Long, do all white lawmen jump to such quick and easy conclusions? Or is it the fact that I'm an Indian so you just sort of figure us all the same? You know, one color skin, one uniform mentality?"

"Don't play that game with me," Longarm warned. "I may not be as long in the tooth as you are, but I've made it my business to read men of *every* color. You're tough or you'd be dead. You're smart and confident or you wouldn't have the money to buy that suit and the nerve to ride in third class. But you've also got a chip the size of a barn

26

door on your shoulder. *That* is what concerns me, Big Chief Ochoa. To tell you the truth, I think you're sort of an arrogant sonofabitch."

"How interesting. Anything else you want to tell me about myself?"

"Just that I've met Indian police before and so I have some idea of how you think and operate. The difference between us is that I have to follow more clearly defined rules of law. You, on the other hand, are often *the* law on your reservation. So you have a tendency to be judge, jury, and even executioner."

"Sometimes justice needs to be swift and simple, Marshal." Ochoa's voice hardened. "We've both seen how the guilty often evade justice. They get a smart, expensive lawyer. Or they intimidate the witness who then refuses to testify. Or they *murder* the witness and destroy the evidence. Am I wrong?"

"Not at all."

"On the Navajo Reservation, we sometimes do serve as judge and executioner. But we do so with great respect for life, and I have never in all my years as an officer, ever taken the life of an innocent man."

"I believe you," Longarm said. "But I also hold to what I said before and that is that I have the feeling you might decide to take the law into your own hands when we reach Pagosa Springs . . . if you see fit. And, if you did that, then I'd have to arrest you."

"That would be very bad," Ochoa said, managing a thin smile.

"Look, Chief, this case is going to be plenty difficult enough without us working at cross purposes. So why don't we just stop jousting and come to a fair and friendly agreement?"

"I'm listening."

"First, I'm the one with the authority . . . not you. There-

fore, you will stay the hell out of this unless asked."

"That's it?" Ochoa asked.

"Yep."

"I don't like your idea of an agreement, Marshal. So I'll suggest a better one. You leave me alone unless I break the law. In return, I'll stay out of the thick of things, but you must keep me up to date on anything that has to do with Liberty. Where he is, what evidence they have against him. That sort of thing."

Longarm turned his head and gazed out the window while giving Ochoa's words careful thought. He didn't have to do a thing for this man. Not one damned thing. On the other hand, Big Chief wasn't just going to disappear. If he did, it would be to find the fugitive Ute before he was lynched. And so, Longarm could either agree to the Navajo's terms, or create a thorn in his side.

"All right," Longarm agreed. "I'll keep you up to date on everything in return for you keeping your distance."

"Agreed."

They shook hands.

"Pueblo is coming up," Longarm said. "There will be a doctor there that can suture that arm."

Ochoa just shrugged. "Marshal, I've already told you that I'm not getting off the train until it reaches Trinidad. Then, I'm headed straight for Pagosa Springs. Would you like to come along with me or, given the mood of your people, would that be a major risk and an inconvenience?"

"I can live with it," Longarm replied. "How did you plan to get from Trinidad to Pagosa?"

"Stagecoach?"

"I don't think there is one."

Ochoa shrugged. "Then we buy horses."

"Beats walking."

The Navajo grinned. "This old Indian hates walking. All right, we buy horses."

"Or rent them," Longarm said.

"I own what I ride," Ochoa replied. "And I always carry a clean bill of sale."

"Then that's what we'll do," Longarm agreed, thinking that this trip was going to be even more of a challenge than he'd expected.

Chapter 4

Trinidad, Colorado, had begun as a supply center for the westward trail and was now firmly established not only as an important southwestern railhead but also as a coal mining and ranching town. Also, farmers as well as cattle and sheep ranchers for hundreds of miles south and east depended on the stockyards to buy and load their livestock for transport to Denver. And finally, Trinidad was the hub of a logging industry as well as a jumping off place for miners entering the southern gold fields. You could buy about anything in Trinidad, but the costs were higher than in Denver while the selection and quality were generally not as good.

Longarm had been through the town many times, and as he and Chief Ochoa stepped down from the train he could see that Trinidad was bustling with activity. He turned to the conductor and said, "Looks to have grown by at least a few hundred every time I pass through."

"Oh, she's growing and can thank The Denver and Rio Grande."

"Mike, I wish you a quiet and uneventful return to Den-

ver. I talked to Riley a few minutes ago and he seems to have made a complete recovery."

"Thanks be to God. I wouldn't work the third-class coach for the life of me," O'Connor confided. "And Marshal, I'm sorry about being so stiff-backed over that Indian. I was wrong about him because he behaved like a white gentleman."

Longarm opened his mouth to speak, then decided not to waste his words. "Take care," he said, grabbing his bag and heading after Ochoa who was already half a block ahead and marching off to where Longarm had no idea.

He hurried after the Navajo and, because his legs were far longer, caught up with him two blocks later. "Slow down! What's your big hurry?"

"I don't like this town. I had trouble here about eight years ago. The men who attacked me are probably all gone or dead by now. I killed two and left a third hanging on for his life . . . but you never know. The local marshal was not interested in the facts of the situation so I had to light out on the run."

"Let's hope he's gone."

"Yes, let's do," Ochoa agreed. "And the sooner we buy a couple horses and our outfits and leave, the happier I'll be. I seem to remember that the liveries were up at the end of this street."

"Maybe we ought to buy our supplies first."

"No," Ochoa said. "If the horse dealer realizes we have to have animals that will cross the Rockies, he'll hold us up for too high a price. Let's just act like we are going to stick around these parts and are either interested in renting a buggy or a couple of swaybacked nags."

Longarm wasn't sure he agreed. "I'm not going to lie to the man about being a federal officer of the law."

"Then why don't you go into that general store and buy

31

us blankets, rain slickers, ammunition, and food. I'll pick out the horses and start dickering."

"Now jest a minute," Longarm said. "Maybe I'd like to pick out my own damned horse."

"Trust me, when it comes to judging horseflesh, you can't beat the Navajo. I'll make the deal but hold off until you arrive to make payment."

"But just for *my* horse, saddle, and outfit. I'm not paying your way, Chief."

"Of course you're not!" Ochoa looked offended. "Marshal, I thought it was understood that the United States Government is paying our way."

"What!"

"You heard me."

"Big Chief, let's get something straight. Sure, I've got travel funds—"

"Given to you by the government."

"Yeah, to *me*. Not you!"

The distinguished Navajo smiled patiently, then replied, "Marshal Long, you need to understand that I've been paid by your government most of my life, in one form or manner or the other. I'm going to back you up as a voluntary assistant. Why are you making such a big deal over this matter of a few federal dollars?"

Before Longarm could answer, Ochoa demanded, "How much money do you make a month?"

"Huh?"

"What's your monthly pay?"

"What business is it of yours?" Longarm snapped.

"As Chief of Police of the entire Navajo Reservation, I finally made fifty-seven dollars a month. I'll bet you make more than that right now. Don't you!"

"Maybe I do . . . and maybe I don't," Longarm answered, getting more exasperated by the moment. "But that is neither here nor there."

"A man of your age with your experience working for the Navajo Reservation Police doesn't make but about thirty dollars a month. Now what kind of fairness is that when you make twice as much?"

"Look, I can't help that your people are underpaid."

"Underpaid!" Ochoa rolled his eyes and made a sour face. "That's quite an understatement. And what are we talking about here but you putting up a few extra bucks so that I can ride with you over to Pagosa Springs? I'd think that, given the mess we are about to step in . . . you'd want to hire me on your *own* hook. Marshal Long, one thing I've learned in this life is that being penny wise and pound foolish is one of the biggest mistakes you can commit in any professional arrangement."

"I didn't ask for your help . . . in fact, I asked not to have it! And I never paid anybody out of my own pocket in my life. I can take care of the Hawk murder investigation just fine without you."

"You might jolly well *think* you can, but what if you can't? Have you ever heard of the Black Widow?"

"As a matter of fact, I have."

"Then you ought to know that she alone could settle your hash . . . not to mention her murderous son or daughter."

Longarm took a deep breath. "I've been fully briefed on the whole family."

"Then you should know that you'll need all the help you can get when we arrive at Pagosa Springs."

"Ochoa, I just can't figure you out. You're dressed like a wealthy cattleman and now you're trying to weasel funds outta me."

"I'm not asking for cash, just supply me with my needs."

"No, dammit!" Longarm shouted. "I'll not pay one thin dime of your bill. You either pay your own freight . . . or get lost! Is that understood?"

"Perfectly." The former Chief of the Navajo Police didn't

33

seem upset or angry. But he added, "The day will come, Marshal Long, when you will wind up paying far more for my services than the price of a nag and a few pitiful supplies. Yes, the day will come when you will be willing to pay for far, far more than I have just asked."

"Hell will freeze over first."

The Navajo turned and started to leave, then halted and slowly pivoted around on his boot heel. "I can't do it."

"Can't do what?" Longarm asked suspiciously.

"I can't leave you to your own foolishness. You'll need me and, later on, you'll gladly pay me. I have no room in my heart for anger or retribution for your present foolish and unkind words."

"They weren't—"

"So I'm going to travel to Pagosa Springs and remain in the background as we previously agreed. When the time comes for me to act in your behalf and that of the Ute boy, Liberty, then you will be more than willing to offer me a just compensation."

"I don't believe what I'm hearing."

Ochoa shrugged his powerful shoulders and raised his palms to the sky. "I won't gloat when you beg me to help. Indians don't gloat like whites."

"Get out of here."

"I'll find us a good deal on the horses. I'll pay for my own."

"You bet you will," Longarm said. "And you'll pay me for the grub and supplies that you'll use on the way over to Pagosa Springs."

"Of course, but I expect a very profitable return on my current investment."

Before Longarm could think of a retort, Ochoa turned and headed up the street looking for a couple of horses to buy. Longarm stomped off in the opposite direction feeling exasperated. "Never met anyone that brassy. He's going to

drive me crazy before we reach Pagosa Springs."

And yet, even before he came to the general store, Longarm had to admit that there was something kinda special about Big Chief Ochoa. The Navajo didn't carry a gun that was visible, but Longarm would bet anything that he had at least a couple of them hidden on his person and that the ex-Navajo Chief of Police could use them well and in a hurry. He was probably an excellent tracker. If the Ute kid was on the run, Ochoa might be invaluable.

"But I'll pay him nothing," Longarm muttered as he entered the general store. "Not till hell freezes over."

It took Longarm about half an hour to select the purchases that he and Ochoa would need for their difficult trek over the imposing Continental Divide. He asked the stoic and unsmiling storekeeper, "How far and how long will it take us to ride over to Pagosa Springs?"

"As the crow flies, it's only about a hundred and fifty miles. But even this far south you'll still have to ride over very high passes."

"About ten thousand feet in elevation?"

"Higher. You'll need good horseflesh under your saddle blankets and it'll get cold at night so you'd best buy an extra heavy woolen blanket or two which I just happen to have on a special sale."

"How much?"

"Ten dollars each."

"Ten dollars for *one* lousy blanket?"

"They're not lousy. They're made of hand woven Navajo wool . . . there's nothing finer or warmer. And you'll need rain slickers . . . that's for certain. If you get wet and chilled up in that high country you'll get pneumonia and die of a fever. I seen it happen aplenty."

Longarm was at the man's mercy. He knew that everything in Trinidad was high priced and he cussed himself for not buying what he'd needed before leaving Denver. He

could have saved the government at least twenty or thirty dollars.

"How much does my bill add up to?" Longarm asked when the supplies were stacked up high on the counter.

The merchant tallied the sum using a stub pencil and writing pad. He must have added the column up at least three times, "Grand total is just one-ninety-eight-sixty-three. Though I really do think you ought to stock up on a little more food. The high mountains give a man a ferocious appetite. And you didn't buy a rope or halter for your animal or any oats for your horses. Animals can't find enough grass up there to meet the demands on their bodies. A horse needs grain to climb those mountains and I just happen to have horse oats on sale. A bag will only run you—"

"Two hundred dollars," Longarm interrupted with a growl. "And you are going to throw in fifty pounds of oats, two new halters, and lead ropes for free."

The merchant was a tall, thin man with a hangdog expression perfectly suited for gaining the upper hand in financial negotiations. "I couldn't possibly do something like that!"

"I am a federal marshal and I am expecting a government discount."

"What?"

"You heard me. Longarm flashed his badge in the man's homely face. "Mister, at the rates you charge for store merchandise, I ought to call you Jesse James and arrest you for robbery! Now get the damned grain and I'll be back to pay for everything pretty quick. And you had better not have taken one thing from this pile or I *will* have you arrested!"

"Don't be ridiculous, Marshal. Just because you are accustomed to dealing with thieves and worse doesn't give you the right to be insulting to us honest, hard-working folks."

Longarm bit back a caustic reply and headed up the

street. He didn't really trust the Navajo and he wanted to be on hand when their mounts were chosen and their prices negotiated.

"Hey, Marshal! Look what I bought for us!"

Custis spun around and saw Big Chief Ochoa leading two saddled horses in his direction. One was a very fine-looking bay mare with four white stockings and a blaze down its forehead. The animal showed both spirit and breeding. But the gelding was a disaster! At least sixteen hands tall, with a jug head, crooked legs, pencil-thin neck and prominent hips, the strawberry roan ought to have been put out of its misery at birth.

Longarm's mouth formed a hard line of disapproval, and when they met, he yelled, "Chief, if you think I'm buying that jug-headed offspring of a camel and a mule, you've got another thing coming!"

"But Marshal Long," Ochoa said, faking shock and distress, "I'm sure that you would prefer the gelding to the mare. I've ridden both and the gelding has by far the easier gait. It's also a more trustworthy and sensible animal and the seller told me that it possessed incredible stamina. He said it was a real Rocky Mountain trail horse that would never let you down."

"No thanks."

"But—"

"You can take that ugly bastard back to the guy who sold him to you for a refund, which I'm sure you won't get, or maybe you'll get lucky and sell him to a blind man. I don't care what you do with that horse, but I'm not buying him."

"But I paid seventy dollars for this roan . . . with this good saddle, blanket, and bridle included as part of the deal!"

"Then you *ride* him to Pagosa Springs!" Longarm tore

the reins attached to the pretty bay mare from Ochoa's fist. "How much did this horse cost me?"

"Fifty-five dollars with saddle, blanket, and bridle."

Longarm's jaw dropped. "Are you telling me that you paid *more* for that jug-head roan gelding than you did for this mare!"

"Sure. He's a far better trail horse. He's an animal with more sense, strength, and stamina."

Longarm laughed out loud. "Boy did you get fleeced on that big, ugly bastard! Some Navajo judge of horseflesh you are!"

"How much were the supplies?"

"A hundred each. And so, subtracting what you paid for this mare and her outfit, that means you still owe me forty-five dollars."

"Wait a minute! I had to drive quite a bargain to get that mare for fifty-five. The man started out asking eighty. So that means you owe me!"

Longarm groaned. "Look," he said, "pay me forty dollars and we're square."

"Twenty dollars because I also got an exceptional deal on your saddle."

"I'm beginning to hate you," Longarm said, taking the twenty that had suddenly appeared in the Navajo's hand. "I really am."

"That will change," Ochoa promised. "Let's get our supplies and get out of Trinidad before our luck runs out."

" 'Luck'? What luck? I've really gotten skinned on this horse deal and I couldn't do much better on our traveling supplies."

"What a shame. You should have let me do the bargaining at the mercantile. I'm sure that I could have done much better."

Longarm mounted the mare seeing no need to lead it all the way back to the general store. But no sooner was his

right leg swinging over the cantle than the horse commenced to bucking like a demon. Longarm never even managed to get his seat and set his stirrups before he was flying over the mare's head and landing hard in the middle of the street.

Ochoa caught the mare's reins and led her back to Longarm saying, "I forgot to say that this mare bucks a little at first. I'd have thought a federal marshal of your size and experience would be able to handle her."

"Gawdammit," Longarm hissed. "Why'd you buy a horse that bucks!"

"I bought her for myself. I thought that you'd want the gelding being as how you are a larger man and he is a far larger horse."

"Let me give this mare another try!" Longarm said, struggling to his feet and brushing off his pants.

This time he did manage to get both boots in the stirrup before the bay mare exploded into the air. Longarm tried to drag her head up from between her knees but he was a little late and the mare got to bucking so hard he lost his stirrups as well as his balance and went tumbling. He struck the ground and smashed up against a water trough, fighting to regain his breath.

Rolling up to his hands and knees, he watched the Navajo catch up the mare, swing onto her back and ride her around so that she acted just as gentle as a kid's pony.

"She must not like you," Ochoa called. "I think that she feels you are too big and heavy a man to be carried over those mountains."

"Bull! I don't outweigh you by more than thirty pounds!"

"But you *look* a lot heavier. And I think you are very heavy-handed."

Ochoa began to rein the mare around in figure-eights, then he dismounted and remounted twice while she stood

as calm as a diary cow. "Nothing wrong with this pretty gal . . . if she takes a shine to you."

"She will soon enough!"

Ochoa pointed out several bystanders who were chortling and obviously enjoying Longarm's sorry predicament. "Marshal, wouldn't it be better to tackle this little problem you and the mare have later when we don't have an audience? I've already adjusted the gelding's stirrups for the length of your legs."

Longarm stood up and a sharp pain deep in his backside brought a gasp to his lips. He did not think he was up to being bucked off a third time. "All right," he hissed, limping over to take the jug-head's reins. "Let's get our gear and just leave!"

"Wise decision," Big Chief Ochoa said with a tolerant smile.

Chapter 5

They rode right up into the high mountains and Longarm soon realized that he really did have the stronger of the two horses. His jug-headed strawberry roan stuck its long, skinny neck straight out like a mallard in flight and attacked the steep grades with a vengeance that left Ochoa and the pretty bay mare far behind. The Navajo kept shouting at him to slow the killing pace, but the roan had the bit in its teeth and fire in its eyes.

"This thing doesn't want to slow down!" Longarm yelled over his shoulder.

"You have to slow down or this mare is going to die!" the Indian cried.

Longarm had to really bear down on the reins in order to make the gelding ease off on its horrendous pace. And when they finally topped the first of what would prove to be many passes, he jumped off the big horse and discovered that it had hardly broken a sweat and its breathing was barely labored.

"Well Ugly, I guess you've made a believer of me," he said. "You've more heart and stamina than any horse I ever rode."

The animal affectionately knocked him backward with its huge head, then jerked the reins out of Longarm's fist and started devouring the local vegetation while they waited for Ochoa and his mare to finally catch up.

"This isn't going to work," the Navajo complained as he dismounted his heavily lathered and breathing mount. "I've never killed a horse yet and I'll not kill this one trying to keep up with that roan."

"What do you suggest?" Longarm asked. "Do you want me to tie a rope from your saddle horn to mine so that we drag your pretty mare over the Rockies?"

"That might be the only answer," the Indian answered a little sullenly.

They let the mare blow for about fifteen minutes, and when her sweaty flanks had stopped heaving, they continued upward along a rutted freight road that seemed to Longarm to be impossible for any wagon to ascend. But soon enough, they saw a big logging wagon come skidding around a corner with the driver shouting at a span of six mules and leaning hard on the brake.

"Outta my way you stupid sonsabitches!" he screamed. "I can't stop!"

Longarm and Ochoa had to really scramble to get off the road and avoid being killed. This seemed to thoroughly anger Ugly who took a hunk of hide off the back of one of the passing mules with a single bite from his long yellow teeth. The mule bawled in pain and the driver tried to grab his whip and lay it on the strawberry roan, but he wasn't quick enough to get the job done so he applied a vile cussing instead.

"I hope all the drivers aren't that ill-tempered," Longarm remarked as they passed by.

"If you had to drive a team and a freight wagon up and down this goat trail for a living I expect you'd have the same poor attitude," was Ochoa's answer.

42

They didn't see anyone else on the road until late that afternoon when they came upon a pair of rough-looking prospectors headed down the mountains to Trinidad. The prospectors blocked the road and the bigger of them shouted, "We could use some food! We ain't et in two days!"

"Marshal, they look awful thin," Ochoa said. "Mean, too. Maybe we ought to give them a little sourdough bread or something."

"Not me," Longarm said. "They can buy their own food."

"Come on! Just a can of peaches or beans."

"Not at two dollars a can!" Longarm gave Ugly his head and the roan nearly trampled the pair before they could jump aside.

"Cheap bastards!"

"Deadbeats!" Longarm yelled back.

One of the miners had a gun. He yanked it out of his pants and fired twice, causing Ugly to start bucking. Longarm managed to grab the saddle horn and stay in his seat, but it was a close call, and when he got Ugly under control, he drew his own pistol and went charging back down the road after the prospectors. When they scattered into the trees, he decided that they weren't worth arresting so he galloped back up to rejoin Ochoa.

"Sometimes it's better to be generous than stingy," the Navajo said in a voice dripping with reproach.

"They'd have just wanted more and more and probably would have tried to get the drop on us and take everything we had," Longarm replied. "I consider myself a fair judge of men and that was a bad bunch."

"I'd have thrown 'em a few tins of food and kept moving."

"Then next time, you're buying the food," Longarm snapped.

43

They rode in silence until nearly dark when they came upon a small mountain mining camp called Gold Gulch. It wasn't much, but there was a hotel and a restaurant, which Ochoa eyed hopefully.

"I think we ought to put up here and get a room and a hot meal," the Navajo suggested.

"Not me," Longarm said. "We've got blankets and food. Let's ride on through town and find a place to camp for the night."

"I dunno," Ochoa replied, looking up at the clouds. "I feel a rainstorm coming in on us. I think we'll get drenched tonight. Might be better to just bite the bullet and pay for a good room and a soft bed."

"You go right ahead and do that," Longarm told the Indian. "I'm riding on and not spending another unnecessary cent until we get to Pagosa Springs."

"Well, what about all those rain clouds!" Ochoa pointed to the north. "Look like thunderheads to me."

"Don't look anything to worry about from where I'm setting," Longarm told the man. "But you do what you want."

"If I got a room, you'd be long gone. You know that roan won't hold back and wait for this mare. And I doubt you'd hang around late in the morning and wait for me either."

"You got that right."

"Then I guess I got no choice but to stick with you," the Navajo said, looking pretty unhappy. "But dammit, I just don't know why we have to be so stingy and in such a big hurry."

Longarm gave him a hard look. "I'd think that you'd be just as anxious as myself to get to Pagosa Springs, seeing as you are the one that is interested in saving that Ute kid named Liberty."

"Well, I am!" Ochoa looked offended. "But I expect

44

they've already captured and lynched him. A good week or ten days will have passed since the murder of Senator Hawk and that other fella. That's a long time to arrive after the scene of a crime and expect any of the evidence or participants to still be hanging around just waiting to be either arrested or questioned."

"Yes, it is," Longarm agreed as they rode through the little mining settlement without even stopping for a beer. "So what are you going to do to help me, if anything?"

"I know some people in Pagosa," Ochoa admitted. "In fact, I know *lots* of people that live around there. I used to go to that area to do some hunting and fishing when I had the urge to smell the pines."

"It's a little far from the Navajo Reservation, isn't it?"

"I liked to travel whenever I had the chance. I'd always stop in and pay my respects to the local marshals and constables, explaining my business. I found that, even though I was an Indian, the fact that I was also a lawman like themselves counted the most. I was often invited to stay in their homes with their families for an evening or two, and we'd talk about our profession."

"That's nice."

"It *was* nice," Ochoa said with a smile. "Most white lawmen ordinarily wouldn't give an Indian the time of day. But being as I was the Chief of Police . . . well, it gave me some respect in their eyes. And they were always interested in reservation law and how I handled things among my people. And, of course, I listened and learned from them as well."

"You're a real generous and friendly fella," Longarm said. "I can see that. I can also see that you like to spend someone else's money—or the government's—a whole lot more than you like to spend your own."

"Makes sense, doesn't it?"

"From your point of view, it does."

"From the *Indian* point of view, it does as well," Ochoa explained. "You see, that's the difference between whites and The People. We believe that there is more value in sharing our goods and wealth than in hoarding and accumulating it. The most important among us are often the poorest. That can almost never be said for the whites."

"I'm not entirely sure I buy that," Longarm replied. "I've seen plenty of Indians who made a lifelong effort at trying to accumulate as many cattle, sheep, or horses as possible. I've met Indian ranchers down in Texas and up in Wyoming and they sure watch the dollar trying to stay afloat . . . just like their white counterparts."

"Then they are acting more like whites than Indians," Ochoa said. "Sharing is the real Indian way."

"For a fact?"

"Absolutely."

"If that's how you really feel, then why don't you give the next poor prospector we meet a few dollars. Give *all* the poor prospectors you meet a few dollars."

"Then I'd be poor like them and unable to assist anymore."

Longarm glanced at Ochoa and shook his head. "You know what I think?"

"What?"

"I think you just like to create hot air. To argue for the sheer sake of argument. I believe that you will say damn near anything just to have something to yap about whether you care about it or not. That's what I think."

Ochoa laughed. "Marshal, you have really misunderstood this poor Indian!"

Longarm scoffed. "You're not poor! Be honest. You're worth quite a bit of money."

Ochoa's grin faded. "What makes you think so?"

"The hat, boots, clothes. Your travel to Denver. When I first saw you in that third-class coach dressed the way you

46

were, I thought you looked about as out of place as a duck in a tree. I think you play this poor Indian role to the hilt and get a kick out of trying to make the white man pay more than his share even though you could probably buy and sell him on a whim."

"What a colossal imagination you have, Marshal! Why, if I could make up things like you, I'd be writing those dime novels that are selling so well to the easterners! Yep, I'd be writing a whole bunch of lies and needing a wheelbarrow to haul all my money to the bank!"

Longarm wasn't buying a thing this Indian said anymore. Some men were chronic liars and he was beginning to think Jerome Ochoa was one of them. Might be he wasn't even a Navajo but instead a scheming Ute. It made Longarm think that Ochoa could not be entirely trusted.

"I think we ought to seek some immediate shelter," Ochoa said when he heard the distant boom of thunder. "Or, better yet, return to that last settlement and get a room. I tell you, it's going to rain hard!"

"We've got slickers."

"Yeah, but—"

"You sure are nervous about the weather for an Indian," Longarm complained. "I'm beginning to think you were raised soft."

"I just don't want to get soaked and sleep wet and cold all night. I'm older than you and it affects my rheumatism."

"You've got rheumatism?"

"That's right. And I promise you, Marshal, you'll get it too if you don't take better care of yourself."

"Look," Longarm said as they topped a little hill and looked down into a valley. "That's a mining camp up the road."

"And take a look at the sky. If you don't think that isn't a thunderstorm heading our way, you'd best think twice."

As if to confirm the Navajo's judgment, a jagged bolt of

47

lightning forked down from the heavens and it was followed an instant later by a boom of thunder. Longarm had to admit that the clouds were really massing just to the north.

"Well, Marshal? Are you going to let the government get us a room in this camp, or are you going to be stubborn and insist we brave the elements? You know, we aren't going to do much damn good if we arrive in Pagosa Springs on our deathbeds with pneumonia."

"All right," Longarm relented, feeling a gust of cold, damp air. "Let's see what is available. Maybe we can sleep with our horses in a livery for less than a dollar."

"The livery!"

Longarm chuckled as he put the roan into a gallop. It had a long, easy stride and could cover ground with amazing quickness. The pretty bay mare, however, must have been a harder riding animal because when Longarm glanced back over his shoulder, he saw that the Indian was bouncing pretty high.

The mining settlement was called Vulture Creek and it was a pretty sorry affair. There was a livery, but the ragged and unsavory-looking man who ran the place said that he had no indoor stalls and that the horses would have to be penned along with quite a few head of livestock.

"I take no responsibility for your stock," he warned, chewing on a stem of dry grass. "Your horses will probably get the shit kicked out 'em tonight by some of the mules or the bigger animals. Might turn up lame or even worse."

"Then what the hell do we need you for?" Longarm growled as the first cold drops of rain began to pelt them. "We might as well tie our horses under a tree somewhere and save ourselves some money."

"Well," the liveryman drawled, pulling up his baggy overalls and kicking the dirt with the toe of his shoe, "you

could do that all right. But you'd have to leave 'em out back and they could get stolen."

"How about we tie them right here to the outside of this pen?" Ochoa suggested.

"Oh no," the liveryman protested, vigorously shaking his head back and forth.

"Well, why not?" Longarm demanded.

"Because they get to fightin' between the poles and then one of 'em rears back and takes my whole pen down, that's why not. No, either tie 'em up out in the forest and take your chances of 'em gettin' stolen, or pen 'em and take your chances they get kicked, bit, and beat to shit."

It was all that Longarm could do not to grab the skinny, filthy fool and throttle him by the neck. But Ochoa intervened. "We'll pen them. But I insist we keep our saddles and outfits in the barn where they'll stay dry."

"Cost you extra and I ain't takin' no responsibility for your gear. No sir! Thieves are thicker'n ticks on a hound hereabouts. I was you, I'd get a hotel room and carry all my stuff up to it and watch over it good."

"Pay the man," Ochoa said to Longarm, then, twisting back around to the liveryman added, "but we expect you to grain these horses well."

"Cost you extra."

"Fine!" Longarm was getting so exasperated he had to walk away. Grabbing up his saddle and gear, he started up the street to the town's only hotel. It started to rain harder and he hoped that the place had a room to rent.

"Hold up, dammit!" Ochoa cried, dragging his own saddle and outfit. "I'm not as young and strong as you are."

Longarm didn't break stride but bulled into the little hotel. It had a big cast-iron stove in the lobby and the clerk behind the counter didn't even glance up from his newspaper when Longarm marched over and dropped his wet gear.

"Mister, I'm sorry to interrupt your reading, but do you have a room to rent tonight?"

"I might," the clerk muttered around a big wad of chewing tobacco.

Longarm pounded his fist on the counter so hard that the guest book flew up into the air. "Make a damned decision!"

Now he had the man's full attention. Longarm spun the guest registration book around and started to sign in, but the clerk said with unconcealed satisfaction, "Got a room, but it's gonna cost you two dollars."

"What!"

"It's the Presidential Suite."

Longarm almost burst out into derisive laughter. He looked around at the shabbiness of the establishment and said, "President of *what*?"

"Don't matter. It's about three feet longer and four wider than the other rooms so we rent it for more. Take it . . . or leave it. I don't care because I don't own the place."

"That's obvious. Does it have two beds, or one?"

"Two . . . with plenty of blankets."

"We'll take it," Ochoa said, slogging in behind and dropping his already sopping wet saddle. "Just pay this good man, Marshal."

Longarm felt the hotel shiver as the storm really began to intensify. That made him feel a little more agreeable. Ochoa had been right, it would have been a miserable night camping out in the woods.

"Presidential Suite is up the stairs, first door on your right."

"Where can we get some hot food . . . lots and lots of it?" Ochoa asked gazing over at the stove and a rough-looking bunch that huddled close to it for warmth. "I'm afraid I didn't see a cafe or restaurant."

"Saloon next door serves food as well as drinks. Ain't cheap, though. Everything up here has to be freighted in,

you see. It's hard and expensive. The stew is good, but you better avoid the chili or you'll be spending a lot of time on the chamber pot tonight."

"What about a steak?"

"Cost you almost as much as the whole cow were you eating in Denver."

Longarm lugged his gear upstairs. The Presidential Suite wasn't much more than two beds and a washstand, but it did have an original oil painting on the wall. The painting was of one of the past American presidents but of such poor quality that Longarm couldn't decide if it was President Grant . . . or Abraham Lincoln. He just knew it wasn't old George Washington because the figure had black hair and a beard instead of a white wig.

"Not bad, huh?" Ochoa said, pushing into the room and dropping his saddle and gear in the middle of the floor. "Custis, we *really* got lucky."

"Yeah," Longarm said without enthusiasm. "But there are no locks on the door."

"So?" Ochoa asked. "We got guns don't we? And you'll notice that I announced you were a marshal in a rather loud voice down below. That really grabbed their attention in a hurry. I said it to discourage anyone from breaking in here and trying to steal from us while we are out filling our bellies."

"I see."

"Ready to eat?"

Longarm was famished. "Okay. Let's go."

He tromped back on down the stairs and, as they passed the registration counter, Longarm slowed his step and said to the clerk, "If anyone steals our belongings, I'll hold you personally responsible."

"Not me!"

"Yes, you," Longarm snapped. "It'll come out of your hide or your pay."

"But I can't watch—"

"If I were you, I'd haul myself up those stairs and read my damned newspaper sitting watch outside the Presidential Suite until we return. Understand?"

"But—"

"Here," Ochoa said, dragging a dollar out of his pocket. "We ought to be back in an hour. That should compensate you for your time."

"Thank you," the clerk said, giving Longarm a nasty look. "You, at least, are a gentleman."

Longarm hurried outside and was assaulted by the storm. He ducked into the saloon and found it crowded. Along one wall was the bar and it had men standing in front of it shoulder to shoulder. In the middle of the room were tables and in the back, there was a counter behind which an employee was cooking and serving meals.

"Why don't we order whiskey first?" Ochoa asked. "It might help to ward off the chills."

Longarm agreed. "Lead the way."

Ochoa marched across the saloon, then shouldered between a couple of miners and tried to catch the overworked bartender's attention. But one of the miners, a large and unkempt looking fellow, shoved Ochoa back and spat, "They don't serve Indians in here, so make tracks."

Longarm started to intervene, but he needn't have bothered because Ochoa grabbed the miner's chin whiskers and jerked them down hard as he brought up his left knee. It happened so fast that, unless you'd really been watching, you'd never have understood how or why the big miner collapsed holding his bloody face.

"He broke my damned nose!" the man wailed, gazing up at Big Chief with tears in his murderous eyes. "You Indian sonofabitch, I'm going to kill you!"

A pistol materialized in Ochoa's fist almost like magic. Longarm thought it must have come from up the Navajo's

sleeve because it happened so suddenly. The pistol cocked and Ochoa pressed it against the miner's forehead.

"And just *how* were you planning to kill me?" he asked the man whose life he held in his fist.

The miner began to shake. One of his friends made a move for his gun but Longarm jumped forward and put a viselike grip on his forearm saying, "I believe you would be wise not to interfere."

"But he broke Johnny's nose!"

"Maybe it will teach your friend some manners."

Longarm reached for his badge. He held it up for everyone in the saloon to see and yelled, "I'm a federal marshal and this Navajo is a chief of police so let's have no more trouble. Bartender!"

"Yes sir!"

"Two whiskeys . . . your *good* stuff."

"And make 'em doubles!" Ochoa called, slowly removing the muzzle of his pistol from the miner's forehead and slipping it into a shoulder holster that even Longarm hadn't detected.

The whiskey was not up to Denver standards, but it was probably the best in the camp so they paid the bartender and went over to order something to eat.

"I'd like a steak," Ochoa told the busy cook who was working over a stove whose pipe ran up through the ceiling. "Thick, juicy, and red."

"I got steaks. They'll cost you a dollar-fifty, but it comes with all the beans and bread you can eat."

"Fine." Ochoa turned to Longarm. "How about you, big spender?"

"The same," Longarm replied to the cook, "only burn mine a little longer."

"Be three dollars."

Ochoa held out his hand. "Marshal Long?"

"I'm paying mine . . . but not yours."

53

"Cheapskate."

They paid and the cook looked at Ochoa and said, "Haven't I seen you in here before?"

"It's possible."

"I think you shot a man down, right over there by that old piano." The cook's eyes widened with complete recognition. "In fact, you shot the piano first, then the fella that was trying to drill you. I heard you took his body out across the back of a horse."

"That's right. I felt bad about the piano."

The cook grinned. "You just sort of make trouble wherever you go, is that it, Chief?"

"No, I just don't take any shit from bigoted people."

The cook looked confused. "What kind, Chief?"

"The kind that hates others because they're of a different color."

"You mean like me hating you because you're an Indian."

"That's right. How soon will our steaks be ready?"

"Right away," the cook said, going to work.

Longarm followed Ochoa to an empty table. When they were both seated, the Indian said, "Thanks for backing me up with that other fella. I might have had to kill him if you hadn't been around."

"No problem." Longarm sipped his whiskey. It ran hot down his gullet into his gut and he felt its heat spread. "Did you really kill a man here?"

"I'm afraid I did."

"How many others have you killed in your lifetime?"

"I don't keep count."

"More than ten?" Longarm asked.

Ochoa sampled his whiskey. "As a matter of professional courtesy, you should know better than to ask such a question."

"I think I've just figured it out," Longarm said, snapping his fingers. "I understand your game now."

"Oh?"

"You're a professional bounty hunter."

"Congratulations," Ochoa told him. "I do accept reward money, something that was never offered on the Navajo Reservation."

"I think," Longarm told him, "that we need to part ways tomorrow. You see, I don't like bounty hunters. They have no interest in the law, only in money."

"That's not true," Ochoa protested without passion. "I always try to bring in the worst of the worst."

"Oh? So who are you going after when we get to Pagosa Springs?"

"I'll go after the man that killed Senator Hawk and the federal dispatcher, of course."

"Not with my help you won't."

"I'm sorry to hear that," Ochoa replied. "I really was beginning to think we could become an outstanding team."

"Think again," Longarm told the Navajo as they raised their glasses and studied each other thoughtfully.

Finally, Ochoa said, "Marshal Long, you are making a big mistake. We both want the guilty to be arrested and brought to justice."

"That's right, but the difference is you do it for the money."

"And you don't?" Ochoa scoffed. "Are you trying to tell me that you'd do this for free?"

"That's not what I meant."

"I *know* what you meant," Ochoa said. "And let's have some honesty between us. You are well paid and have a job to do. I, on the other hand, get no pay other than what I can pick up in reward money."

"You," Longarm said, "get paid for bringing in an outlaw or fugitive of the law alive . . . or dead. Bounty hunters prefer to bring their people in dead, while I want to bring mine

in alive to face a judge or jury. Which means, while we both get paid, we have entirely different aims."

"Too bad you feel that way," Ochoa said. "I was just starting to like you."

"You'll get over it," Longarm told Ochoa as his bloody steak arrived.

They had a good dinner and a second glass of whiskey before they retired back to the hotel. The desk clerk had fallen asleep guarding their room. They awakened him and went to bed with the rain still coming down hard.

The storm passed in the night and after breakfast, they checked out of the Presidential Suite and headed for the livery. The man who owned the place was standing at the horse corral wringing his hands in anxiety.

"I'm afraid someone stole your horse last night!" he cried even before they reached him. "I can't be responsible for that, though. I told you—"

"*Which* horse?" Ochoa shouted in anger.

"Why that pretty bay mare, of course! Who'd steal that ugly roan?"

Ochoa ran up, grabbed the liveryman by the front of his coat and shook him like a terrier would a rat. Shook him so hard that Longarm had to jump in or else the Navajo might have snapped the man's turkey-thin neck.

"Take it easy!"

Ochoa backed off. He took a deep breath, slung his saddle over the top rail, and studied the horses inside the pen. "Mister, which ones are for sale?"

"Why . . . them three bays and that big pinto. And that mule and that runty buckskin."

"Which is the cheapest?"

"The buckskin. He probably don't weigh six hundred pounds. He's a real runt and an ornery little sonofabitch."

"How much?" Ochoa grated.

"I could give him to you for thirty—" the liveryman

56

saw Ochoa stiffen and start to come at him and gulped, "—for just twenty dollars he's yours, mister!"

"I'll take him," the Navajo said. "Catch and saddle up the little sonofabitch."

"Mister, I really don't want to have anything to do with him. Like I said, he's an ornery little bugger for certain."

"Get him," the Navajo said, "because, if I have to slop around in that corral with my good boots, I'm going to take him for *free!*"

The liveryman looked to Longarm for help but got none. "Aw, okay," he whined, grabbing a rope and heading into the corral.

The buckskin pony proved to be a mean little bastard. He almost kicked the liveryman's head off and did manage to bite him on the arm. But when he was finally dragged outside and Ochoa took the halter rope, the little beast had a change of heart. Longarm didn't know what the Navajo did, but he did see the Indian speak into the buckskin pony's ear and look him straight in the eye. The conversation was short, no more than a minute or two, but when it was over, the buckskin was ready to behave.

"What'd you do to him!" the liveryman blurted as they were saddling the roan and buckskin. "I can't believe my eyes!"

Ochoa didn't bother to reply. Instead, he mounted the pony and reined it around in a large circle until he found the tracks of his pretty bay mare. Longarm rode up to join the Navajo and stared at the tracks. "Looks like he's heading up into the mountains same as we are, huh?"

"Yep," Ochoa said, voice tight with anger. "But even if he wasn't, I'd catch and find him. A horse thief is a *dead* thief."

"Now wait a minute. There's no money in this."

"No money?" Ochoa echoed. "I just spent twenty dollars for this pony!"

"But no bounty, dammit!"

Ochoa smiled. "Who says? If he's just stolen my horse, you can bet your ass he's stolen others before it and probably done a lot worse. My money says that we are after more than just a onetime horse thief. And I'll bet you anything that there is a bounty on his head. Might be a pretty good-sized one, too!"

Longarm studied the Navajo in silence and then, together, they headed east.

Chapter 6

They rode out of town with Ochoa pushing the buckskin pony as hard and fast as he could travel. Longarm, on the other hand, had to fight to keep the strawberry roan from running over the top of his partner's much smaller mount.

"Marshal, how old are these tracks!" Ochoa shouted after they'd ridden for about five miles.

"Not more than three hours," Longarm replied.

"You're right," the Navajo said, twisting around in his saddle. "It didn't stop raining until about four o'clock this morning. I think our horse thief took my mare out of that livery corral at first light. He's pushing her hard and probably hoping that it will start to rain some more this morning in order to wash out his tracks."

"I wonder if he has any idea he stole a horse that belongs to a law officer," Longarm called out.

"*Former* law officer. I'm just a greedy, money-grabbing bounty hunter now. Right?"

"I don't care what or who you are," Longarm said irritably. "Just remember that when we overtake the man who stole that mare, I'll be the one that will make the arrest. Is that clear?"

"Very clear!"

Ochoa didn't say anything more the remainder of the morning. The footing was treacherous as they climbed ever higher. Several times the scrambling little buckskin lost its footing and fell. Each time, Ochoa kicked out of his stirrups to keep from injuring himself. Longarm had it much better because Ugly had huge feet and great balance. He slipped sometimes, but he never fell. Because of all the mud, tracking the horse thief proved very easy until they were joined by a busy logging road; then there was a lot of wagon traffic cutting through the soft mud, which slowed the Navajo's progress.

"You see a man riding a pretty bay mare pass you an hour or two ago?" Ochoa shouted at one point up at a mule skinner whose big freight wagon was loaded with heavy logs.

"Yeah, I seen a fella like that."

"What'd he look like?"

"Like he was in a helluva hurry," the driver answered, setting his brake and rolling a smoke. "He was a big galoot wearing a red flannel shirt and black hat. Had a gun strapped to his hip and he was whippin' his mare fairly to a nubbin', I tell you. What you want him for?"

"He stole that horse from me."

"He'll kill her if he don't slow down," the mule skinner said, twin plumes of smoke filtering lazily out of his nostrils. "I passed a couple of riders but I remember this one because I thought it was a real waste of fine horseflesh. Yes sir! No need to ruin a good animal like that bay mare. She was blowin' mighty hard and he was whippin' her ass for all he was worth. I doubt that mare will even get him all the way to Bear Creek."

"Thanks!" Ochoa shouted, unable to avoid the churning mud being slung up in the air by the heavy iron wheels that plastered his shirt and hat.

Longarm heard the Navajo cussing as Ochoa scraped away the offending mud. The man had a certain fastidiousness about himself and he definitely did not like to be unclean. However, staying clean on a road this sloppy after a rain was impossible.

They passed several more wagons coming down from the mountains, all headed for Trinidad and it was the Navajo who called up to every one of them and got pretty much the same story. Yes, they'd seen the big man and the handsome mare he seemed bound to run to death. Each report caused Ochoa more anxiety, although Longarm could not be sure if the Indian was thinking about the mare's welfare . . . or his pocketbook.

"Bear Creek!" Ochoa shouted.

Longarm gave the strawberry roan its head and the tall horse easily overtook the buckskin pony. They galloped side by side, but the pony was having a tough time of it so they slowed to a walk about a mile before they reached the outskirts of town.

"Just remember," Longarm said once again, "I'm in charge. If your man is here, we'll arrest him for stealing the mare."

"Fine," Ochoa said looking satisfied with the arrangement. "You are the front man. I'll back you up if there's trouble."

"I doubt there will be," Longarm said. "We've gotten a pretty good description of the man and he shouldn't be hard to spot. I'll pretend like I'm a regular guy and just walk up and get the drop on him. No trouble. No shooting. Understood?"

"Understood. But this town won't have a marshal. It's too small. So what are you going to do with our horse thief?"

"I'll take him with us and turn him over to the first marshal we come upon. We'll write up the arrest papers and continue on to Pagosa Springs."

"Whatever you say."

Longarm heard the Navajo . . . but he didn't really believe him.

They rode into Bear Creek at a walk, not wanting to attract any attention or to give their man any reason to think he'd been followed. The town was bigger than most in this part of Colorado with several businesses constructed of logs. It sat in a small valley among the pines and there were three lumber mills in full operation. Longarm also saw evidence of mining.

"There!" Ochoa hissed. "That's my mare tied up in front of that general store up the street on the right. See her?"

Longarm might not even have recognized the mare because her head was down low and her once shiny coat, mane, and tail were clotted with reddish colored mud. The mare looked like an old wagon horse that was ready to be put out of her misery.

Longarm glanced sideways at the Navajo and said, "You just take it easy. The mare will clean up. You did get us bills of sale on these horses, didn't you?"

"Of course. With full descriptions."

"Good. Let's mosey up the street past the mare a few doors and then wander back to the general store. I'll go in first. If I see someone that fits the description of our man, I'll get the drop on him and bring him outside for questioning. Okay?"

"You're the boss."

"Just try and remember that and we'll do fine," Longarm replied.

They tied their horses in front of a gun shop and pretended to be looking the town over like new arrivals interested in maybe a business opportunity or a job as they strolled down to the general store. "Okay," Longarm said, "if our man is inside, I'll make the arrest."

"I'll be right here," Ochoa promised.

Longarm went inside. There was a clerk stationed by the door and he was ringing up some goods for an older woman. He nodded to Longarm and went about his business. Longarm pretended to gaze around at the dry goods but he was really searching for the man who'd stolen the bay mare. The store was busy and there were at least a half dozen men shopping inside.

I'll bet that's him, Longarm thought, spotting a rough-looking man wearing a red flannel shirt. The man's clothes were spattered with mud and he appeared to have just climbed down from a horse or a wagon

Taking a deep breath, and easing his gun out of its holster, Longarm slipped the gun inside his jacket, then casually walked down to the suspect. "Howdy."

The big man stared at him, then turned away without speaking. He reached for a can of horse liniment and that's when Longarm poked him in the back with his gun and said, "Mister, I'm a United States deputy marshal. You're under arrest for horse thieving. Don't make a fuss and you won't get hurt."

"What the hell are you talking about!" the man shouted, starting to spin around in anger.

"I said not to move!" Longarm grated, pushing the muzzle of his gun harder into the man's ribs and also clamping his hand on his shoulder. "Now we're going outside to have a private conversation."

"I ain't going nowhere with no gawdamn lawman!"

Longarm had been in this situation many times and he'd learned that this kind of man, while unusual, best understood force. And so, without a moment's hesitation, he pistol-whipped him across the back of the head, right behind his left ear. The big man's knees folded but Longarm held him erect.

"All right," he said, "that was just a little tap. You either

do as I say or so help me I'll crack your thick skull with the next one."

"You sonofabitch! I didn't steal no damn horse! I been working all morning and just came in here to get something for my team."

"Sure you did. The mare you took is right outside. We're going to pay her a visit and then you're going to confess."

"I'll go to hell if I'll confess to horse thievin'!" the man raged. "And I don't care who the hell you are, mister."

"What is going on here!" the clerk shouted, hurrying down the aisle in his white apron, waving a broom. "I demand to know the meaning of this trouble!"

"I'm a United States marshal and I'm questioning this man in the matter of a horse theft. Now step aside because we're leaving."

"My name is J. T. Edwards and I certainly don't appreciate you coming in here and causing a disruption in my establishment. No sir, I certainly do not! And furthermore, I insist on seeing your officer's badge this very instant."

"Later!"

"Right now!"

"I'm busy," Longarm said between clenched teeth. "And, if you don't get out of our way, I'll also arrest *you*."

Edwards jumped back. Assuming an expression of extreme outrage, he shouted, "For what criminal offense!"

"Obstructing justice. Now step aside!"

The store owner considered making a stand in the aisle, but when Longarm shoved his prisoner forward, Edwards jumped aside. The other customers had gathered around and one of them cried, "Jim, he's got a gun in your back. What do you want us to do?"

"Just . . . just don't do anything yet," Longarm's prisoner replied. "This stupid bastard has made a bad, bad mistake and it's going to cost him plenty."

"But there's blood pouring down your cheek!"

Longarm could see that this was not going well and he knew that he had to get outside and put some space between him and these angry customers, so he pushed Jim forward with the gun still pressed to his back. When several of the man's friends tried to crowd him, Longarm shouted, "Everyone stay back! This is an arrest!"

"Who the hell are you!" the store owner screeched, waving that broom handle. "I demand to see your badge!"

Longarm wanted to shove the badge down the man's throat sideways but, instead, he pushed Jim up the aisle and onto the sidewalk. "All right," he said stopping at the hitching rail where the bay mare was tied, "that's the horse you stole from my partner early this morning."

"You're crazy! I've been working at the freight yard since sunup!" With blood still trickling down his cheek and the back of his head, Jim added, "You pistol-whipped the wrong man, Marshal! And gawdamn it hurts!"

Out of the corner of his eye, Longarm saw Ochoa step away from the storefront. The general store emptied and men formed a half circle around Longarm and his prisoner. Most of them were armed and all looked mad as a bucket of teased snakes.

Longarm shouted, "You men go back inside like before and tend to your own business!"

"Jim is our friend and this is our business," one of them swore. "I was with him all morning. He ain't stole that damn sorry mare. Jim is a good family man and he works for the Acme Freighting Company . . . same as I do! Who the hell do you think you are, mister!"

Longarm was beginning to feel that he'd made an awful mistake. Everyone around him was shouting and standing up in defense of the man he'd just arrested, but he had to stay in control or things could quickly get out of hand. "Quiet!" he shouted. "Has anyone else seen Jim this morning?"

"I have," another mud-spattered man said. "I helped him hitch the teams in our freight yard. Then we had a quick cup of coffee about an hour ago in the cafe up the street and came over here to get a few company supplies. What right do you have to come here and pistol-whip a hard-working man? I don't care who you are, mister, you can't act like this against working men!"

A chorus of shouts filled the air and the crowd seemed to be feeding on its own anger and outrage. Longarm could feel the situation spiraling completely out of control. It was time to admit his mistake and then try and make amends before he and Ochoa continued to hunt for the horse thief.

Longarm holstered his gun but kept a fistful of Jim's coat material clenched in his big fist. "That mare was stolen this morning and belongs to my friend."

"What damned friend!"

Longarm looked for Big Chief Ochoa but the Indian had vanished.

"What friend?" another echoed.

"Mister," Jim hissed before Longarm could think of an answer, "you'd better have a badge, an apology, and the money for a doc. Otherwise, you better git your ass out of Bear Creek or we might just lynch *you* for stupidity!"

The air was cool but Longarm could feel perspiration breaking out all over his body. "Who saw the man that rode this mare into town not more than two hours ago!"

Nobody said a word.

Longarm pushed Jim away and confronted the hostile crowd. "Answer up! Someone must have seen the fella that rode that mare into town."

"I think you'd best show us your badge," the store owner demanded without trying to hide his contempt.

Longarm decided that was probably the best thing to do so he reached into his coat pocket and showed them his authority.

"Gawdamn dumb-assed lawmen," someone close to Longarm swore. "Bastards think they can just come into a town and do whatever they want because someone pinned a piece of tin on their chest."

Longarm swung on the man and said, "If I were you, mister, I'd watch my mouth or it will land you in big trouble."

"What are you going to do, pistol-whip me like you did poor Jim?"

"I might."

"I think you need to leave our town immediately," the store owner said. "I think you ought to just climb on your horse and ride like hell before you find yourself in serious trouble."

"No," Longarm told them. "Someone here stole this mare in Vulture's Nest early this morning. There is a horse thief in this town that I mean to apprehend and arrest before I leave."

"We don't even know if that mare belongs to you," a man said, looking around for support. "Boys, this jasper might have found or stole the badge. Why, he might be a horse thief his own damn self!"

Where the hell was that Navajo! Longarm raged inwardly. *Where is he right now when I really need him?*

"Ask him for a bill of sale on that bay mare, Mr. Edwards!"

Edwards drew himself up, untied his apron, and handed it to a man. "I think that would be in order, Marshal. Also, I'd like to see more proof as to your identity. Like Morris said, you could have found or stolen it yourself."

"I don't have the bill of sale on that mare," Longarm said, feeling his position eroding as surely as if he stood on a sandy riverbank.

"Well, in that case, we have a problem," Jim said. "You come barging into the store, pistol-whip me and you don't have proof you even are a lawman, much less that you own

that mare. Boys, I think we need to teach this uppity stranger a hard lesson!"

The crowd started to advance on Longarm, who backed into the muddy street, drawing his gun. "I am a United States deputy marshal working out of Denver. And, if anyone tries to lay a hand on me, I'll shoot to kill."

They believed him. Longarm could see that they were all just waiting for someone else to make the first stupid move. Any move. Longarm took a deep breath. Sometimes, discretion really was the better part of valor and he would have been content to get out of this scrape even if it meant letting the horse thief remain free.

He was just about to say something to that general effect when a volley of gunshots sliced through the tension causing everyone to spin around just in time to see another big man wearing a flannel shirt crash through the bat-wing doors of a nearby saloon. He staggered, tried to lift his smoking pistol, and two more shots pierced the swinging doors and sent him crashing into the mud.

"Holy cow!" someone breathed. "What the—"

Longarm swallowed and then shook his head as Big Chief appeared. Not a word was spoken as the Navajo studiously reloaded his gun, then glanced up at Longarm standing in the muddy street surrounded by the angry citizens of Bear Creek.

"Marshal Long, this is the one," Ochoa said matter-of-factly but loud enough for everyone to overhear. "The bartender inside saw him climb off my bay mare. Saw him tie her up and come for whiskey. The dead fella even bragged about how he'd gotten a new horse over in Vulture's Nest. Naturally, I tried to arrest him but he drew his gun and just had to shoot it out."

Longarm cleared his throat and faked great enthusiasm. "Nice work, Chief Ochoa! Well, we'd better be on our way

to Pagosa Springs to settle that murder case. No time to waste."

"Yes, sir!"

Ochoa holstered his gun and marched down the boardwalk as if he'd just had a nice visit with a minister instead of having just shot a horse thief to death. Acting very careful not to step into the muddy street, he sort of reached over the hitch rail and untied the bay mare. He led her over to the little buckskin pony, then mounted the mare and tied the pony's reins to his saddle horn.

"Ready when you are, Marshal."

"Then let's ride," Longarm ordered, hurrying through the mud to his own horse, untying then mounting the tall gelding.

"Hey, wait just a minute!" Jim shouted an objection. "What about the damages to my head!"

Longarm took it to the limit when he wagged his forefinger at the man and scolded, "Next time an officer of the law gives you a reasonable order, you'd better move your feet a lot quicker."

"But I was innocent!"

Longarm reached into his pocket and counted out three silver dollars. He pitched them to Jim. "That ought to pay the doc for his trouble."

"That ain't fair, gawdammit!"

"The man can send a request for remuneration to Denver, can't he Marshal Long?" Ochoa asked solicitously.

"That's right."

Longarm nodded his good-bye, reined his big strawberry roan about, and then sent it paddling through the mud, knowing that Big Chief would be following right behind.

"Hey," Edwards shouted, running into the street. "Marshal, what about *funeral* expenses!"

Longarm twisted around in his saddle. "I give you permission to sell the deceased's gun and whatever other be-

longings he has for expenses and giving the rest to a worthy charity."

"Shit!" Edwards screamed in frustration.

"Tough shit," Ochoa added under his breath.

"Damn you, Ochoa," Longarm complained as they made their way quickly to the end of the business district, "why didn't you come back into the general store and get me to arrest the right man?"

"I meant to! Really. But you were in a bad fix already and I was afraid that the real horse thief was going to get away. So I just had to take action, Marshal. Otherwise, who knows but what he'd have gotten away clean!"

They rode wide around a big freight wagon and the little buckskin pony took a bite out of the weary bay mare's rump hide. She was so exhausted she barely flinched. But Longarm's roan wasn't going to let the infraction pass without a reprisal. His mouth opened wide and his yellow teeth clamped down on the ornery pony's neck. The pony squealed in terror and attempted to pull away but Ugly bit harder until Longarm kicked him in the jaw with the toe of his boot.

"Stop that!" he shouted.

The roan laid its ears back flat and the pony got as far away as possible from the gelding.

Longarm shook his head. "Ain't nothin' is going right."

"We're fine," Ochoa said, sounding surprisingly cheerful for someone who'd just shot another to death. "I'll admit having my mare stolen was bad luck, but it all worked out."

"How do you figure?"

Ochoa shrugged. "We rid the world of a horse thief and you taught the citizens of Bear Creek a little respect for law and order. What's so bad about that?"

"I wouldn't even try to explain it to you," Longarm told him as they rode on toward Pagosa Springs.

Chapter 7

"There it is," Longarm said, reining in Ugly and gazing down at Pagosa Springs. "It's as pretty a town as you'll find anywhere. It would be a fine place to live."

"Oh, I don't know if I'd say that," Ochoa replied skeptically. "I've heard that the winters up here are pretty rough and the snow gets mighty deep."

"I except that is true," Longarm replied. "Point me toward the Hawk Ranch."

Ochoa stood up in his stirrups and gestured toward the north end of the valley. "You see that cut in the hills?"

"Yeah?"

"That's where you'll find Hawk ranch headquarters. But aren't you coming into town first?"

"I don't see any point of it," Longarm replied. "There's no marshal to report to, is there?"

"Nope. You'll be the big chief as far as lawmen go in these parts."

"What are you going to do?"

The Navajo frowned. "I'm going to drift on into town and see some of my friends. I'll hear all the local gossip and find out whatever I can about Liberty."

"I hope he isn't lynched," Longarm said. " 'Cause if that were the case, I'd be expected to make some arrests."

"If the Ute kid was lynched, no one would tell you anything. This town owes a lot to Senator Hawk, and the Hawk family rules the roost. You can be sure that no one would dare point any fingers in their direction."

"Might be a good idea to pretend that we aren't even acquainted," Longarm said. "That way, we each gather our own independent facts and get together and compare notes when no one is the wiser."

"I agree. Just as long as you share with me as much information as I share with you. That was our agreement. Remember?"

"I remember. I just wanted to make sure that you did."

"What are you going to do with two horses?" Longarm asked.

"I'll sell the pony and keep the mare. The way she looks right now I couldn't even get my money out of her. But in a few weeks, she'll look all shiny again. But don't you be selling that big strawberry roan without giving me the first chance to buy him. Okay?"

"Okay." Longarm stuck his hand out and they shook. "You keep your nose clean, Big Chief. I don't want to have to arrest you for gunning someone down."

"Not a chance. And watch out for yourself at the Hawk Ranch. Mrs. Hawk isn't called the Black Widow without good reason. I wouldn't put it past her to have murdered her own husband. And she'd think nothing of doing the very same to you, Marshal."

"They sound like a bad bunch, all right."

"They are."

"One last question," Longarm said. "What do you know about the sale of thirty thousand acres of Ute land to the state of Colorado?"

Ochoa thought about that for a moment, then replied, "I

know that someone is going to profit big and you can bet your life it won't be the Ute people."

"I expect not. Do you think that the senator's murder had anything to do with that reservation land sale?"

"Wouldn't surprise me." Ochoa shook his head. "Look. I could tell you all sorts of things about the family but you need to find them out yourself. The important thing is not to trust them or believe a word they say. And most of all, don't let your guard down because, if old lady Hawk and her daughter get the slightest hint that you might suspect them of killing the senator, you're in mortal danger."

"All right," Longarm agreed. "I'll be coming into town after my visit at the ranch and probably run into you tonight."

"That would be smart. They'll no doubt offer you their hospitality . . . but turn it down flat."

"I will."

Longarm reined Ugly toward the north, and when he had ridden about a mile, he twisted around in the saddle expecting to see the Navajo heading directly for Pagosa, but the man had disappeared.

He's a real strange and crafty one, Longarm thought. *I'm just glad that we ride the same side of the fence.*

As he headed toward Hawk Ranch, Longarm reviewed everything that he'd learned so far about the family. He recalled that Nettie had been an only child whose first husband had died suddenly, then whose parents had both died so that she had inherited a cattle kingdom before marrying the ambitious John Hawk. Now, Senator Hawk was dead . . . the fourth one to die of mysterious causes. Or maybe the fifth one, if you counted the federal dispatcher. Five people dead and the Black Widow was still alive. Nettie Hawk, once a widely recognized beauty, was now an old woman with a lovely daughter and a son that Longarm still didn't know much about.

Poisoning. That's what it sounds like to me.

Longarm knew that, as a federal officer, he'd be offered a room and meals at the Hawk Ranch. He was determined to refuse that hospitality at any cost.

Two hours later, the wagon track he'd been following ended at a gate. And beside the gate waited a cowboy with a carbine resting across his saddle horn.

"Afternoon," Longarm said in greeting.

The cowboy managed to nod his head, but he didn't return the greeting.

"Nice day."

No response.

Longarm flashed his badge. "I'm United States Deputy Custis Long. I've come all the way from Denver to see Mrs. Hawk."

"Well, then you've wasted your time and money. Mrs. Hawk gave me orders that she did not want to see anyone."

"But I'm—"

"No exceptions," the cowboy told him. "Might as well turn that mule-headed horse around and ride back to Denver."

Longarm bit back an angry response. Better to try and reason with the man. "Look. I'm sure that, if Mrs. Hawk knew I was sent here by the governor himself, then she'd be willing to see me."

"I don't think she'd care if you were sent here by Jesus Christ hisself." The cowboy shifted the barrel of his rifle ever so slightly toward Longarm and growled, "Now turn that ugly horse around and git!"

Longarm had two choices. He could call the fool's bluff or do as he was ordered and return under more favorable circumstances. He decided on the latter course of action.

"Okay, Cowboy. But I'll be back."

"Not without Mrs. Hawk or her daughter's say-so."

"What about Jake Hawk? Is he home, too?"

"I'm done jawin' with you, Marshal. I never cared much for lawmen. Most of you bastards are as crooked as a dog's hind leg. So you just turn around and go away because I have a real itchy trigger finger and no patience for you, lawman."

"What's your name?"

"Huh?"

"You heard me! What is your name?"

"Elden. Elden Hoag."

"Elden, you haven't seen the last of me."

Elden spit a stream of thick, brown tobacco juice across the fence and scoffed with derision. "Any man who'd own a horse that ugly can't have much sense or be taken seriously. Now, git!"

Longarm reined the roan about and headed back the way he'd come. He was seething and frustrated but there was no sense in getting shot over something that could wait a little while longer.

When he rode into Pagosa Springs, Longarm saw Big Chief Ochoa sitting in a wooden rocking chair in front of a bank. The Navajo was surrounded by several other Indians and they were laughing. Longarm wondered what Ochoa had discovered so far but knew better than to ride up and ask. They'd agreed to act as strangers to each other and try to communicate in secret.

Longarm spotted a livery and pointed the strawberry roan in that direction. He was tired and a little saddle sore. If Liberty had been caught, tried, and lynched, he knew he'd be starting back real soon. But if the Ute kid was still on the run Longarm figured this job was just beginning.

"Howdy, mister!" a friendly looking man in his early thirties called out from a stack of straw he was pitchforking into a wagon. "Jeezus, I never seen such a big, ugly horse! Where in the hell did you find him!"

"I bought him in Trinidad."

"They should have paid *you*!"

"He's a lot better animal than you'd expect." Longarm dismounted and led the roan over to a tie rail. "I'd like to put him up here for a day or two."

"Why sure. Cost you a dollar a day. If you add just one extra dime per day I'll grain the sorry critter. He needs to put some flesh on his bones, although nothing will do much to make him look any better."

"Like I said, he's a lot better mount than he appears. Never quits. He's a demon in the mountains."

"He's a demon all right. You want the extra grain?"

"Sure."

The liveryman took Longarm's reins, and the roan laid his ears back and snapped at the man who practically jumped out of his skin before tossing the reins back to Longarm and yelling, "Sonofabitch! Did you see the size of his teeth!"

"Yeah."

"Why's he so mean?"

"He gets tired of being insulted."

"I'd shoot that horse and feed him to the dogs," the liveryman said, fists doubled at his sides.

"Look. I like the roan and we get along fine. Now, do you want to put him up or shall I find someone else? I'm not leaving him with a man who'll mistreat or starve him, that's for certain."

"I'll do neither," the liveryman said. "I'll take your money, I'll feed and care for him well. You've the word of Horace Walker on that matter."

"Fair enough, Horace. Where shall I put him?"

"In that pen yonder. There's a bay mare and a buckskin pony in there already but I think they will get along."

"I expect so," Longarm said.

He unsaddled Ugly and led him over to the pen. When

76

the big gelding saw his old friends, he whinnied and seemed very happy. But then the pony got in his way and he kicked it in the head and chased it around the pen for several minutes.

"I never seen such a mean-tempered animal! You think he'll kill that pony when we turn our backs?"

"Nope. He just wants to settle who is the boss."

Longarm paid Horace for two days' board. The man offered to lock up his saddle and bridle for free. "Hotel just up the street called the Bonner House. Rooms are clean and the price is good."

"What about food?"

"There are three cafes in town, all forgettable but they won't ruin your stomach. You here for business . . . or pleasure?"

"Maybe a little of both." Longarm started to leave, then turned and said, "Excuse me but I was trying to remember something. Wasn't there a murder here a week or two ago that was important?"

"That's right. Senator John Hawk and a federal dispatcher named Jason Snyder were murdered by a Ute Indian kid. Terrible thing! We just had the funeral a few days ago and everyone in Pagosa Springs attended. Senator Hawk was a very popular man in these parts and I guess there isn't a businessman in this town that hasn't received some favor or other from him."

"Including yourself?"

"That's right. He'd buy a horse from me when I had a good one. He also rented some animals when he had a lot of guests visiting. I liked the senator. Damned shame that he was murdered by that Indian kid."

"Did they catch him in the act?"

"No, but they found evidence and there wasn't much doubt he's the guilty one. After he murdered the senator

77

and that Snyder fella, the kid was seen riding away as if the devil were hounding his tail."

"Didn't a posse go after him?"

"Sure, but he's an Indian and they know how to disappear in these mountains. That, and they got a lot of friends. Jake Hawk and some of the locals have combed these mountains every day since the kid vanished but haven't found his hideout yet."

"Maybe he headed for Mexico."

"Naw," Horace said. "An Indian can't survive far from his own kind. I never knew one to travel more than forty or fifty miles from the reservation."

Longarm thought of Big Chief but didn't say anything about the Navajo. "Isn't there any law in these parts?"

"Nope."

"Well," Longarm said, "there is now."

"What does that mean?"

"I'm a deputy marshal on assignment from Denver."

"No!"

"Yes, I am."

"Well, why didn't you own up and say so from the start?"

"Because I wanted to find out what you knew about the murder. Lots of times, when people learn I'm a lawman, they'll clam up."

"Show me your badge."

Longarm pulled it out of his coat pocket.

"Well I'll be damned!" Horace said. "You sure fooled me. I guess I figured a lawman wouldn't be caught dead on a horse that ugly."

"Like I told you, he's a good mount. He'll outrun and outwalk any horse I've ever ridden and he never tires. But I didn't come here to talk about horses. I came to find out who really killed the senator and the dispatcher."

"I told you . . . the Ute kid named Liberty."

"You told me that no one actually saw him commit the act of murder . . . only that he was seen making tracks from the ranch."

Horace frowned. "I'd think that would be a pretty darned good indicator of his guilt."

"Not in my mind and not in a Denver courtroom, it wouldn't."

"Well," Horace said with a sigh, "there is talk that the pair were killed by Mrs. Hawk. They call her the Black Widow, you know."

"So I've heard. Did you see the bodies?"

"No one did. They were laid out in closed caskets at the funeral. The senator's casket was the finest thing you'll ever see. Snyder's wasn't bad, but it sure took second place to the one they laid the senator out in."

"Who laid them out?"

"You mean who is the undertaker?"

"That's right."

Horace pointed up the street. "He's also the local saw-bones and the dentist. Name is Porter. Gideon B. Porter. He was called out right after both murders and then he came back to town. The bodies stayed at the ranch until it was time to load 'em into Porter's hearse and haul them to the cemetery just west of town. Big funeral. I didn't think there were that many folks in these parts. I'll bet three hundred people were in attendance. I was there and it was quite a show."

"So the only one that saw the bodies was Mr. Porter?"

"And the Hawk family, of course."

"All right," Longarm said, "I'll get a room and pay Mr. Porter a visit."

"I'm afraid that won't be possible," Horace said. "Mr. Porter was so upset that he went off on vacation right after the funeral. He was a bachelor. Drank a bit, he did. Any-way, he looked kinda sick at the funeral and he told every-

one that he was leaving town. Might be gone for quite a spell. Don't know what we're going to do the next time one of us needs a tooth pulled or a bone set or worse."

"I can understand why that would be quite a problem," Longarm said absently. "Did Mr. Porter give any indication where he was going for a vacation?"

"No sir. But I happen to know he has a son that lives east of here in a town called Mancos. It's clear over near the Utah border."

"I've been through Mancos."

"Well, that's where the younger Porter lives. Not that I'm saying his father went to see him but I heard that they were close. Mancos would be my guess as to where Mr. Porter went on his vacation."

"Thanks."

"You'll be comfortable at the Bonner House. I just sent an Indian over there a few hours back, but they won't let him a room."

"Because he is an Indian."

"That's right. He was a nice-looking man wearing nice clothes. But an Indian is an Indian."

Longarm had his own opinion on that but he kept it to himself, saying, "I guess I'll have to start asking questions at the Hawk Ranch."

"You can try."

"What does that mean?"

"Senator Hawk liked company. He'd invite damn near anybody out to his ranch when he was there. He was proud of the place and liked to show it off at every chance. And, once you see it, you'll know why. But Mrs. Hawk, she don't like company at all."

"What about her son and daughter?"

"Della and Jake always do what Mrs. Hawk tells them."

"What are they like?"

"I don't know. Della hardly ever comes to town, but

when she does the men can't keep their eyes off of her. Jake is fine. He struts around and likes to spend his family's money. He's . . . well, he can get a little crazy with the whiskey. I just try to stay out of his way . . . especially when he's drinking, which is almost always."

"But you said he's been hunting the Ute kid every day."

"Yeah. He starts out looking for him in the Dutchman's Saloon, then looks for him in the Bulldog Saloon, then the Gold Strike Bar. After he and his 'posse' friends get plenty lubricated up, they all get on their horses and go thundering out of Pagosa. It's a joke! People are laughing and at the same time worried that the 'posse' will come upon some innocent Ute and lynch him just for the hell of it."

"I understand."

"Jake isn't a thing like his father, the senator. He's been raised with too much and he acts like he is some kind of royalty in these parts. No one likes him except the ones that he buys whiskey for and they might not like him either, if he didn't have the name and the money."

"Thanks for the information."

"You be careful," Horace solemnly warned. "When Jake Hawk discovers that there is a *real* law officer in town, he's not going to be very happy. He's appointed himself as the sheriff and he won't like you telling him he's nothing but a wild sonofabitch that needs to stay at the ranch and let a professional handle things."

"I'll keep your warning in mind," Longarm replied, starting off for the hotel carrying his rifle and saddlebags, with his mind on the missing undertaker.

Had Gideon B. Porter been threatened or . . . paid to disappear? Had he seen something when he'd prepared the bodies to indicate that all was not as it seemed? Had he even seen evidence that would either prove or disprove the guilt of a kid named Liberty?

Longarm didn't know the answers to any of those questions and he wasn't too excited about riding Ugly all the way over to Mancos on what very well might prove to be a wild-goose chase.

Chapter 8

The Bonner House was exceptionally nice and quite unusual for a town the size of Pagosa Springs. A large oil portrait of Senator John Hawk was the centerpiece and it hung over the mantel of an enormous rock fireplace. The lobby floor was polished oak, the furniture as nice as you'd find in Denver's finest hotels. There were even crystal chandeliers and a very impressive Persian rug to give the establishment a look of unexpected refinement and elegance.

A small bronze plaque caught Longarm's eye as he moved across the lobby and it read: WELCOME TO THE BONNER HOUSE FOUNDED AND OWNED BY SENATOR JOHN HAWK AND FAMILY.

So, Longarm thought, *this is the place where the senator escaped when he needed to get away from the Black Widow. It was probably also where he wined and dined important politicians and wealthy supporters who preferred a citified atmosphere to that of the ranch.*

The desk clerk wore a suit and tie. He was an older gentleman and smiled as if Longarm were his best friend.

"Good afternoon, sir! Welcome to Bonner House. How can we accommodate you?"

"I'd like a room."

"We would be extremely honored to have you as our special guest," the clerk told him. "Room rates come with supper, which requires a suit and tie for our gentlemen guests."

"I don't have a suit and tie. Can't I save a little money and get just a room without meals?"

The clerk's smile slipped. "We can do that, of course. It would mean that you would be lodged in our older, west wing." He covered his mouth and coughed daintily. "Uh-hem. It is a little more . . . spartan. Clean, but no frills."

"If it has a bed, nightstand, and thunder pot, that's good enough for me."

"Of course. But no private bathtub. Are you aware that we have natural hot springs?"

"Yes."

"West wing guests are not allowed in them but there are some public baths just outside of town."

"Fine," Longarm said, becoming annoyed. "How much will it cost me a night?"

"Four dollars."

"That's pretty steep."

To the clerk's credit, he managed to smile before saying, "You can find other hotels and we sincerely invite you to do so."

Longarm was tempted to walk. "Four dollars without supper?"

"That is correct. Five *with* supper . . . if you have a coat and tie, which you informed me you do not. What is your pleasure?"

Longarm's "pleasure" would have been to choke this arrogant old fossil into genuine humility but he couldn't do that so he said, "The west wing will do."

"Please sign your name . . . or an X if you—"

"I can read and write." Longarm snatched up the pen and

signed into the guest book. He watched as the stuffy old codger read his name and then saw the man's eyes widen as he read the tag: United States deputy marshal.

The clerk glanced up and said without warmth, "Welcome to Pagosa Springs, Marshal Long. We don't often have the pleasure of hosting a federal marshal. Most of them are forced to lodge at lesser establishments."

Longarm was doing a slow burn as he placed four dollars on the counter. "My key, please."

"Of course. Oh, one more thing, Marshal. We don't allow our unmarried guests to invite lady guests into their rooms. This is a very respectable hotel and I'm sure that you can understand the need for that rule."

"Sure. You don't want a gaggle of whores parading through this fancy lobby upsetting the genteel folks. No problem."

The clerk managed to look properly offended as he pointed Longarm toward his room in the "west wing," whatever that meant.

Actually, the room was quite nice despite its second-class status. It had rugs, a large mahogany dresser, a handsome four-poster bed, nightstand, and a porcelain pitcher and wash basin. On the nightstand was a pad of free hotel stationery. Best of all there was a copper bathtub in the corner of the room and everything was fresh and spotless. Longarm grunted his approval, unpacked his few belongings, and stretched out on the bed for a few minutes. Without intending to, he fell asleep.

It was sundown when Longarm awakened. He poured water into the pitcher and washed the sleep from his eyes, then wet his hair and combed it straight back with his fingers. Chagrined that he had fallen asleep and hearing the rumble of his empty belly, he left the room, locking it, and then went out to find something to eat. Longarm wasn't sure

about his plans, but he figured that, after supper, he would spend a few hours in the saloons learning whatever he could about the murders. With luck, he would discover a great deal without anyone even knowing he was a newly arrived Denver lawman.

That hope was soon dashed, however, when a passerby stopped him to say, "Good evening, Marshal. Hope you can put an end to the craziness that has taken over Pagosa Springs."

"I'll . . . I'll certainly try."

"Jake Hawk and his friends have been raising Cain in Pagosa for almost two weeks. Some innocent Indian is going to get shot down if you don't put a stop to the nonsense. No one wants to see Pagosa Springs get a black eye."

"Of course not."

"I own the Maverick Saddle and Boot Shop just up the street. I support a wife and two sons. Now, I don't know if Liberty killed Senator Hawk or not . . . but even an Indian deserves a fair trial."

"Absolutely."

"I mean, they *are* humans."

"That's right."

"Jake Hawk and his friends have scared most of the Utes back to their reservation. They're all afraid that he or one of his friends are gonna get drunk and shoot them down like rabid dogs. We just can't have that sort of thing going on. It isn't good for business. I sell saddles and other tack and harness to the Utes and they pay cash. All this hot talk about rope justice gives outsiders the wrong impression of Pagosa Springs and I believe it is unhealthy for this town's bright future."

"I'll do what I can."

"My name is Evan Forrest."

"Marshal Custis Long."

"I expect this double murder is why you have been sent

here. Everyone is glad you came. Everyone except Jake Hawk and his cronies. Watch out for them. When they get drunk and rowdy, there is no telling what they might say or do. As far as they are concerned, they don't need or want outside interference."

"Is Jake Hawk in town now?"

"I'm afraid so," Forrest replied unable to hide his anger. "From sundown to midnight, he's nearly always at the White Lightning Saloon."

"Thanks."

Longarm spotted a cafe across the street. "Is that place any good to eat?"

"No better or worse than any other in Pagosa. I recommend their beef stew. For the money, you can't go wrong."

"Fine."

"Good luck, Marshal."

A few minutes later when Longarm entered the cafe, all conversation died. There were about ten tables and all but two were taken. Longarm nodded and went to the empty table at the far end of the room. He sat down with his back to the wall and waited for someone to take his order.

"What'll it be, Marshal!" a smiling brunette who looked to be in her mid-thirties asked.

"I hear your beef stew is delicious."

"Steaks are even better."

"I'll have the stew, coffee, and sourdough bread. Are your pies fresh?"

"I made them myself this morning. We have apple and cherry."

"I'll take apple."

"The whole pie?"

Longarm grinned. This gal had sparkle and she was pretty. About five-six and padded in all the right places with dimples in her rosy cheeks. She wasn't wearing a wedding ring, either. "I guess half the pie would do me fine."

"Okay. You can have seconds on everything and it will only cost you . . . thirty-five cents for the stew, bread, and coffee. Half an apple pie will cost you an extra six bits but you won't be sorry."

The woman sashayed off, gently swinging her hips and Longarm couldn't help but stare. It'd been a while since . . . well, never mind. He was up to his neck in trouble here and needed to keep focused on business . . . not pleasure.

"Hey, Marshal!"

Longarm looked over at a nearby table occupied by four loggers.

"We was wondering if you are going to need any help when you go onto the reservation and ferret out that murdering sonofabitch, Liberty."

"No."

"But you might!" They all nodded as the one kept talking. "You see, those Utes have made it clear that they don't want us coming on their reservation. Of course, once a big chunk of it is sold to the state of Colorado, they won't have any more to say about that."

"This piece of reservation property that the Indians are being forced to sell," Longarm asked. "Is it valuable?"

"Hell, yes! Got lots of timber on it," another of the loggers said with excitement in his voice. "Be worth a fortune. Once we get it in private hands, you can bet we'll have enough work to last us about twenty years."

"Jobs are important."

"You bet they are and we don't want this murder to foul up the land sale. I mean, everyone knew that Senator Hawk was our friend. He was pushing this deal so we'd have jobs and our kids would have our jobs. I figure that's why that yellow-bellied bastard Liberty killed him."

"To queer the land sale?"

"Why else?"

"I still have no idea."

"Well, Marshal, if you need deputies to go with you and get that little murderer, then all you have to do is put the word out and you'll have a couple hundred men in no time, all armed and ready to go to war against them damned Indians."

"I'll keep it in mind," Longarm said as his bowl of stew, platter of bread, and coffee arrived.

"You do that, Marshal! Just don't be trying to go on the reservation without an army or you'll get yourself scalped for certain."

"Sure."

"By the way. I forgot to mention that my name is *Miss* Milly," the waitress said. "Just holler out when you need seconds and I'll come runnin'." She turned to the table full of loggers and when she spoke, her voice held a mild reproof. "You boys let the marshal eat in peace. Just pay up and go have some fun."

"We would if you'd come along, Milly!"

She made a face at them that brought smiles. "That'll be the day when I go with the likes of you rough boys."

They liked her teasing, tipped handsomely, and tromped out of the cafe leaving laughter in their wake.

"Don't mind them, Marshal. And don't take 'em too serious. They're hardworking men, but they aren't the kind you'd want in your posse."

"That's true enough."

"Just call out if you need me," she said, walking away swinging her hips.

Longarm enjoyed his supper, having seconds and then managing to consume half a pie. "Milly," he said, preparing to leave, "that was excellent."

"I'm glad that you liked it." She eyed him up and down. "You staying in town long?"

"I have no idea."

"Found a room at one of the boardinghouses, I expect?"

"Bonner House."

Her eyebrows lifted with mild surprise. "I hear that place is real elegant."

"I rented a room in the 'west wing,' which is supposed to be a cut below the rest of the place."

"I've never been in any of those rooms. Too high-toned and expensive for the likes of this working gal."

"Maybe you'd like to see what the rooms are like?"

"Is that an invitation?"

"It is."

Her hands smoothed the front of her apron. "Marshal, I'm afraid I have to close and then clean up the kitchen and do dishes. I won't be able to leave until ten."

"I'll be by then. The only thing is, you either have to be a man or I have to sneak you in through the window."

"Are you serious?"

"Yep. Bonner House rules."

"I guess the high and mighty Bonner House don't want no trash coming in the front door, huh?"

"You're not trash."

"Let's be honest, Marshal. I'm not exactly a member of the high society."

"Do you own a big winter coat, bandana, and hat?"

"Sure, but—"

"Wear them and we'll hurry past the desk clerk without any problem."

Milly flushed with excitement. "Would you like me to bring a little something in that coat to drink?"

"That'd be great."

She leaned close and whispered, "I could use a little help on the bottle, Marshal. No one gets rich in this line of work and I don't get paid until next week."

Longarm got the message. He added two silver dollars to his bill. "See you at ten."

"I can't wait."

Longarm sauntered outside wondering if he'd done the right thing or not. Milly was definitely attractive and he knew that she wasn't a tramp. Tramps didn't work as hard as he'd seen Milly work the past hour and he suspected she did very well with her tips despite the poor-mouthing. *Well, have a few drinks with her and let it go at that. You haven't enjoyed a woman's company since Denver. What's the harm?*

Longarm headed down the street to the White Lightning Saloon. When he entered the place was filled with loud conversation, laughter, and music, but his unexpected appearance changed that and the saloon fell silent.

"Well, well," a tall, square-jawed man with long black hair said loud enough for everyone in the saloon to hear. "If it isn't the marshal from Denver. What a surprise!"

Ignoring the man whom he figured was Jake Hawk, Longarm said, "Bartender, I'll have whiskey."

The bartender was a wizened fellow with a bad limp. He looked to Jake Hawk for permission and it must have been given because he poured Longarm a shot, then whispered, "Marshal, you better get out of here!"

"I'm in no hurry."

Longarm sipped the whiskey, then placed his back to the rail and saw that Jake had attracted four look-alikes, all heavily armed. "You must be Jake Hawk."

"That's right."

Longarm studied the senator's only son. The man's clothes were tailor made, his boots of the highest quality and his cartridge belt was beautifully hand tooled. In it rested a pearl-handled Colt that would have cost at least a hundred dollars in any Denver gun shop.

"Sorry about the death of your father," Longarm said. "But we'll get to the bottom of it before I leave Pagosa Springs."

Hawk was a strikingly handsome man. His face was un-

marked by fists or weather and his lips turned downward at the corners with a definite touch of arrogance. He had broad shoulders, but his eyes were red-rimmed with exhaustion. "Marshal," he said, "I don't want anything from you or any other lawman. We can handle our own affairs."

"That's right," echoed a man that Longarm judged a professional gunfighter. "We think you ought to go back to Denver tomorrow."

"Sorry," Longarm told them. "But I've got my orders and they are to find out who murdered Senator Hawk and Jason Snyder, the federal dispatcher. Once I do that, I'll arrest them and take them back to Denver for trial."

"Uh-uh," Hawk said. "You got it all wrong."

"Really?" Longarm casually shifted his whiskey into his left hand and hooked his right thumb on his gun belt. "How is that, Jake?"

"We know that Liberty killed them both and we're gonna hold a big necktie party for this town. So you can just leave Pagosa and go tell whoever gives you orders that everything is taken care of."

"I can't do that."

Jake barked a hoarse laugh. He looked to his right at the two men flanking him and then to his left. "Boys," he said, "I don't think that the marshal is very intelligent. Didn't I tell him to leave Pagosa Springs?"

They all nodded.

"But didn't he say he was staying?"

Again, the four nodded in agreement.

"Well then, I guess we'll just have to teach him a hard lesson."

"Hold on now," Longarm warned, finishing his whiskey and dropping the glass at his feet. "In the first place, you might get killed yourself. In the second place, my death would only bring more like me and you'd be charged with

murder and most certainly taken off in manacles, tried, and hanged."

Longarm let that one sink in for a few moments then added, "Now who is sounding smart or stupid?"

The gunfighter whispered something under his breath that Longarm was unable to hear. But it must have been a caution because Jake Hawk's face flushed with anger and he said, "Okay, Marshal. We won't kill you tonight. But the warning still holds. Get out of town and let us take care of our own affair."

"I won't do that."

"Then you might not be breathing very long."

Longarm walked up to Jake Hawk, looked into his bloodshot eyes, and whispered, "Is that a threat on my life?"

"Take it as you want."

"You've been drinking hard since your father was killed and it's taking a toll on your good sense," Longarm told the man. "I'm going to take that into consideration and let your words pass. But don't ever threaten me again. Are you wanted for any crimes?"

"Hell no!"

"I think you are a liar."

"You look like you are a walking dead man to me," the gunfighter said softly as his hand shaded his pistol.

"Mister," Longarm asked, "what is your name?"

"Casey."

"Full name!"

"George Casey."

"Well, George, my advice to you is to find a rock and hide under it before I step on you like a damned bug."

"Get out of here, George," Hawk said.

"But—"

"I said get out!"

Casey swallowed hard, spun on his heel, and left the saloon.

"He doesn't like you," Hawk said, "and neither do I."

"Too bad. I'm going to want to talk to your mother and sister tomorrow. Tell that man at your gate I'm coming back, and if he tries to stop me, I'll either kill or arrest him, I really don't care which."

Hawk nodded. "Marshal, my father would have contacted your boss and sent you packing. I can't do that but I have my own ways."

"Are you a back shooter, Hawk?"

"Hell no!"

"Then either make a move or shut up. I'm tired of your threats."

Jake Hawk stiffened and his face flushed with anger. He lowered his hand toward his gun and might even have drawn if the men beside him hadn't grabbed and hauled him out of the saloon.

The tension suddenly died and Longarm relaxed "Bartender, I'll have a refill."

"Marshal, I—"

"Now."

"Yes, sir."

Longarm got his refill and the bartender shouted, "Music!"

The music began to play, and when Longarm finally had a real good look at all the people in the saloon, he realized that Big Chief Ochoa was sitting at a back table with a gun in his fist. For just an instant, their eyes met and the Navajo smiled. Then, Ochoa finished his drink and headed outside.

Chapter 9

Longarm left the saloon about an hour later with a pretty good bottle of whiskey resting in his coat pocket. He was heading for the cafe to meet Milly and she was on his mind when someone suddenly appeared from the shadows, catching him off guard. Longarm reached for his gun, knowing he was too late if the shadowy figure's weapon was cocked and ready to fire.

"Relax, Marshal," Ochoa told him. "You'd already be dead if I intended to kill you."

Longarm took a deep breath. "I don't appreciate being startled."

"Sorry, Custis, but you need to understand that you've just become a very unpopular fella in Pagosa Springs. And, if you don't pay more attention to what is going on, you won't last long."

"What have you learned about the murders?"

"Not much," Ochoa admitted. "Liberty is out there but no one knows where he is hiding. My guess is that he is still on the Ute Reservation."

"What makes you think so?"

"Think about it, Marshal. Liberty is just a kid. Where

else can an Indian run to for help other than his own people?"

"Any chance that the Utes would turn him over to us?"

"Nope."

"Even to you?"

Ochoa smiled. "Which is to say that one Indian is the same as another, even if I am Navajo."

"That's *not* what I meant."

"I think it is, Marshal. But I'm thick-skinned so it doesn't matter. The fact is that they'd no more trust me than you."

"So where does that leave us?"

"You're the high-paid federal marshal. You tell me."

Longarm expelled a deep breath. "I'm going out to the Hawk Ranch and have a talk with the widow and the daughter."

"They won't tell you a damned thing."

"I've got to try."

"If you ask me, I think we ought to be concentrating on who would benefit the most from holding up—or even killing—that land sale. And once we've figured that out, talk to them."

Longarm could see the logic but also the problems. "I don't believe anyone would benefit except the Utes."

"If that is true, then Liberty probably did kill Senator Hawk and the dispatcher. But I'm not prepared to believe that without proof."

"Why not?"

Ochoa frowned. "This probably won't seem like much of an answer to your question, but the simple fact of the matter is that Indians aren't as conniving and devious as white people. If you told me that the kid got into a fight and killed someone . . . well, I'd accept that as the truth. But the idea that he hatched up a plan to kill the senator and that dispatcher just doesn't wash."

"What if someone put him up to the idea?" Longarm asked. "Someone like Jake Hawk."

"I dunno," Ochoa said. "As you discovered just a few minutes ago in the White Lightning Saloon, Jake Hawk is a hothead. And because of it, he doesn't strike me as the kind that would get anyone else to do his killing."

"I disagree. He has George Casey on his payroll and the man is definitely a hired gunfighter."

"Good point. But you also saw how Jake was ready to fight. He's not the kind that would stab his father and the dispatcher. Instead, he'd have shot them both full of bullet holes."

"What makes you think that the senator was stabbed?"

"Not 'think'," Ochoa corrected. "I *know* they were stabbed to death."

"How do you know?"

"I got lucky. The undertaker didn't run off to Mancos after all."

"You found him here in Pagosa?"

"Not exactly, but he didn't run very far."

"What did he say?"

"After plying him with a full bottle of whiskey, he confessed that both the senator and the dispatcher died of multiple stab wounds. And there's one other little thing you ought to know."

"I'm listening."

"Porter is scared."

"Of who?"

"Jake Hawk. The Black Widow. Even Della."

"Did he say that they threatened his life?"

"No. They're too smart to make that kind of boneheaded mistake. But Porter is no fool and he refuses to talk with you."

"Too bad," Longarm said. "I'm going to talk to him anyway."

"You might be signing his death warrant."

Longarm removed a cigar from his coat pocket. "All right, Big Chief, I'll stay away from the man . . . for now. But see if he can give you any more details."

"Such as?"

"Were they killed together? Or were they murdered in different rooms? And was there evidence of a fight?"

"Porter wouldn't know about that. The undertaker said that when he arrived, both bodies were already cleaned up, dressed in fresh suits, and laid out in separate upstairs bedrooms."

"Fine," Longarm said, "But ask your friend if their knuckles were bruised. Also, did either man have any other physical injuries?"

Ochoa frowned. "I just told you that they were both stabbed many times. What else could have happened to them?"

"They could have been shot first and then stabbed *in* the bullet wound. But more likely, they might have been poisoned and then stabbed to throw us off the track."

"I see what you mean. Okay, I'll ask Porter if he really inspected the corpses or just placed them in caskets. Anything else you want to know?"

"Not that I can think of at the moment. I'm going out to the Hawk Ranch tomorrow."

"So I overheard. Be careful."

"If I don't come back by tomorrow night then you can assume that I've been murdered," Longarm said. "In that case, telegraph my boss, Marshal Billy Vail. He works at the U.S. Federal Marshal's office. It's near the Denver Mint on Colfax Avenue."

"I know. I've been there to see how the big-time boys live," Ochoa said. "I was impressed with them, but I don't think the feeling was mutual."

Longarm glanced at his pocket watch. "It's ten o'clock and I've got an appointment."

"Oh?"

"Keep in touch."

"It would help if I knew who you were going to see at this time of the night."

"Why?

"Because, if you turn up dead in the morning, I'd have some idea of who to interrogate."

"She's a waitress named Milly."

"I remember her. She used to be Jake Hawk's woman but they had a falling out sometime back. Jake never was one to stay true to a woman and the word that I got was that he beat Milly up real bad a couple of times."

"Is that right?"

"Yep. Be careful what you say to her, Marshal. For that matter, be careful what you do to her!" Ochoa laughed. "But she is a looker. Good night and good luck when you go to the Hawk Ranch."

"Thanks."

Longarm went across the street to the cafe. He peeked through the window and saw Milly sitting all alone at a table. Rapping on the glass, he caught her attention and she hurried to the door.

"I wasn't sure that you would come," she told him.

"Why not?"

"Because I'm sure someone must have told you about Jake and me."

"That's history . . . isn't it?"

"Yes, and I don't know what I ever saw in Jake."

"How about rich and handsome?" Longarm offered.

"Sure, he's that." Milly put her hands on her hips. "But he's also the meanest man I ever met. He's arrogant and cruel, just like his mother and his sister, who never gave

me so much as a hello, even when Jake and I were talking about getting hitched."

"It went that far, huh?"

"I was a complete fool and Jake can be real charming. He had me wrapped around his little finger. And sure, I am poor and he is rich. He bought me some nice things and he took me to the best places in town. All of a sudden, I was a somebody in Pagosa Springs and I liked the feeling."

Milly stared up at Longarm. "Anything so terrible about that?"

"Nope. I'm just glad that you saw the light."

"Well, I did the day that Jake almost beat poor Arnie Andersen to death just for talking to me."

"Who is he?"

"Arnie was a nobody . . . just a big Swede from Minnesota and handsome as anything. He had blue eyes and this big square jaw and the cutest dimples in his cheeks. He liked to flirt, too. And that was his big mistake."

"Jake whipped him?"

"Not in a fair fight. Arnie was beating the hell out of Jake when George Casey interfered. George tripped Arnie from behind, then kicked him in the head when he fell. After that, Jake had the fight all his way. I never seen any man beat so bad as poor Arnie."

Milly's voice cracked and tears filled her eyes. "Jake broke Arnie's nose and one of his legs. Couple of ribs, too. When he finished, you couldn't even recognize the Swede. I tried to stop Jake, but he turned on me and I got whipped almost as bad as Arnie. Jake called me a whore. He loosened my teeth and blackened both eyes."

"And no one in this town tried to stop it?"

"Not even Senator Hawk, who watched the whole thing. You see, everyone in Pagosa Springs is afraid of the Hawks and their hired bullies. They'd have been crazy to try and stop the beating . . . especially with the senator watching."

"I wish that I'd have been there," Longarm told her. "What happened to the Swede?"

"Arnie disappeared just as soon as he could crawl out of the sickbed." Milly shrugged. "I don't know where he went, but I'm pretty sure it was far away. Jake stood over him with his gun drawn and I thought he was going to shoot Arnie to death right in front of everyone. But the senator yelled at Jake and the fight was over."

"So Senator Hawk saved Arnie's life."

"Maybe." Milly's expression was bitter. "But to my way of thinking, he let Jake and Casey do their damage. I doubt that Arnie will ever be quite the same after that kind of a beating. It would change almost any man, wouldn't it?"

"Maybe, but maybe not."

"I hope not. Arnie was sweet and fun loving." Milly waved her hand in front of her face as if to dispel a bad dream and took Longarm's hand. "Let's stop talking about what happened to Arnie Andersen. Let's talk about *us* and what we have on our minds for tonight."

"What do we have on our minds?"

"Did you bring a bottle?"

"Yes. It's right here in my pocket. The bartender at the White Lightning Saloon said it's the best he could offer."

"Good. Now do you still want to try and sneak me past the desk clerk at the Bonner House?"

"Yes. Did you find a heavy coat and hat?"

"I'll be right back," Milly said, her voice now gay and excited.

A few minutes later, she appeared wearing a floppy old felt hat, heavy workman's jacket, and dirty wool trousers and boots that Longarm was sure were much too large for her feet. "Marshal, what do you think? Will I finally make it into the respectable Bonner House?"

"Without a doubt."

"Then let's go."

Longarm started to put his arm around Milly's slender waist, but she pulled away. "Not yet," she said with a laugh. "I'm supposed to be a working*man*, remember?"

"You're right."

Longarm and Milly were laughing when they reached the Bonner House, then climbed the front steps, crossed the porch, and entered the lobby. They separated a little and both strolled across the floor without gaining the least bit of attention until they reached the staircase.

"Marshal Long?" the desk clerk called.

Longarm turned and asked, "What?"

"Apparently, you are inviting a friend up to your room."

"That's right."

The clerk studied Milly with disapproval. She kept her head down a little and Longarm was sure her face was hidden, but the clerk seemed curious and displeased so Longarm stomped over to his desk. "Don't tell me that there is a rule for taking a man upstairs to share a drink."

"No, but . . . well, he looks rather disreputable and—"

"But that's none of your business, is it?"

"No, but—"

"Then don't make me angry," Longarm growled. "I'm a federal marshal investigating the murder of Senator Hawk and a man named Jason Snyder. In the course of my investigation during the next few days, I'll interview anyone I choose in my own room. Is that perfectly clear?"

The clerk gulped and his Adam's apple bobbed up and down. "Of course, Marshal Long, it's just that this hotel—"

Longarm raised his finger and pointed it between the man's eyes. "Not another word or I will make your life very difficult. Is that understood?"

"Certainly."

"Good!"

Longarm turned and led Milly up the stairs to his room. Once inside, she threw off her hat and coat exclaiming,

"Custis, you sure put that uppity bastard in his place!"

"He was way out of line."

She hugged Longarm, and when their lips met he felt her hunger and desire all the way down to the tips of his toes. Pulling away, he said, "How about a glass of whiskey?"

"How about going to bed first?"

"You don't believe in wasting any time."

"No," she said, unbuttoning her blouse, "I do not."

Longarm watched Milly undress. She held him with her eyes, which were bold and provocative. It had been Longarm's intention to ask her a few questions about Jake Hawk and see if she could tell him anything important, but he guessed the questions could wait a little longer.

"Well," she asked, raising her arms overhead so that her large breasts rose enticingly, "What do you think?"

"I like it."

"Honestly?"

Longarm unbuckled his cartridge belt and draped it over the bedpost. Then he unbuttoned his pants and proved to Milly that he was telling her the truth because his manhood was already stiffening.

"Oh my gosh!" she exclaimed. "I've hit the jackpot."

Milly came over and dropped to her knees. She took his manhood into her mouth and sucked on it until Longarm was hard and trembling. Then he kicked off his boots, finished undressing, and pushed Milly down on the bed.

"This going to be very good," she panted.

"I know."

"Take me quick this first time," she hoarsely pleaded, raising her hips and spreading her legs.

Longarm mounted her and sighed with pleasure as the woman wiggled her bottom and pulled him even deeper into herself. When Longarm began to move his hips ever so slightly, she stuck her tongue in his ear and he felt her

hot breath and the words, "Come on Marshal, use me harder!"

Longarm was more than happy to oblige. He pistoned his big rod in and out, then around and around until Milly was moaning and her heels were wildly spurring the bedspread.

"Oh, Custis, you are making me feel so fine!"

"Come on, honey!"

Milly worked her bottom even harder and soon she was shivering and clawing his back in ecstasy, her legs gripping Longarm's thrusting hips, her body extracting every drop of his spurting seed.

It took them several minutes to catch their breath and when Longarm kissed her mouth and held her tight, Milly murmured, "This is the way I always thought lovemaking should really feel."

"Don't try and tell me you've never done it so good before," Longarm said.

"All right, I won't. But it was about the best I can remember in a long, long while. I think I need a drink now."

Longarm climbed off the woman and poured the whiskey. When they'd had a couple of swallows, he said, "You know why I'm here. Is there anything you can tell me that might help me figure out who killed the senator and that other fella?"

"Everyone thinks the Ute kid killed them, but not me."

"Why not?"

"I think Jake is your man."

"Why . . . other than the fact that he beat Arnie Andersen and you half to death?"

"Jake despised and feared the senator." Milly looked deep into Longarm's eyes. "I know that isn't real evidence, but he hated the senator worse than you can imagine."

"Why?"

Milly shrugged. "The senator was always humiliating

Jake. He'd put him down every chance he got . . . especially in front of important people."

"Any particular reason?"

"Jake got drunk once and told me that the senator didn't think he was capable of having children."

Longarm's eyebrows shot up in question. "Are you saying that Senator Hawk thought Jake was illegitimate?"

"That's it exactly."

"What did Jake think?"

"He agreed." Milly sighed. "The two didn't even look like father and son. Oh sure, they were both tall men with black hair, but the senator has a hooked nose and Jake's nose is dipped."

"Maybe Jake inherited his nose from his mother."

"No, hers is hooked, too. And Jake has high cheekbones and a square jaw unlike either the Black Widow or the senator. If you ask me, Senator Hawk not only thought Jake was a bastard, but he also thought he'd someday be his executioner."

"I see. But what if the senator was poisoned by the Black Widow . . . or even by Della?"

Milly shook her head emphatically "Della loved the senator. I mean, really loved her father."

"What makes you think so?"

"Because she would wait on him hand and foot. Because when they were together, you could just see the love between them. I never once saw Nettie Hawk show her husband the least bit of affection and Jake would practically break out in a sweat whenever his father was close because he hated the man so much. But Della was different from either of them."

Longarm thought of Billy Vail's story of how cruel Della could be and said, "From what I've heard, Della is as bad as her mother."

"She might have had to be to stay alive."

"I hadn't thought of that," Longarm admitted.

Milly took his hands in her own and pulled his body close to her own. "I don't want to talk about them anymore tonight. I just wish you could stay with me and avoid that family."

"I can't do that. I'm going to ride out to the Hawk Ranch and speak with Mrs. Hawk and her daughter tomorrow."

Milly hugged him tightly. "Then you might not come back."

"I'll come back and I'll bring you here tomorrow night."

"Promise?"

"Yes."

Milly reached down and began to massage his manhood. "How long do I have to wait for seconds?" she asked.

"Let's finish our drink and see what happens?" he suggested, thinking he needed just a little more time.

She giggled. "Marshal I feel it growing big again!"

"It remembers what it just did and it wants more of the same."

"Then," Milly whispered spreading her legs wide apart and guiding Longarm's stiffening manhood back into her honey pot, "it shall have all that it wants!"

Longarm groaned with pleasure and buried himself deep into her still hungry body.

Chapter 10

"Well, Ugly, this could get sticky," Longarm said to the strawberry roan as he drew near the pair of horsemen guarding the entrance to the Hawk Ranch. He recognized both men. One was Elden Hoag and the other was George Casey, the gunfighter he'd confronted last evening in the White Lightning Saloon. They were armed but not holding their weapons. Still, Longarm knew that both men were ready and eager to use them.

"Morning!" he cheerfully called out to the pair. "Nice weather we are having, isn't it!"

Neither of the Hawk riders said a word or offered a smile. Longarm took a deep breath and expelled it slowly. He kept Ugly moving forward at an easy trot and when he was within fifteen feet of the gate, he reined the gelding up and said, "I come to see Mrs. Hawk and her daughter."

"We know that," Casey told him with an edge in his voice.

"Well, then," Longarm replied. "What's our next move?"

"I'd like to put a bullet through your belly," Casey growled, "but we have orders to bring you up to the ranch. So come on through the open gate."

Longarm rode his horse onto the ranch. Still smiling, he said, "You can lead the way, boys."

"You ride ahead, we'll follow," Hoag hissed.

"Nope. I mean no offense, but I just don't trust you boys. Besides, I don't know the way to the house."

"You can almost see it from here," Casey hissed. "Just do as we tell you or we might forget our orders and kill you just for fun."

"Say, do either of you fellas know what time of day it is?"

Longarm's unexpected question caught both riders by surprise and the gunfighter snapped, "Who cares!"

"I do," Longarm replied, reaching for his pocket watch that seemed to be attached to his watch chain. Only instead of the watch, Longarm produced his twin-barreled,.44 caliber derringer, catching both men off guard.

Casey instinctively made a move for his sidearm, but when Longarm extended the little derringer outward, cocking it all in one smooth motion, the professional gunman froze.

"Smart move," Longarm told him as he drew his Colt and returned the derringer to his vest pocket. "Now both of you put your hands on your saddle horns and keep them there."

"You'll never get away with that one again," Casey snarled.

"I'll always outsmart you," Longarm told him. "And, if you try to draw on me, I'll put a bullet through your craw before you clear leather."

"Big talk!"

"The talk is over. Boys, turn your horses around and lead me to the ranch."

The pair had no choice except to do as Longarm told them, but they muttered obscenities all the way into the ranch yard.

"Thanks for your escort, fellas!" Longarm called as they trotted over to the bunkhouse.

The Black Widow and her daughter were standing on a wide veranda that belonged to one of the handsomest mansions that Longarm had ever seen in the West. It was a white, two-storied affair complete with pillars reminding Longarm of the many southern mansions he'd seen while growing up in Virginia. That seemed like a long time ago and he'd been a poor boy, but he'd seen the mansions and admired them even as he now did this one.

The Hawk mansion was a fitting backdrop for the pair of women who waited on its porch. They were both tall and statuesque, with Della being about five-ten and her mother maybe a couple of inches shorter. Their hair was the color of a raven's wing and the Black Widow's was streaked with silver. Even so, she was still handsome, although Longarm saw hardness and resolution in the deep lines of her once classically beautiful face. Della had no such lines marking her true character and Longarm judged her to be about thirty. He remembered that Billy had thought her addled—criminally insane, actually—but she appeared perfectly normal on this fine day. Her arms were folded across her bosom and she was wearing an expensive-looking riding habit while her mother wore a calico dress.

Touching the brim of his snuff-brown hat, Longarm smiled and said, "Good morning, ladies!"

"Hello, Marshal," Della said with a smile as her brown eyes measured him closely. "I hope you were welcomed to the Hawk Ranch properly by George and Elden."

"I was," Longarm replied. "Although I doubt that we are going to become good friends."

Della laughed and the sound of it was deep and a little strange. Longarm did not dismount because, out West, waiting for an invitation was always the polite thing to do.

"What is the purpose of your visit?" Mrs. Hawk demanded.

"I'd like to extend my condolences for the death of Senator Hawk. I am sure that he was well loved and respected not only by your family and friends, but by everyone who knew him."

The notorious old woman snorted with derision. "My late husband was a hard . . . but a good man. He sure wasn't a saint and he was hated by a lot of the people that knew him, you can be sure of that."

"Mother!" Della scolded.

"Well, you know that it's true. Your father would have admitted as much, so why should I stand here and lie to this damned lawman?" She looked right into Longarm's eyes and said, "I do not like small talk, Marshal. So state your intentions and then leave this ranch."

"I came to investigate the senator's sudden death."

Her eyes flashed and her chin lifted in a defiant posture. "My husband died of natural causes."

Longarm shook his head. "Uh-uh," he countered. "I know that isn't the case and so do you."

"Marshal, are you calling me a liar?"

Longarm knew that he was on very thin ice. Knew that even now Jake or someone else probably had him in their gunsights. "No ma'am."

Nettie Hawk's chest heaved up and down as if she had been running. Finally, she asked, "Then who says my husband died of any other cause?"

Longarm wanted to name the town undertaker, Gideon Porter, but understood doing that would probably be signing the man's death warrant. So instead, he smiled and told her, "Mrs. Hawk, I just think that the odds of your husband and that federal dispatcher dying together of natural causes is highly unlikely."

The Black Widow trembled with fury.

"Mr. Snyder had a bad heart and consumption among other chronic ailments," Della offered. "My father had also been feeling poorly for several weeks. He had frequent and severe fevers from an unknown disease. It is quite possible that my dear father gave Mr. Snyder his disease, which killed him within hours of their first meeting. Tragic, but hardly uncommon."

Longarm wasn't buying a word of that nonsense and replied, "I understand that neither man underwent an autopsy."

"That's right," the older woman said through clenched teeth. "If you were any kind of investigator, then you'd know we have no qualified physician in Pagosa Springs."

"What about the undertaker?"

"What about him!"

Longarm could see that this interview was going to be even more difficult than expected. It was equally clear that Mrs. Hawk was in no mood to offer him her hospitality. "Ma'am, would you mind if I watered my horse and stretched my legs? I would also appreciate a drink of cool water or whatever you have to offer from your kitchen."

Nettie Hawk said nothing.

"Mother?" Della asked, looking at her. "We may have lost Father, but we haven't yet lost all our manners."

"Phhtt!" the Black Widow hissed. "This stupid sonofabitch is here because he believes I murdered my husband and that sickly Mr. Snyder. I'm not going to offer him a thing except a way off my ranch before someone blows his silly ass out of the saddle!"

"Mother!"

But the older woman lifted her chin defiantly, turned, and stomped back into the house leaving Della Hawk and Longarm locked in an uncomfortable silence.

"Miss, my horse really is thirsty."

Della looked at the gelding and said, "Marshal, it would

be a mercy to let an animal that ugly die in the quickest manner possible."

Longarm had to laugh and so did Della, breaking their stiff silence. "I guess he is ugly. In fact, I *know* he's ugly! But it is equally true that he possesses the heart of a lion. He carried me over the Rockies hardly breaking a sweat or taking a deep breath. I never seen a horse like this one that could go so hard all day and still be fresh."

Della cocked her head a little to one side, pursed her lips, and said, "Marshal Long, aren't you exaggerating a little?"

He was not surprised that she knew his name. "No, Miss Hawk, I am not. Ugly is a remarkable animal."

"Well," she replied, "remarkable or not, he is too ugly to live."

Her response reminded Longarm of the chilling story Billy Vail had related concerning this person and the baby bird she had allowed the ranch cats to torment and finally devour. He couldn't help but wonder if Della was still as twisted as she had been at age fifteen. Looking at her now, it simply did not seem possible. Miss Hawk appeared to be intelligent, sociable, and she certainly was beautiful. Recalling Billy's dire warnings and seeing her now, Longarm had to conclude that the young woman was a complete enigma. Somehow, that made him all the more attracted to her in a way that he did not completely understand or even appreciate.

"Why don't you step down?" she asked. "The nearest water trough is right over there by the barn. I'll go in the house and get you a glass of cold lemonade. I'm afraid that you won't be invited inside. My mother is not very sociable under the very best of circumstances and the loss of my father has been hard."

"I'm sure it has been equally hard on you."

"In some ways it has been harder," the beautiful woman

admitted. "My father and I were very close."

"And was the senator also real close to your brother?"

Della smiled. "Are you already trying to wheedle information out of me about the Hawk family?"

"I was just curious."

"Then you will hear it said all over town that Jake and my father were not on good terms."

"Is that true?"

"Yes . . . I'm afraid so."

"May I ask why?"

"Why don't you either shoot that ugly horse or go give it a drink? Then come back and we'll sit on the porch and talk awhile, so long as you don't ask any real personal questions."

"Fine," Longarm told her. "But I am a federal lawman investigating the death of two men so you'd better understand that I didn't come all the way from Denver to talk about cattle prices and your fine mountain weather."

"I know that, and you should know in return that I'm not going to tell you anything different than my mother would say if she was sitting next to us both on the porch. I just couldn't."

Longarm nodded his acceptance and then led his roan off toward the water trough. Ugly wasn't really all that thirsty but the horse did drink. In the meanwhile, Longarm was trying to think of what to say to Della that would give him some fresh insights or information, yet not cause her to run him off in anger. After their conversation, he was of the opinion that riding out to this ranch was probably a big waste of time. The Black Widow was going to make sure that nothing important about the senator or Liberty would be divulged.

"Lawman," a thunderous and menacing voice said from behind. "Anybody who would ride that ugly a horse can't have any good sense."

Longarm turned to confront a giant. A man so huge that he could have found employment in a carnival freak show. The man stood at least a half foot taller than himself and probably weighed in the neighborhood of two hundred and eighty pounds, all of it muscle and bone. He had deep scars on his face and his nose had been busted so many times it looked like a cabbage, but Longarm could easily imagine the damage this ox of a man's opponents had suffered.

"My horse is ugly, all right."

"*You're* ugly. Your face looks like the butt of a mule."

"Right," Longarm answered, furious about the fact that the strawberry roan had suddenly gotten real thirsty and wouldn't raise its head from the trough.

"Lawman, I think you ought to kiss my bare butt," the giant announced.

"What?"

The giant turned around, unbuttoned his pants and dropped his drawers. "Kiss it!" he demanded. "Kiss it good or I'm gonna turn around and then I'll break your gawdamn neck."

Longarm couldn't believe what he was hearing from this oaf. But he did believe the man would button up his pants and then commence to break his neck. So there seemed to be no choice but to hit first and hit hard.

"Okay, Buster."

The giant laughed, then made the cackling sound of a chicken as he spread his legs and bent over at the waist.

Longarm dropped his reins, walked toward the huge man and then kicked with all his might so that his boot struck the giant where his legs forked, probably crushing his horse-sized gonads.

"Awhhhh!" the giant screamed, grabbing his crotch and hopping up and down like a fella in a sack race. When the huge fool hopped around with murder in his eyes then

114

reached for Longarm's throat, he got a second dose of the boot leather. "Awhhhhh!"

Longarm jabbed the screaming giant in the nose and then punched with a straight right cross to the neck. The huge man collapsed to his knees with blood streaming out of his nostrils and his mouth open, sucking for air. When he tried to stand up, Longarm kicked him in the jaw and sent him crashing over backward, laid out cold as a frozen fish.

George Casey, Elden Hoag, and two other rough-looking men came piling out of a huge wagon barn and Longarm drew his pistol, cocked it, and yelled, "This isn't your fight, boys! No reason to die over something that's not your concern."

The four Hawk cowboys skidded to a halt then looked past Longarm who heard Della shout, "Boys, stay out of it! Otto had a whipping coming to him that was long overdue."

"But Miss Della," Casey complained. "The marshal damn near killed him."

"I saw the fight and Otto got what was coming. Go back to work."

Longarm holstered his gun. "Thanks."

She looked at Otto and then at him with unconcealed admiration growing in her eyes. "You didn't need my help, Marshal. Otto has whipped a lot of men, sometimes as many as three or even four at a time. But you handled him like he was a baby. You're a real dirty fighter."

"I fight to win because I can't stand the pain of losing."

"I can see that."

"And the truth is, Miss Hawk, I—"

"Della. Call me plain old Della. But call my mother Mrs. Hawk or she'll have you skinned alive."

"Okay. Like I was saying, the truth is that I caught Otto completely by surprise. Next time, he'll be harder."

"I'll see that there isn't a 'next time' on this ranch."

"Much obliged."

"Lemonade on the porch is cold. Why don't you come up and rest yourself. Any man that can whip Otto deserves something stronger than lemonade, though."

"That will do for now."

"You married?"

"Beg your pardon?"

"I asked if you were married," Della said, leading him back to the house.

"No."

"That's good."

"Why?"

Della climbed the front steps and said, "Because you interest me."

Longarm tied Ugly and tried to think of a response. Finally, he looked up at the woman and asked, "Interest you how?"

"I'm not sure yet myself," she replied. "But I'd like to find out. Leave that ugly horse and come on up here to sit awhile with me. You are the most interesting man I have met in quite a long time. Maybe . . . maybe ever."

"I'm flattered."

"Don't be. Instead, beware."

Longarm raised his eyebrows in question and mounted the stairs. He took a seat in a white wicker chair and said, "That's an odd thing to say, Della. What do you mean?"

"I mean that I don't believe you are quite as dense as you'd like me to think. Mother said the same. You came here with your mind probably already made up about what happened to my father and Mr. Snyder."

"Really?"

"Yes. You came with the notion that either Mother or myself killed them."

Longarm shook his head. "Most people in these parts are pretty sure that the Ute Indian kid—what was his name?"

"Don't play stupid with me. You know his name."

"Oh yes, Liberty," Longarm said, forcing a disarming smile. "I heard that he worked here and that your father was quite fond of the kid."

"Treated him better than he ever treated my brother."

"So why would the Ute kill your father?"

"I'm sure you have heard of the land sale deal."

"I have, and that brings me to the question of where are those documents?"

"Mother burned them."

Longarm concentrated on his lemonade for a moment, then raised his eyes to hers and said, "Why?"

"We didn't agree with my father on the land sale."

"Why not?"

"We were interested in leasing some of that land for its timber."

"Without your father's permission?"

Della turned away for a moment and, as Longarm studied her face, he could see that she was under some inner conflict. "I need the answer to that question. Can you help me?"

"My father was hard underneath that outward appearance," she said, not speaking directly to Longarm. "He could smile at you and at the very same time be wanting to nail your hide to the barn door. He was best at hiding his feelings of anyone I ever knew and I was probably the only one who really ever understood him fully."

"And still liked and admired him."

"Not liked. *Loved* and admired him. But he was very stubborn about things and no one could change his mind. Not even me."

"Was the land deal fair for the Utes?"

"Hell, no! We'd have leased just a part of it from them for fifty years and then given it back. We'd have paid a

fair price for their timber and they'd still have owned the land forever."

"I don't understand why your father—"

"Like I said, he treated that Ute like a son. You see, in his younger days, when he'd come up here there was some trouble and he was one of a posse that caught and hanged a Ute for stealing cattle. But later, my father learned that the Indian they'd hanged was innocent and that one of the posse was the true cattle thief."

"I see."

"My father—and I can tell you this now—killed that man. Shot him from ambush with a rifle then buried his body under a rockslide. The body was never found and my father never told me where it was hidden. But I believed him about the hanging and I knew he lived in guilt about the innocent Ute he'd helped hang."

"Are you trying to tell me that was the real reason why he took Liberty into this house and treated him like a son?"

"It was a big part of it."

"Did Liberty kill your father and the dispatcher?"

"I think so."

"But you're not sure."

"No," Della said. "The house was empty. Mother and I were away when they died."

"How did they die?" There was a long silence and then Longarm pushed harder saying, "Stella, please don't tell me it was of natural causes because, if you do, I'll be sure that you or your mother killed them."

"All right," she finally answered. "My father and that other fella were stabbed to death."

"I see." Longarm sipped his lemonade and it was sweet. "Did Liberty have a knife?"

"Sure. A big hunting knife. And he knew how to use it."

"What does that mean?"

"People around here mostly hate Indians. We protected

118

Liberty from that as much as possible, but he would go off to Pagosa by himself sometimes. He liked to smoke and drink like most men and that's when he would get into trouble. Anyone from around here would know to lay off because he worked for us and was looked out for by my father when he was around. But sometimes, newcomers would try to pick a fight with Liberty."

"And succeed."

"Yes. He got beat up fairly regularly because he isn't a big man. I'd say Liberty doesn't weigh a whole lot more than myself. But he was very agile and quick. You know that game where you put your hands on the other person's hands and then try to slap him before he can pull back?"

"Yes."

"Liberty never lost. He was that quick. He bought a gun, but my father insisted he never wear it, much less practice on this ranch. But Father did allow him a hunting knife and the day came that some newcomer picked a fight and died for his mistake."

"Liberty stabbed him to death?"

"That's right. It's common enough knowledge. Happened about five years ago, so you'd have to ask someone that's been in town at least that long."

"I will." Longarm frowned. "What did you, Jake, and your mother think of Liberty?"

"I liked him. Mom and Jake hated him."

"Why?"

"Jake, because he was jealous of the way my father treated Liberty better than his own flesh and blood. Mother, because she just hates all Indians . . . especially Utes. She was a Kilbane when she grew up and a lot of her relatives were killed by Utes while they tried to tame this country and build this cattle ranch. She'll hate the Utes until the day that she dies."

"But you don't?"

"No. I think they got a real bad deal. It was me that talked Mother and Jake into seeing if we could block the land deal and lease Ute land. And believe me, that wasn't easy."

"I expect not, seeing as how your mother hated the Utes."

"Jake hated Liberty but he sort of admired him, too. Especially after he killed that fella in a knife fight. The man was from Arkansas and bragged that he was a bad knife fighter himself. Said that he was a cousin to Jim Bowie but I never believed that talk. No matter. Liberty carved a hole in that man's belly big enough to hide a cat."

"So, Della, what do you think will happen now with the proposed land sale?"

"I have no idea."

"I see." Longarm finished his lemonade and carefully placed it on the table. "Where do you think Liberty is hiding?"

"Marshal Long, I'm afraid that I haven't a clue."

"That sort of leaves me up a creek without a paddle, doesn't it?"

"I expect so." Della smiled, reached over, and placed her hand on Longarm's hand. "What's your first name?"

"Custis."

"Nice and strong . . . like you are."

"Thanks. And that's all you have to tell me?"

"For the time being."

"What does that mean?"

"It means that I might think of something more that you'd find interesting." Della looked over her shoulder at the front window. "But I don't think I could tell you sitting here."

"Then where?"

"Why don't we meet in three days up in the pines?"

Longarm stood up. "I don't have time for games, Della.

If you don't have something for me . . . then say so."

"I'll have something for you. Something good and important."

"Are you sure?"

"Positive."

"Then I'll see you in three days, unless I get a lead on Liberty and head off to find and arrest him."

"You'll never find Liberty unless he wants to be found. See that rocky outcropping to the west?"

"That one?" he asked, pointing.

"Yes. I'll meet you at its base about mid-morning three days from now. Come alone."

Longarm went down and mounted Ugly. "Della, you aren't plotting to kill me, are you?"

She laughed and there was nothing he could do but rein his roan about and ride away wondering.

Chapter 11

It was nearly sundown when Longarm rode back into Pagosa Springs. He put his roan up at the livery and started for the cafe when he spied Big Chief Ochoa coming in his direction.

"Well, Marshal, I see you survived the Black Widow and her daughter. What did you find out?"

"I'm hungry. Let's go eat and I'll tell you."

"Be better if we're not seen hanging around much together."

"All right." Longarm turned around and went back to the livery. He skirted the barn and wound up by a pile of hay where they could talk privately. "The truth is, I didn't find out a whole lot."

Ochoa scoffed. "Come on! We're both lawmen, remember?"

"Mrs. Hawk wasn't even civil. She employs a giant named Otto that wanted me to kiss his butt. Instead, I kicked him in the balls and he is going to be out of action for a while."

"You *whipped* Otto Klinger!"

"Yeah. The fool really did drop his pants and that made

him easy pickings. I expect he is still in a lot of pain."

Ochoa laughed. "Well, I didn't think anyone could whip that big bastard. If it'd been me, I'd have just shot him. What about Della?"

"She's as beautiful as her mother must have been at one time."

"And as deadly."

"I'm not so sure of that," Longarm replied. "She gave me lemonade on her front porch and—"

"And it wasn't even poisoned?" Ochoa teased.

"Nope. At least, I don't feel anything yet."

"You've more guts than good sense. And, I suppose while Della was acting like a proper lady and telling you how much she loved her poor old father, she also said that Liberty really did kill the senator and the federal dispatcher."

"That's right."

"Bet she even told you about the man that Liberty stabbed to death in a knife fight some years ago."

"She said he was from Arkansas and probably got exactly what he deserved. Della told me that people picked on Liberty all the time when he came here to town."

Ochoa wasn't smiling anymore. "At least that much is true. What else did she say?"

Longarm thought a moment, then answered, "Would you believe she told me that she and her mother and brother opposed the Ute land sale?"

"No!" The Navajo's smile slipped. "I wouldn't believe that for a minute."

"Why not?"

"Because it makes no sense."

"Della said that they wanted a fifty-year *lease* on the Ute timberland and were willing to give the Indians a fair price."

"Oh, sure!" Ochoa snorted with derision. "They are just

a bunch of good Samaritans out to right the past full of wrongs."

Longarm didn't appreciate the man's heavy dose of sarcasm. "Look. I don't know what to believe . . . yet. But Della struck me as someone who was telling the truth."

"I thought you were smarter than that, Marshal! Don't you know that the whole family *hated* Indians? The senator even helped to hang an innocent one accused of rustling a couple of old cows years ago."

"Della told me about that and how much guilt it caused Senator Hawk for the rest of his life. She said that was the primary reason he took Liberty into the house and treated him like a son."

"Bullshit!"

"Then why did the senator adopt the boy?"

"How should I know? Maybe Liberty is his son . . . or even his grandson."

"What is that supposed to mean?"

"You haven't seen our prime suspect and sweet Della probably didn't bother to tell you that Liberty is not a pure-blooded Ute."

"That's news to me."

"There's still a lot you don't know about what is going on around here. But I have a suggestion."

"Spit it out."

"Let's meet outside of town tomorrow morning about eight and ride over to the Ute Reservation. We can talk to their chief and get another side of the story."

"But you told me they wouldn't talk to either of us."

"Maybe I was wrong. I actually have made a few mistakes in my life."

"Have you found out anything more to shed light on things?"

"I spoke to the undertaker again. He said that there were no obvious signs of a fight. No bruises on the senator's

knuckles. No evidence of any other cause of death."

"No bullets and no poison?"

"Not that he could detect." Ochoa frowned. "He's real scared, though. I'm not sure he will ever tell the complete story, but I believe what he's told me so far."

"Is Liberty a hothead like Jake?"

The Navajo frowned. "I really didn't know the young man but I've seen him a few times. My impression is that he's withdrawn until he's chugged a few drinks and then he starts to feel like a big man. Liberty is about five-feet-ten-inches, but slender and he probably doesn't weigh one-fifty. I heard he was whipped a lot when he was a kid and I think it made him bitter toward most whites . . . not that that is so unusual."

"I suppose not."

"I also know that he finally learned to take care of himself."

"You mean with a Bowie knife?"

"Yes. And his fists. He has very quick hands and is a lot stronger than he appears. When sober, he could give anyone a good fight."

"Della thinks that he suddenly got mad at the senator and stabbed him to death, then turned on Snyder just to eliminate any witnesses."

"Yeah, she'd say that," Ochoa agreed, not bothering to hide his disgust. "Did Miss Hawk also happen to mention where she, Jake, and the Black Widow were at the time of the murder?"

"They were off someplace."

"How convenient. No outside witness I'd expect."

"That's right."

"I don't buy a word of it. Della is trying to protect herself and her mother. Can't you see that?"

"I can see that she isn't crazy. I can also see that you

125

are probably as interested in saving another Indian as she is her family."

"I'm a bounty hunter. I don't play favorites."

"I hope not. Anything else?"

"Watch out for Otto Klinger. He is definitely crazy."

"I'll see you in the morning," Longarm told the Navajo. "Which end of town?"

"West end. The reservation stretches all over the place but we can find out where Liberty came from easy enough."

"But not where he is hiding."

"That's right."

Longarm headed back toward the cafe. He wasn't a bit sure what good it would do to visit the Utes, but he had no other ideas of how to start unraveling the mystery of two murders, so he guessed a visit to the reservation was as good a place to start as any.

"Why hello, Marshal!" Milly cried, hurrying over to his table. "You look kind of discouraged."

"I am." Longarm smiled at some of the other customers who were listening. "Why don't you get me a big, juicy steak with lots of potatoes and then I'll finish with a piece of cherry pie . . . but only if you baked it."

"I sure did."

Milly's fingers brushed his sleeve and then she moved away to fill another customer's empty coffee cup and go give someone in the kitchen Longarm's dinner order.

"Say Marshal, you got any leads on where we can find that murderin' Injun yet?" a man asked from the next table.

"Nope."

"When you find Liberty . . . you find the senator's killer. And, if I was you, I'd start on the bastard's reservation. That's for sure where he's hiding out."

"Maybe I'll pay them a visit."

"You'll want to form a posse first. I'll pass the word around and tomorrow morning we can—"

126

"Never mind," Longarm said quickly. "I'd just as soon handle it myself."

"Marshal, if you go out there alone," another customer said, throwing in his opinion, "you ain't likely ever to be seen again. Them Indians don't like white men and they positively hate a white lawman. You better form that posse, Marshal, or you'll end up facedown in the pines with a bunch of damned arrows stickin' out of your back!"

Longarm was in no mood for this kind of talk. "I appreciate your advice, boys. But I'd also appreciate if you let me eat in peace and kept your opinions to yourself."

They were offended but he didn't give a damn.

"Coffee, tea, water, beer, or whiskey?" Milly asked coming over to his table.

"I'll have a beer while I'm waiting for my steak and potatoes."

"Coming right up."

Milly gave him a smile that cheered Longarm considerably and when the beer arrived, his mood lightened even more. "Thanks."

"Same time, same place after work?" she whispered low so that the other customers couldn't overhear.

"I'm a little wore out tonight. How about another time?"

Milly's smile faded. "Custis, are you giving me the brush?"

"All right. Same time. Same place."

"Not if you have to force yourself."

Longarm drained his beer and held out the empty glass for a refill. "I'll be here at ten. You be ready."

Her radiant smile returned. "Yes, sir!"

There were snickers all around the room but Longarm didn't care. He would enjoy Milly but get more sleep tonight. And who knows what tomorrow might be when they went out on the Ute Reservation.

• • •

It was about eleven o'clock and Longarm was worn out. Their lovemaking had been long and passionate, so he was ready for sleep.

"Close your eyes," she told him as she began to dress. "I'm going back to my place."

"You can stay here all night."

"I know. But I'm also tired and I can sleep a little later if I leave now. Anyway, our date was very nice."

Longarm laced his fingers behind his head and stared up at her. "You're a fine-looking woman, Milly."

"Do you mind if I consider that as your idea of a marriage proposal?"

Longarm stammered, "I . . . I—"

"I was only kidding. It's all right. I know that you'll be leaving when you've solved this murder case. But maybe I'll be leaving with you."

"Oh?"

"I've a sister who lives in Denver. We always got along well together and she's been urging me for years to come there and start over with my life. Custis, wouldn't it be nice to see each other on a regular basis!"

"Sure would," he said, knowing that would not square too well with Karen Lacy.

"I'm leaving now. Shall I turn out this lamp?"

"Thanks and good night."

Milly was fully dressed and Longarm was naked as he lay on the top of the bed. Studying him, she clucked her tongue with appreciation and said, "You are a fine specimen of manhood."

"I'm glad you think so, Milly."

She kissed him tenderly, then went over to the nightstand. "Custis, do you want me to open this window a little more? It feels kind of stuffy in here."

"Go ahead."

Milly reached for the window and as she raised it up, a bullet crashed through the glass. Longarm vaulted off the

128

bed, grabbing his pistol and kneeling beside her. The only apparent injury he could see was a scratch on her cheek. "Stay down! Are you hit anywhere bad!"

"No," she whispered, her body trembling. "I think a piece of flying glass nicked my cheek. What happened?"

Longarm grabbed his pants and pulled them on, then he sneaked over to the busted window and gazed out into the dimly lit street and saw a huge silhouette with a pronounced limp hurrying away. Longarm swore, "Otto Klinger!"

There was no time to finish getting dressed and no time to go downstairs through the lobby if he wanted to apprehend the man that had mistakenly fired on poor Milly. Longarm rushed over to the washbasin, wet a towel and wiped away her blood.

"Press this to your cheek."

"Where are you going?"

Longarm shoved one leg through the window. He would drop to a porch only a few feet below, then be able to jump to the street without much difficulty. "I'm not letting that big sonofabitch get away with an ambush. Everyone downstairs will be coming out to see what all the excitement is about. That's when you should sneak out through the lobby."

"Okay, but be careful!"

Longarm landed on the roof of the porch, then vaulted to the empty street below. He took off running in the direction that the giant had been moving and ran as hard as he could until he saw big Otto struggling up into his saddle. The giant was riding a draft horse.

"Hold it!" he shouted, raising his weapon. "You are under arrest for attempted murder!"

Longarm couldn't see the giant's expression but he heard the roar of his curses and then Otto was sawing on his reins and bringing his own gun up as he sent the draft horse lumbering toward his hated enemy.

129

"Stop or I'll shoot!"

Otto opened fire, but even an expert marksman would have found it almost impossible to shoot accurately while that big draft horse was trotting forward. Longarm raised his pistol and took careful aim, knowing that he was not in any great danger from being shot, but only from being trampled.

His first bullet caused the giant to throw up his arms and raise himself in his stirrups. Longarm drilled the easy target four more times before Otto Klinger somersaulted off the back of his draft horse. Longarm heard the air whoosh from Otto's lungs and the solid "thunk" of his head as it struck the hard-packed earth.

The big horse finally lurched into a gallop and lumbered past Longarm, who calmly reloaded his pistol. There was no hurry because he knew without even examining the corpse that Otto was dead.

"Good riddance," he said aloud.

Now that the danger was past, Longarm was aware of the sharp rocks bruising the bottoms of his tender feet as he advanced to examine the giant's blood-stained body. He searched Otto's pockets but didn't find anything of interest or value. As he finished, several guests and employees of the Bonner House ran up looking all excited.

"Holy Hannah!" one yelled. "It's Otto!"

"He tried to shoot me through my bedroom window," Longarm explained. "Fortunately, he missed."

"Bad mistake," another onlooker said, eyes fixed on the giant. "But I do have to say that Otto Klinger was the stupidest man I ever met and plenty ornery. He beat up a lot of men here in Pagosa and enjoyed every minute of it, so I say good riddance!"

"My sentiments exactly," Longarm replied, walking back to the hotel and seeing Milly dash outside without anyone noticing.

Longarm waved to the woman and she blew him a hurried kiss. Then he went inside and fell into bed. There was glass scattered all over the floor, but he wasn't about to clean it up.

Had Klinger really planned to ambush him and escape? Or had the idiot been put up to the job by the Black Widow . . . or Jake or Della? Longarm had no idea, but it seemed possible the giant had conceived the plan by himself. After all, he had been beaten quite badly and had probably suffered the brunt of cowboy humor back at the bunkhouse. Longarm figured there was no way of even knowing if Otto Klinger had been instructed to kill him or not.

But he would ask that question of Della when he met her in a couple of days.

Chapter 12

"Hey!" Ochoa called, galloping up on his little buckskin pony, "I heard about all the excitement last evening. Looks like the fun has already started."

"You call my gunning down a would-be assassin 'fun'?"

"I expect that it was a lot more enjoyable for you than it was for that idiot Otto, wasn't it?"

"Sure, but he almost killed Milly by mistake."

"You would be wise not to mess with that pretty gal anymore," Ochoa said. "You could infect her with a sudden and terminal case of lead poisoning."

"We'll be more careful in the future."

"I've heard that one before."

"Let's talk about the Utes," Longarm told him. "I've been on their reservation before."

"Liberty comes from this northwest corner and his people don't live but about twenty miles away."

"Do you think they know where he's hiding?"

"Of course. And I'd also be willing to bet that they are supplying him with food and shelter and are prepared to do so until we give up the chase."

"This is a big and a tough country," Longarm said. "I don't see how we could ever find him."

"We couldn't," Ochoa agreed. "Jake Hawk and his people know this country better than we do and they couldn't catch Liberty. The only way that we can find him is to either convince his family that we mean to help or if Liberty gets stupid and makes a mistake."

"What kind of a mistake?"

"Maybe he decides to come in and drink a little whiskey."

"He wouldn't do that, would he?"

"Probably not," Ochoa conceded. "So that means we have to convince his family and people that he'll get a fair deal . . . if he surrenders to you."

"If he's innocent, he just might surrender, but if he's guilty of those murders, he'll never give himself up," Longarm said.

"Well, at least that tells us something important."

Longarm saw the truth in that and nodded his head. "Why don't we pick up the pace a bit and see if we can get there by noon."

"What's the hurry?"

"The hurry is that we didn't bring any supplies to stay overnight on the trail. I mean, unless the Utes invite us into their tepees, we're going to be in the saddle half the night, aren't we?"

"There's a trading post located at the edge of the reservation. It's run by a friend of mine and he'll take care of us tonight."

"That's good to hear," Longarm replied, pushing Ugly into an easy gallop that left Ochoa and the buckskin struggling to keep up the pace.

Three hours later, they dismounted at a log cabin and tied their horses to a hitching rail, then stomped inside

where Longarm met Ochoa's friend, the Indian trader named Boone. He was a small man who looked to be in his fifties but was spry and of good humor. Boone greeted them warmly and invited them into his little trading post.

"It's good to see you, Big Chief. I suppose that you're here on account of the senator and that other poor bastard gettin' murdered."

"I am."

"And you're looking for that Ute named Liberty that everyone thinks killed the senator and that other fella."

"Right again," Ochoa said. "Do you know where we can find him?"

"If I knew that," Boone answered, "I could sell the information and retire to a rocking chair. Jake Hawk and his boys have offered me quite a lot of money to lead them to the Ute but I couldn't help them either."

Longarm stepped forward. "Do you know Liberty?"

"Sure. And I know his family, too. They're all real decent people. I've been trading with them for years. Knew Liberty when he was just a little shaver and liked him even then."

"It sounds like you don't think he is our murderer," Longarm offered.

Boone scratched his scraggly beard. "I can't say one way or the other. You probably heard about how the senator took him into the Hawk mansion and treated him like a son. More than a son, in fact. And I'm sure that you've heard everyone in Pagosa Springs say that they *know* Liberty is a murderer."

"That's right."

"Don't be too quick to believe it," Boone advised. "Liberty did kill a man in a pretty ugly knife fight so I ain't sayin' he for sure isn't your man. All I'm sayin' is that there are a lot of folks at the Hawk Ranch who might have killed the senator, starting with his wife, his daughter, and

his son. Any or all of them could have committed the murders."

"Boone," Ochoa said, "let's have a drink and then you tell us who *you* think killed Senator Hawk and the dispatcher."

"Good idea."

Boone led them into his crowded little post and through a maze of merchandise piled nearly to the ceiling. Longarm saw blankets, traps, cases of tinned goods, boots, clothes, and dresses among other things. There were also some old saddles hanging from the ceiling and a few rifles that looked as if they'd come right off a Civil War battlefield. All in all, it was quite a collection.

"You've got some trading post," Longarm remarked.

"Wanna buy it?"

"No."

Boone hooked his thumbs through his suspenders. "I'd part with the post and everything under this roof for . . . oh, two thousand dollars. You can't go wrong with a price like that. Make you a good and an easy livin'."

"What's the matter," Ochoa said, "business been a little poor lately?"

"Why you ask me a fool question like that!" the trader demanded.

"Because the last time I was here, which was less than three or four months ago, you told me you wanted four thousand dollars. I just wonder why the price went down by half."

"I didn't think you'd remember that figure, Big Chief. And, to be honest, business has been real poor. The Utes are upset, and even though I had nothing to do with any of that vigilante stuff that Jake and his friends are doing, they've cooled toward all us white . . . me included!"

Boone looked hurt and a little outraged, Longarm thought as they bellied up to a rough plank laid across a

pair of empty whiskey barrels. Boone grabbed a bottle and asked, "Whiskey?"

"What else?" Ochoa replied, looking at Longarm, who nodded his approval.

Boone filled three dirty water glasses and raised a toast. "To finding and hanging the real killer of Senator Hawk and that other poor bastard."

They drank and Boone smacked his lips. "You boys can spread a couple of my trading blankets on the floor and rest easy tonight. I expect you've come to talk to Liberty's family."

"We have," Ochoa said. "Now tell us who you think is the *real* murderer?"

"I think it's the Black Widow and her daughter. They are both capable of the foul deed."

"I don't think Della would have murdered her father," Longarm said. "Everyone says she loved him very much."

"Yeah, I expect that she did," Boone agreed. "But she would do it if her own life or welfare depended on it."

Longarm leaned forward, elbows on the plank. "Meaning?"

"Meaning that it would not surprise me if the Black Widow forced Della to do in her father and that dispatcher."

"For what reason?"

"Money." Boone looked from one to the other. "Or didn't you boys bother to learn all about that land sale deal that the state was trying to push?"

"We heard about it," Longarm replied. "Mrs. Hawk even admitted that she burned the documents."

"Oh?" Boone's eyebrows raised and his brow furrowed. He was a filthy little man and his facial creases formed black lines. "Well, from what I heard, it was a good deal for the state of Colorado and a real bad deal for the Utes."

"That seems to be the general consensus," Longarm remarked. "Della told me that she and her mother tried to

talk the senator into killing the deal so they could lease some of the Ute land for the valuable timber."

"Well, there you have it! The senator wouldn't cave in and them two women had him killed or maybe even did it their own selves."

Longarm glanced at Ochoa and he could tell from the Navajo's expression that he wasn't buying that explanation either. But there was no sense in arguing so Longarm choked down his rotgut whiskey and said, "We'd better get going if we plan on seeing Liberty's family today."

"They only live about ten miles south of here," Boone said. "I don't see any big hurry."

"Let's go," Longarm insisted, dropping some coins on the plank and heading for the door.

"Your big friend sure is restless," Boone said.

"I know," Ochoa agreed. "We'll see you this evening."

"Be careful on the reservation. Jake, George Casey, and some of the other men from Pagosa have really stirred them up like a nest of hornets. They're real touchy right now and you'll have to be careful how you ask your questions."

"I will be," Ochoa promised, following Longarm back out to their horses.

"There it is, Marshal, the Ute village."

Longarm stared down at the miserable collection of wooden huts and tepees. He could see Indians resting in front of their places while their kids enjoyed the afternoon warmth. Some of the older boys were riding off to hunt and a large group of women were tanning hides over near a small stream. The Utes had a horse herd, but it was small, numbering less than twenty animals.

"Not too prosperous looking, is it?" Ochoa asked.

"Nope."

"Before the white man came and penned them onto this reservation, the Utes were a hunting people like my own.

They went over the mountains and hunted the buffalo. There were even some mountain buffalo up in the surrounding big valleys. But, of course, they were all wiped out by the hunters."

"Did you trade with the Ute?"

"Sure. We generally got along well, although they were the worst horse thieves I ever saw. The Ute took a lot of pride in having more horses than they could ever use. They'd steal a horse they traded to you the day after you owned him. Then, the next year, they'd ride that horse onto Navajo land and try to sell him to us all over again. Now, they don't have many horses and the buffalo are gone, finished off by the prospectors that poured into this country. Today, these people just sit around and live off your government. This land isn't any much good for farming, so the only thing they can do is trap, raise horses and sheep, and take odd jobs in town that are too hard or disagreeable for white men. It's a sad ending for the Ute."

"Who is the leader of this bunch?"

Ochoa pointed. "You see that ramble shack with the tepee sitting right by the front door?"

"Yeah."

"That's their headman's house. It was also Liberty's."

Longarm blinked. "Liberty was the son of a chief?"

"No big deal anymore in that," Ochoa responded. "You see, since Chief Ouray died, these people have no real leadership and they are too poor to live together. Not enough game or grass for that so they live a small bunch here and there all over the reservation. Maybe once a year, they try to get together, but they're a defeated and bitter people."

"All right," Longarm said, "let's go down there and see what we can find out."

"My guess is that we won't find out much. What I think might be important, however, is to tell the chief that we aren't so sure that Liberty is a murderer."

"Can he speak English?"

"Some." Ochoa frowned. "You show him your badge. That won't impress him very much, but at least he will know that you have some authority. The Ute respect authority. Tell them that, if they turn over Liberty to us, he will be taken away and get a fair chance to speak his peace."

"I will," Longarm vowed, nudging Ugly with his boot heels and starting down the long slope into the valley.

When they were spotted by the children, everyone stopped what they'd been doing and came to their feet. They gathered by the chief's wooden shack and waited as Longarm and Ochoa rode into their squalid village with dogs barking and nipping at their horse's heels. Both Ugly and Ochoa's runty little buckskin pony kicked a couple of them hard and that sent the pack off to keep their distance.

"We come to speak to Chief Moy-ahni," Ochoa announced to an old woman dressed in buckskins and beads.

Longarm decided that the woman was the chief's wife and she went into the shack and in about five minutes, Moy-ahni appeared. He was not a tall man but he was dressed in fine white buckskins with beaded moccasins and an eagle feather in his silver hair. Longarm had no idea how old the man might be, but he looked to have lived a good many years.

"Great Chief Moy-ahni," Ochoa began, after dismounting and making a slight bow to the stoic old man, "we come to speak of very serious matters concerning your son, Liberty."

"Speak, Navajo."

"I would like you to meet my friend, United States Deputy Marshal Custis Long. He has come a long way to see that justice is done for your son and for Senator Hawk and the other dead man."

The chief turned the focus of his attention on Longarm

who also dismounted and made a slight bow of respect.

"Show him your big, shiny badge," Ochoa hissed under his breath.

Longarm produced his badge and the chief stepped forward to study it closely. He even seemed to be reading it, although Longarm doubted that was the case. Finally, the chief stepped back and made a sweeping gesture with his arm to indicate that he was willing to speak inside the tepee.

The old woman opened the flap and the chief entered first followed by Ochoa and then Longarm. The floor was covered with more buffalo robes and there were a number of bows and quivers of arrows, some decorated with eagle's feathers, stacked on one side of the tepee. On the other were several woven reed baskets in various stages of construction.

"Great Chief Moy-ahni," Ochoa began. "I am sad about the grief that these killings has caused for you and your people. I do not believe that your son, Liberty, killed those two white men. However, by hiding, he points the finger at himself."

Ochoa pointed his own index finger to his chest. "When a man is guilty, he runs. When he is innocent, he stands before all who will listen and tells them of his innocence. We believe Liberty is innocent."

"He is innocent," Moy-ahni said slowly. "Liberty no kill senator or other mans. Only kill one mans with big knife."

"I need to ask him questions," Longarm said. "I have to find out who did kill those men and then take them away to a jail where they will speak their peace and be judged by other white men. This is called a trial by jury."

"I know this," the old chief replied. "Liberty be hanged."

"Not if he is innocent."

"He innocent." The chief raised his forefinger and pointed it first at Longarm then at the Navajo. "You mens

find mens who kill senator and other mens. Then my son come to speak his peace."

"Maybe your son knows who these men are," Longarm persisted. "We need his help if he is to be judged innocent. Unless we can find the men guilty of these murders, I must find and take Liberty far away to a jail."

"White mens judge my son guilty and hang him. Choke by neck until blue in face."

The chief tilted his head to one side, stuck his tongue out, and made a strangling sound as he rolled his eyes. It was, Longarm thought, too accurate and vivid a pantomime to be guessed at. Clearly, Chief Moy-ahni had been witness to at least one hanging and quite probably a good many more, and Longarm was willing to bet they had been Utes who had been lynched by white vigilantes.

"Talk to him in Indian or something," Longarm whispered. "We aren't getting anywhere this way."

"I don't know Ute very well."

"Try!"

Ochoa began to converse haltingly. Soon, the two Indians were having a lively conversation. There was much nodding of chins but even more shaking of heads. At times, their voices took on anger and then changed to reason. After what must have been a good hour of negotiations, both men stopped speaking.

"Well?" Longarm asked quietly.

"The chief wants to know if you can be trusted."

"And you told him?"

"I told him I thought so, but was not sure."

"What!"

"If I had said anything else, he might have thought me dishonest."

"Then—"

"He has agreed to bring Liberty to trading post tomorrow at about noon. There is to be only ourselves and Boone.

141

No one else. If there are any more white men even close to the trading post, they will run away and promise that they will never bring Liberty out of hiding again. Instead, he will live in the high mountains and grow old there until he goes to the Spirit World."

"That's great news! Tell Chief Moy-ahni that I agree to his terms."

"He also says that Liberty will not go away with us and that, if we try to take him by force, there will be much bloodshed and we will die."

Longarm's spirits dropped. "Tell the chief that I agree to this. But also tell him—"

"Speak to me!" Moy-ahni angrily demanded. "I am old but I can still hear forked tongues wag!"

"I am sorry, Great Chief of the Ute people," Longarm apologized. "I have forgotten my manners and was disrespectful." He dug into his pocket and found a gold coin. Handing it to the chief, he added, "Please take this as a gift and a sign of my respect for yourself."

"Excellent!" Ochoa whispered.

The chief was clearly impressed and pleased by the gold, but suspicious enough of its worth that he bit into it to test its mettle. Satisfied that the coin was real gold, he grinned and then reached for his peace pipe.

"Don't start choking on the smoke," Ochoa warned.

"Don't worry."

They smoked the peace pipe until the tepee became extremely smoky and then their meeting was past. Longarm and Ochoa mounted their horses and rode away, waving good-bye. The adults just stared at them, but the children laughed and waved back in return.

"What do you think?" Longarm asked.

"I was surprised that he would agree to do that."

Longarm took a deep breath. "This could mean we finally get to the bottom of the murder."

"Liberty will not give himself up . . . even if he is guilty," Ochoa said. "And you cannot break your word to Chief Moy-ahni and try to arrest him."

"I know that."

"Well, then, where does that get us?"

Longarm shrugged. "I'm not sure, but whatever happens, it will be a step forward and not backward."

"We hope."

Longarm heard the skepticism in Ochoa's voice but refused to be discouraged by it. As far as he was concerned, a door had been opened and they were finally about to make some real progress in the murder case.

Chapter 13

Longarm slept well that night and didn't wake up until midmorning when some boisterous miners barged into the trading post hooting and hollering for whiskey. In the poor light of the room, they almost trampled on him as they hurried toward the back bar shouting and carrying on at the top of their lungs.

"Holy hogfat!" one of them yelled, "there's a damned dead man layin' at my feet! He musta drunk too much of Boone's firewater!"

Longarm roused and sat bolt upright. "I'm Marshal Long," he told the man, "go up another aisle and simmer that noise down."

The prospector stared at him. "You're the marshal?"

"That's right."

"That big fella that gunned down Otto Klinger?"

"That's me."

"Well what—"

"Never mind," Longarm told him, pushing to his feet. "Just tone that yelling down and go about your own business and let me go about mine."

"Well now," the prospector said, "I never saw a lawman

144

whose business it was to sleep all day on the floor of a trading post!"

Longarm was still a little groggy and his head was hammering from the whiskey he'd drunk last night with Boone and Ochoa. Without bothering to try to further his explanation, he shoved past the prospectors and stumbled outside. He went over to a nearby creek, knelt and doused his face in the cold, clear water, immediately feeling better.

"Rough morning?" Ochoa asked with a big grin.

Longarm turned and looked at the Navajo, who did not seem much fresher than himself. "What time is it?"

"Midmorning. You sure got your beauty sleep, Marshal."

Longarm was in no mood for small talk. "Coffee?"

"Yeah, there's some on that fire yonder. Boone likes to cook in the open. It's a habit from his trapper days. But I'll warn you it is strong enough to burn the bark off a pine tree."

"Then it's exactly what I need," Longarm replied.

Two hours later, Longarm had eaten all the food and drunk all the coffee his gut could stand. He was ready and waiting for Chief Moy-ahni and Liberty to appear and then he remembered that the chief had insisted there be no other white men nearby when they arrived.

"Ochoa!" he yelled. "We've forgotten our promise to the chief about no other whites when they arrive with Liberty!"

The Navajo's jaw dropped and then he slapped himself in the side of the head. "Let's get them out of here now."

Longarm and the Navajo burst back inside of the trading post and hurried to the makeshift bar. Longarm shouted, "The saloon has just closed."

"Are you crazy?" Boone yelled over the protests of his shocked customers. "These boys have cash money!"

"Yeah, but the bar is closed anyway. Tell them to come back tomorrow."

"We would have anyway," one of the already drunken prospectors carped. "And we're happy about being here right now. Ain't that right, boys?"

There were four of them and they all enthusiastically agreed.

Longarm pulled out his badge and shouted, "Leave now or I'll arrest the lot of you."

"You and whose army?" a prospector challenged.

"Custis," Ochoa said nervously, "I don't think we want to do this."

"We don't have any choice."

"Choice about what?" a prospector demanded to know.

"They have to go now," Longarm said, drawing his gun and putting a bullet into the dirt floor. His shot sent the prospector scurrying for the door and lest they changed their minds Longarm dogged their heels all the way.

"Dammit, Marshal," one of the prospectors whined, "what in blazes has gotten the matter with you? Ain't drinkin' hard liquor legal here anymore or something?"

"Yeah, something," Longarm told him. "But the good news is that the whiskey will still be here tomorrow when you come back, while I'll be gone."

"Thank gawd fer that!"

The four men left angry and Boone wasn't any too happy, either. "They was just fixin' to get drunk and spend some real money. They'd found a little gold dust and I needed to make some money after the bad time I've been having. Damn, Marshal, couldn't you have—"

"Don't you remember what we told you yesterday about Chief Moy-ahni coming here, but only on the condition that there were no other whites."

"Yeah, but he don't have no gold dust!"

Longarm shook his head. He looked over at Ochoa and said, "Go make sure those fellas don't change their minds and decide to come back and fight."

"All right."

Longarm glanced up at the sun and saw with relief that there was still a little morning left to the day. He expelled a sigh of relief, walked back to the trading post and waited for Liberty.

The sun was straight up when the old chief and two younger Utes appeared on their best ponies. Longarm knew without asking which was Liberty because his paler skin left no doubt that he was of mixed blood. Liberty wore a loose buckskin tunic, pants, and moccasins, and his long hair possessed a hint of auburn. Longarm saw the angry marks where a rope had cut into his neck. There was a Colt strapped around his waist and also a bone-handled Bowie knife. The other warrior was slightly older than Liberty and quite tall. He was missing one ear and had a terrible scar on his left cheek. Longarm wondered if he was Liberty's half brother.

"Marshal," Liberty said, nudging his pony forward with his heels. "My father tells me that you have come from Denver to talk."

"That's right."

"Then I will listen."

"No," Longarm said. "You and your father and this other man must tie your horses and we all talk."

Liberty glanced at the chief, then to the other warrior. He spoke to them in his own language and after several minutes of discussion they nodded in agreement.

"Marshal Long, they'll want free whiskey," Boone announced. "This is your meeting so you gotta pay for it if you want."

"No whiskey," Custis said firmly. "At least, not until *after* the talk."

Ochoa shook his head in disagreement. "Without whiskey, the talks ain't going to last but a few minutes and we'll learn nothing."

147

Longarm frowned. "Okay. Boone, I'll buy one watered-down bottle."

"They'll know the difference and it'll make 'em mad," the trader protested. "Marshal, better no whiskey than watered-down whiskey."

"All right," Longarm reluctantly agreed. "Bring out one bottle."

Boone stomped back into his trading post and Longarm motioned for the three Utes to sit down with him in the front yard. When the Indians shook their heads in refusal, Ochoa whispered, "They don't want to sit in the dirt. Boone will have to bring out some used trade blankets, and they will expect to take them when they leave."

"Dammit, this is starting to get expensive."

"You can afford it. Marshal, don't mess this up over a few lousy government dollars."

"All right. Get the blankets and another bottle."

Ochoa grinned and replied, "I like to see you spend money. I like it because it galls you so much."

"Git!"

When the blankets were presented to the Utes as a present and carefully inspected, they were placed in a circle. Then Longarm, Ochoa, and the three Utes took their places in the yard. Everyone stared at each other for several moments as both whiskey bottles were uncorked and solemnly passed around.

"Liberty," Longarm began after taking a nip of the whiskey, "it is said by many that you killed Senator Hawk and the other man whose name was Jason Snyder."

"Those words are not true."

"It is known that you once stabbed a man to death in a fight. I do not know what to believe so I have come to ask you."

"My brother did not kill these men," the tall Indian said,

148

jaw muscles clenching. "Liberty good Indian! White men bad, not Indian!"

"Amen," Ochoa intoned, taking a deep pull on the whiskey and smacking his lips with satisfaction. "White men speak with forked tongue."

"Shut up," Longarm hissed, "or get lost."

Ochoa's devilish grin slipped. "Sorry, Marshal."

"Liberty, if you did not kill Senator Hawk and the other man at the ranch, who *did* kill them?"

The young Ute turned his head and studied a distant snowcapped peak for a few moments, then turned back to Longarm and finally answered, "I do not know."

"Were you there when the two white men were killed?"

"I was hunting a buck, but his will to live was strong and he still lives. When I came back to the ranch, I put my horse away and then I walked to the house. After I went inside, I called but no one answered. That's when I went into the senator's room and found him and this other man dead."

"How had they been killed?" Longarm asked.

"With a knife."

"A big knife like the one you carry?"

The Ute slowly shook his head back and forth. "Smaller blade. The senator and the other man had been stabbed many times. I decided that I should do something good for that man that had treated me like his son. So I picked the senator up and carried him to his room. I laid him on the bed and went back down to the other man and tried to think of what to do with him."

Longarm detected misery in Liberty's dark eyes. "Did you do anything with the other body?"

"I moved it."

"Why?"

The Ute shrugged. "His wounds were very bad, I took a blanket from a chair and covered the top of his body."

149

"Had the senator and the other man been dead long?"

"No," Liberty said without elaboration. "Not long."

"And then what happened?"

"I went to the corral to get a horse. I would ride and find Mrs. Hawk, Jake, and Della. But when I rode out of the barn, someone I could not see fired a shot. At first, I did not know they were shooting at me. But then I felt a bullet cut my shoulder and another pass my face. I raced the horse into the trees."

"Did you go back to the house?"

"No," Liberty said. "I had no weapon. I decided that the man who killed Senator Hawk also wanted to kill me."

"Did he try to kill you with a rifle . . . or pistol?"

"A pistol, I think."

The chief said something in Ute and the three Indians had a brief, but lively conversation. Finally, the chief said, "I have told my son to show you the bullet wound so that you will know my son speaks the truth."

Longarm glanced sideways at Ochoa, who met his gaze. The both knew that such a wound proved nothing. But Ochoa said, "We would see this wound now."

Liberty slowly removed his buckskin tunic and twisted his lean body to one side so that everyone could see the angry furrow where a bullet had cut across his back. It was mostly healed by now, but there was little doubt in Longarm's mind that it had been caused by a bullet.

"Now," the tall Ute said impatiently, "you will know that my brother speaks the truth."

"I thank you for showing me that and I am sorry. But—"

"Custis," Ochoa whispered urgently, "you had better not try to explain that the wound would not be evidence of innocence in a white man's court of law. This would make them even angrier and they would likely not be willing to see or even speak with either of us again."

Longarm considered the Navajo's words, realized their

150

wisdom and said to the Utes, "I must find out who killed Senator Hawk and Mr. Snyder. Only then will the other white men stop hunting for Liberty. Only then will justice be done. So again, Liberty, do you have any idea who murdered those men?"

"Maybe Jake."

"What about Della?"

Liberty considered this for a moment. "Maybe Della, too."

"But not Mrs. Hawk?"

"No. Too old and slow."

"Why didn't you wait until the danger had passed and then ride back to the house when they arrived home?"

"I did that."

Longarm's brow raised in question. "And what happened?"

"Jake saw the blood on me and drew his gun. He called me a murderer and tried to kill me, but I ran outside and hid. Everyone came out and hunted me, but after dark I went away."

"To your people?"

Liberty nodded.

"But they took you someplace else, knowing that Jake, George Casey, and others would come for you?"

"Yes."

"I'm not going to ask you where you are hiding," Custis said. "I believe your story, but I have to find out who really killed Senator Hawk and Mr. Snyder. Do you understand?"

Liberty nodded.

"I may need to ask you more questions."

Liberty turned to his father who said. "You come to my village. We send for my son. But no arrest."

"All right," Longarm told the old man.

The whiskey bottles were soon emptied and everyone seemed happy again. The three Utes collected their new

blankets and then Liberty went over to the corral and studied the horses.

"Who rides strawberry horse?"

"I do," Longarm answered.

"Ugly horse. Why marshal ride such a horse?"

"I like him. He is strong and surefooted."

"Too ugly to ride," the Ute pronounced before he swung onto his own handsome pony and rode away with his father and brother.

"What do you think?" Ochoa asked when they were gone. "Did we learn anything worth three blankets and two bottles of bad whiskey?"

"Yeah," Longarm replied. "We learned that Liberty didn't kill Senator Hawk and Snyder."

"So, you believed him?"

"I did. Does that surprise you?" Longarm asked.

"I guess not," the Navajo answered. "But then, I've learned better than to second-guess other lawman . . . especially the white ones."

Longarm yawned. The whiskey coupled with the warm afternoon and the hard nights of lovemaking with Milly were beginning to take their toll.

"Boone," he said, "if you don't mind, I think I'll lay over here tonight."

"That's fine, just as long as you don't run off them prospectors and their gold again."

"I promise not to. Big Chief, what are you going to do?"

"Think I'll drink some more whiskey."

"Fine, but don't drink it on my dollar."

"I wouldn't dream of it, Marshal Long." Ochoa winked and headed back inside the trading post.

Chapter 14

Longarm finally got a good night's rest by sleeping in Boone's barn while the prospectors had themselves a party that night. When he awakened the next morning, Longarm went into the trading post and found everyone except Big Chief Ochoa passed out on the floor. He went to the corral and discovered that the Navajo had already left on his runty buckskin pony. Eager to also be on his way, Longarm saddled Ugly and headed back to Pagosa Springs. It was about then that he remembered he had missed his prearranged meeting with Della Hawk. That was bad, and he had no doubt that she would be angry and maybe even refuse to tell him whatever secrets she had promised.

"I'll just have to go see her this afternoon," he said aloud as his belly growled with hunger.

"Howdy, Marshal," the liveryman said in greeting as he took the strawberry roan and led him into the barn to be unsaddled. "Did you find the senator's murderer yet?"

"Afraid not."

"Jake and them boys got pretty rowdy last night. They were saying that if you didn't come up with Liberty . . . by gawd they'd ride out to the reservation and do some arm

153

twisting and maybe even neck stretching if that was what it took to find out where that Ute is hiding."

"If they do that, I'll arrest every damn one of them," Longarm vowed before he headed for the cafe to get something to eat.

"They're ready to bust if you don't get Liberty soon!" the man called.

Longarm didn't even bother to answer. He went to the cafe, which was nearly empty, and smiled as Milly hurried over to say hello.

"Hi," she said, "I've sure missed you."

"I missed you, too," he replied, looking at the nasty scab on her cheek. "How are you feeling?"

"I'm feeling all right, but I don't look so good." She touched her wound. "Everyone has been asking me what happened. Of course, I just made up a story about how I bumbled into something. You wouldn't believe how many men have offered to watch over me at night."

He laughed. "Yes I would. I'm really sorry about what happened. I never expected Otto to ambush me in the hotel room."

"He was always crazy. The undertaker returned and they buried that giant sonofabitch in the pauper's section of our cemetery yesterday. From what I hear, no one from the Hawk Ranch even bothered to attend. Now, isn't that cold-hearted?"

"I have a feeling that Mrs. Hawk and Della are not in the habit of dwelling on the deaths or problems of their employees."

"Jake used to like to egg Otto into saloon fights just to watch the giant stomp them half to death. I thought at least he would attend the bastard's funeral."

"Don't tell anyone," Longarm warned, "but I finally met Liberty."

"You did!"

"Yes, and I'm convinced that he is innocent."

"Did he know who *did* kill the senator and the federal dispatcher?"

"I'm afraid not. When he arrived at the ranch, no one was home. He went inside and found the bodies. When he went out to the barn to saddle a horse, someone opened fire on him."

"From the house?"

"Liberty wasn't sure. The bullets were coming fast and one grazed him on the back. He was unarmed and you can easily understand why he just wanted to escape."

"Whoever shot at Liberty must be the real murderer."

"That would be my guess. Liberty admitted he carried the senator's body upstairs and laid him to rest out of respect. Because of that, he had blood on his clothes. One of the ranch hands might even have opened fire, assuming that Liberty had just committed the murders."

Milly frowned. "I see what you mean. I'm afraid that you seem to be back at the start again."

"Except now I'm sure Liberty is innocent. Whoever opened fire on him probably was our murderer and he might even be under the impression that Liberty saw him and that's why he needs to be caught and hanged."

"I feel sorry for him."

"He must be pretty scared."

"Yes he is, but I'm sure he's also well-protected. Liberty vowed never to surrender. He says that, if he must, he will live out his life in the high mountains."

"That would be sad," Milly said. "How would you like to live way up in those freezing mountains, always watching and wondering if someone was coming to arrest or even kill you?"

"I wouldn't." Longarm removed his hat and combed his long black hair with his fingers.

"Who is your number-one suspect?"

"Jake Hawk."

"Why?"

"Because he seems the most anxious to hang Liberty."

"But wouldn't that be natural, seeing as he thinks Liberty killed his father?"

"Not given the fact that everyone agrees they didn't like each other."

Milly sighed. "I'm glad that you're the one responsible for catching the murderer. All this mystery really is too much for this girl. I'm more comfortable right here cooking and serving good meals. Speaking of which, are we hungry?"

"Famished."

"The steaks look especially good today."

"I'd rather have your stew and sourdough bread, followed by a slab of whatever pie you baked this morning."

"It's apple again. Are we . . . are we getting together tonight?"

"Milly, after what happened in my room a few nights ago, I'm concerned for your welfare. If the murderer is Jake or one of his henchmen, they're going to be watching me closely and trying to nail my hide to the barn door. It would be safer for you if we kept apart for a while."

Milly couldn't hide her disappointment. "I was afraid you were going to say something like that."

"It's just temporary. Only long enough for me to nail this murder case down tight."

"But then you'll be leaving for Denver."

Longarm nodded in agreement.

"I said it before and I'll say it again," Milly told him. "I might be going back with you to Denver. I'm getting real tired of this town and last winter was especially hard on everyone. Our customers always leave me good tips, but everything in Pagosa Springs costs about twice as much as

it would in Denver. No matter what I do, I can't save money or get ahead."

Longarm wasn't too keen on the idea of Milly traveling with him to Denver, but he didn't want to disappoint her any more, so he said nothing.

"If we rented a private railroad coach for the trip to Denver," Milly said, "we could have a lot of fun. Have you ever made love on a moving train?"

Longarm had many times, but shook his head.

"I'll bet it would be great, Custis!"

"With you, it would be great anywhere."

"Aw," she cooed, "you are *such* a sweet talker."

"I'm also hungry. Remember?"

"Ooops! I got so excited that I forgot." Milly hurried off to the kitchen and Longarm settled back to wait for a much-anticipated meal.

The stew was so delicious that Longarm had seconds and then thirds. Milly's apple pie was as good as he could have tasted anywhere in Denver. Custis lingered over his coffee as a few customers began to trickle in, all greeting Milly with genuine warmth, and some with a joke or a flirting compliment. Milly played right back to them and there was no doubt that she could do well in Denver. Maybe even meet a good future husband.

Longarm was just finishing the last of his coffee when Jake Hawk and George Casey entered the cafe. The two men were grim-faced as they strutted up to Longarm's table. Milly saw them from the kitchen and burst out into the dining area yelling, "Jake, you and George leave him alone!"

"Milly," Longarm said, coming to his feet and tossing his napkin on the table, "go back into the kitchen. I'll be fine."

"Custis—"

Jake sneered and his face lit up with mirth. "Custis? Is that what you called him, Milly?"

"Shut up and go away."

"Well, well. Now I clearly see what's going on. Milly is smitten with the big lawman! Casey, what do you think about that?"

The gunfighter snickered and his close-set eyes traveled up and down Milly's body. "It's been all downhill since you sent her packing, Jake."

Longarm reached down and brought his coffee cup to his lips. "Are you boys here to eat . . . or just flap your gums?"

Jake didn't like the question and his leering grin faded. "I came to ask *you* some questions, Marshal."

"You can ask, but I may decide not to answer."

"If I were you," Casey said, hand edging a little nearer to the butt of his six-gun, "I'd be a little more respectful."

"And if I were you," Longarm replied, "I'd back out of here fast."

"I'm not afraid of you."

"Then maybe you ought to be afraid of a hangman, because even if you did manage to kill me, you'd be hunted down and hanged."

Casey blinked and Jake said, "Go outside and wait for me."

"But—"

"When I give you a gawdamn order, jump! Is that understood?"

The gunman's face darkened with humiliation, but he backed out of the cafe into the street. Some of the other customers looked like they also wanted to leave their meals unfinished and run outside.

"What are your questions, Jake?"

"Why didn't you show up today to see my sister? She told me you were coming and she's damned upset."

"You don't care about Della. What do you really want to know?"

"Did you find Liberty?"

"I'm not going to answer that," Longarm replied. "I'm a federal marshal and this is an official murder investigation. But I will say this . . . if you don't quit hunting that kid and start minding your own business, I'll arrest you for interfering with the law."

"Try it," Jake spat. "This ain't Denver. In Pagosa, the Hawk family makes the rules, not the law."

"You're dead wrong on that one," Longarm countered. "And the minute you step out of bounds I'll be on you so fast and hard you won't know what hit you."

"Why don't we just settle this right here and now?" Jake challenged as his hand shaded his holstered gun.

Longarm saw the other customers rise from their chairs, but he said, "Everyone stay where you are. They'll be no fight."

Jake sneered. "What's the problem, Marshal? Have you suddenly contracted a case of the yellow bellies?"

"Back out of here right now while you still can."

"Go to hell!"

Longarm tasted his coffee. "Milly makes a fine cup of coffee. You ought to try some once in a while instead of drinking so much bad whiskey."

"You're real free with advice, Marshal. And you know what people say free advice is worth."

"True," Longarm replied. "But try some anyway."

Before Jake could say another word, Longarm tossed hot coffee in the man's face and then smashed him in the side of his jaw for good measure. Jake struck the floor, rolled, and tried to climb to his feet. Longarm stepped over and disarmed him, then grabbed the man by his cartridge belt and hauled him outside.

"Casey," he said, "I advise you to leave Pagosa Springs."

"It's a free country, Marshal. Are you charging me with any crime?"

"Not yet."

The gunfighter laughed, but it had a cold, humorless sound. "There will come a day when all the talking between us is over. I promise."

"Take your boss back to the ranch. If you see Della, tell her I'll be there tomorrow. Can you remember all that?"

"I never forget anything."

Custis backed into the cafe and watched through the window as the gunfighter helped Jake to his feet and then over to his horse. They rode out together with Jake bent way over his mount's neck.

Maybe, Longarm decided, massaging his knuckles, *I hit him even harder than I thought*.

Chapter 15

The next morning while Longarm was saddling Ugly, Ochoa came riding up on his buckskin pony. He was wearing a side arm and carrying a double-barreled shotgun.

"Morning, Marshal."

"Good morning."

"Going for a ride?"

"That's the general idea."

Ochoa leaned on his saddle horn. "What a coincidence. I was also thinking this is a great day to take a ride. I was heading out to the Hawk Ranch because I still haven't paid my respects. Would you like to come along?"

Longarm almost laughed. "Cut the bull. You know that's where I'm going and you're not welcome."

"Oh? Well I think that Mrs. Hawk will remember me from a few years ago when a couple of her cowboys stole some Indian ponies and decided that they could resell them way down in Arizona. I had to bring them back for trial and Mrs. Hawk was not too pleased by the bad publicity they caused her family. You see, it was an election year and . . . if I recall correctly, she said, 'Miserable timing you Navajo sonofabitch.' "

"She said that to you?"

"Sure did. But I'm sure that time has healed that little animosity and she'll welcome me with the same affection that she'll welcome you."

Longarm finished tightening his cinch. Like Ochoa, he was half-expecting trouble and was well armed. The idea of having a friend at his side was comforting and Longarm knew that this was no time to let foolish pride stand in the way of his good health.

"All right," he agreed. "Let's ride out and see what happens."

As they trotted their horses through Pagosa, some of the shop owners came out to watch in silence. "I'd give a dollar to know what kind of odds they are giving us today," Ochoa commented. "I'll bet they aren't much."

Longarm didn't have anything to say but he supposed the Navajo was right. People would be expecting the Black Widow to turn her men loose on them. Or that Jake and George Casey would decide it was time for a final showdown.

"It's a good day to die," Ochoa said as they neared the Hawk Ranch. "But it is a better day to live."

"Amen," Longarm grunted just before he spotted about five or six cowboys galloping to intercept them. "Looks like we've got a welcoming party."

Ochoa checked his shotgun and Longarm pulled his rifle from its saddle scabbard and levered a shot into the chamber.

"How do you want to play this?" the Navajo asked.

"We can't let them make the play first," Longarm said. "There's too many for that, so we get the drop on them, then take their guns away."

"Easier said than done."

"Let's get steady," he replied. "We can tie our horses up

to that little pine over there and have the advantage if shooting starts."

"Good idea."

As soon as they dismounted and had their horses tied, both men checked their sidearms and then stood their ground as the horsemen drew nearer. Ochoa said, "Jake might seem like a blowhard, but he's very good with his pistol. If words fail and the bullets start flying, don't leave him for last or he'll kill one or maybe even both of us."

"How good is George Casey?"

"I expect he's even better than Jake."

"Are any of the others gunmen?"

Ochoa watched the riders for a few more minutes, sizing them up one by one before he replied. "No. Just Jake and Casey. The others are working cowboys."

"I don't want a gunfight," Longarm said, "but we may have no choice. So I'll take Casey and you go for Jake."

"But he's a lot faster than I am."

"That's why you've got a shotgun."

When the riders drew closer, Longarm raised his rifle and pointed it in their general direction. "That's far enough!"

"You're not welcome here," Jake yelled, dismounting and handing his reins to one of the cowboys. Casey did the same and when the pair came nearer, Longarm said, "I came to talk to your mother."

"She don't want to talk to you."

"She'll have to," was Longarm's blunt reply. "Either that, or I'm going to arrest both you and your mother for murder."

"Over my dead body!" Jake sneered.

"If that's the way it has to be."

Ochoa lowered the barrel of his shotgun and pointed it right at the gunfighter. "Just so I understand. Are you gonna dance with the devil, too?"

Casey gulped, shook his head, and backed away.

"What are you doing!" Jake Hawk screamed. "Get up here beside me."

"I'm not dying for you or anyone else," Casey said, raising his hands. "Let the marshal arrest us. He's got no evidence and we'll be free soon enough."

"No!"

Longarm shook his head. "Think carefully about this, Jake. If you're innocent, you will go free. But, if you're not—"

"Do you really believe I'd murder my own father?"

"As a matter of fact, I do," Longarm told him flatly. "Now slowly reach across your belly with your left hand and drag out that six-gun. Don't let pride turn you into a dead fool."

"Do it!" Casey urged. "This is not how it needs to be. We can—"

"Shut up!" Jake shrieked. "I paid you to stand and fight with me . . . not back down!"

"Jake, I never agreed to commit suicide," Casey replied. "And you don't really want to, either."

Jake Hawk began to tremble. Longarm watched the handsome young man's emotions build, not knowing if his nerve would suddenly dissolve and he'd surrender . . . or if Jake would try to outdraw a loaded rifle pointed at his chest.

"Give it up," Longarm urged. "If you didn't kill them, sooner or later I will find out who did. Don't be a—"

An oath burst from Jake's twisted lips and his hand stabbed downward for his gun. Maybe he was hoping that Longarm would panic and miss. In that case, Longarm would be a dead man. But Longarm didn't miss. He fired from waist level and the rifle bullet struck Jake hard enough to send him staggering backward, gun already in his hand.

Longarm coolly leveled another shell into the breech of

his rifle but needn't have bothered because one of Ochoa's barrels erupted with fire and smoke. The blast struck Jake in the neck and jaw, almost tearing the fool's head off.

Casey threw up his hands shouting, "Don't shoot! Don't shoot!"

It was over. One of the Hawk cowboys leaned out from his saddle and vomited.

"Everyone throw your guns down and dismount!" Longarm shouted. "Big Chief, keep them covered while I make sure they really are unarmed."

Longarm walked past the nearly unrecognizable Jake Hawk, who lay in a spreading pool of blood. He searched all the riders and when he was certain that they were disarmed, he ordered them back in the saddle.

"What are we going to do now?" Ochoa asked.

"We're going to do what we started out to do . . . talk to the Black Widow."

"She didn't do it," Casey offered, lowering his hands.

Longarm's head swiveled around and he stared at the professional gunman. "Keep talking."

"Not much to say," Casey answered, relaxing a bit. "The truth is that Jake killed both his father and that other fella."

"What about Della?"

"She helped and we were all sworn a blood oath to silence."

"Do you have anything to prove what you're saying?" Ochoa asked.

"Can I put my hands down."

"All right," Longarm said, "but keep them in front of you where I can see them."

Casey did as he was told, then said, "Of course, Della won't admit she helped kill the senator and the dispatcher. But she did. Me and Nettie returned from—" Casey's words died on his lips. "Never mind."

"Finish it!" Ochoa demanded.

"No."

The Navajo walked up to the gunman and pressed the shotgun to Casey's chest. "One last time. What were you going to tell us?"

Casey paled. "Before I say anything more, I got to protect Nettie." He glanced over at the other Hawk cowboys. "Tell 'em to get a buckboard and a tarp to cover Jake's body. And order them not to tell the women what happened to Jake."

Longarm thought that was a reasonable request. No mother, not even one as evil as the Black Widow should be allowed to see her dead son with half his face blown away. "All right."

He sent the cowboys off for a buckboard. When they were gone, he turned back to Casey. "Now we're all alone and you're going to tell us what really happened."

"Me and Nettie took a buggy over to Durango."

"What for?" Longarm asked.

"Nettie told the senator she needed some things that couldn't be found in Pagosa. He didn't care. They weren't in love or even friendly anymore. They stayed married only because a divorce would have offended voters. And the senator was facing a tough election this coming fall. I expect he was glad to see us go to Durango."

"What was the purpose of your trip."

"We went over there to see a good attorney."

"What for?"

Casey swallowed. "Nettie and I are in love."

"Say that again," Ochoa asked, staring at the gunman in disbelief.

"I said that me and Nettie. . . . Mrs. Hawk are in love."

"I don't believe it," Longarm said flatly.

"Me neither," Ochoa added.

"Well," Casey said, shrugging his shoulders, "believe it or not, it is the gospel truth."

166

"What kind of a story are you trying to feed us?" Ochoa said.

"Ain't no story. There's still a lot of fire in the old gal. Nettie really knows how to pleasure a younger man in ways that I never even thought of before we started going to bed."

Longarm turned his head to see how Ochoa was accepting this account. Not surprisingly, the Navajo was grinning and he blurted, "Am I to understand that you and that horrible old lady were humping each other!"

"That's a crude way of putting it but . . . yes."

"Well if that don't beat anything I ever heard before."

Casey's face turned crimson with anger. "Nettie has more fire and spirit than most any young woman. What's so funny? I love her, dammit."

Longarm asked, "Did Jake or Della know about you and their mother?"

"Yeah."

"Weren't they a little upset?"

"At first they were. But not for very long. You see, Senator Hawk was always going to bed with other women, though he'd probably slowed down in his old age. Della even admitted to me that she'd caught her father in bed lots of times with the ranch guests."

"Then I'm surprised that Mrs. Hawk didn't kill him."

Casey shook his head. "The truth of the matter is that Nettie tried to keep everyone thinking the great Hawks were just one big, happy family. She never let on that they all hated each other. Well, almost all of them."

"What does that mean?"

"Della loved Jake like a brother."

"What about Liberty?"

"Can I take a leak before I explode?"

"All right."

While Casey stood and made water, Longarm turned to

the Navajo and whispered, "Do you believe any of this?"

"I guess this is going to come as a shock, but the story is so improbable, that yes, I do believe Casey. Mrs. Hawk sure don't look her age. And the other thing is that I think Casey is plenty smart enough to hump hisself into a big pile of money. Hell, he may even get the Hawk Ranch itself when the Black Widow curls up and finally dies."

"Let's ask him about Liberty and exactly how the murders took place."

When Casey had done his urgent business, the gunman buttoned his pants and said, "You'll want to know everything that happened."

"That's right."

"Like I said, Nettie and I were returning from Durango. We'd seen an attorney and I'd given a deposition that the senator was having affairs with other women right under the roof of his wife's house. Don't forget, Nettie's family . . . the Kilbanes . . . owned this ranch long before the senator came into the picture and she figured she ought to get it all back when they divorced and we got married."

"You promised to marry her?" Longarm asked.

"Sure! I love her and she was damn good to me. I don't care what anybody thinks, so why not?"

"No reason," Longarm told him. "Go on."

"Well," Casey continued, looking upset and offended, "when we returned to the Hawk Ranch we found both the senator and that federal dispatcher dead."

"Where was the senator when you saw him?"

"Upstairs on his bed. He'd been stabbed a bunch of times and looked pretty bad."

"And the dispatcher?"

"He was downstairs and had been killed the same way."

"So then what happened?" Longarm asked.

"As you would expect, Nettie was pretty upset and I

wasn't feeling any too cheery myself. I covered the bodies and sent a man to town for the undertaker."

"Then what?"

"Then Jake and Della arrived."

"Where had they been?"

"I don't know and didn't ask. Nettie got real mad when they said they didn't know a thing about the bodies. But finally, they broke down and admitted they'd killed both the senator and that other fella."

"Do you want to tell me why?"

"Sure." Casey took a deep breath and continued. "Jake said he and Della had done them in because they wanted a fifty-year timber lease on the Ute land, which would earn them a fortune. Jake had argued with his father for days and then he just blew up, went crazy, and stabbed the senator to death. He said they had to kill the other man so there wouldn't be a witness."

"He just lost his temper and killed his own father?"

"Sure! When Jake lost his temper, he lost his mind. I don't have to tell you that because you saw what just happened to him. He sure wasn't no professional."

"Not like you, huh?" Ochoa said softly.

"I'm not wanted by the law for anything, anymore. I've served time in prison but I've committed no crimes since I was set free. Marshal, I swear that you'll find no reward posters out for me, George Casey."

"He's telling the truth," Ochoa said. "I looked and there isn't a reward on his head . . . at least one that I could find."

"I tell you," Casey said. "I'm in love and I've changed my ways. Me and Nettie are gonna get married and be respectable folks. Help others less fortunate and just do right. Why, I might even get religion!"

"Don't layer it on too thick," Ochoa warned. "I'd bet a hundred dollars that it would have been just a matter of

time before you crossed the line and broke the law again."

Casey's jaw worked. "Then you'd have lost that hundred."

Longarm changed the subject. "Did Della actually admit to helping Jake kill her father?"

"She said that Jake killed the senator and she stabbed the dispatcher with a kitchen knife. The kind with a long, narrow blade that you use to carve meat off a bone. Della said that Snyder died bad and I remember her saying that the poor bastard was just in the wrong place at the wrong time."

"So then," Ochoa interrupted, "how did Liberty get tagged with the murder?"

"They had to pin it on somebody, didn't they?" Casey asked. "It just so happened that they were upstairs in Della's bedroom trying to figure out who to pin the murder on when they heard the front door slam. Later, when Liberty carried the senator's body upstairs, they stayed in the bedroom, realizing they'd found the perfect murder suspect."

"Why didn't they kill him in the house?"

"They were going to, but Liberty ran out too fast. When that Ute headed for the barn he was covered with the senator's blood and that's when they opened fire on him out of Della's window . . . but they missed."

"Then what?" Longarm asked.

"Jake and Della told me how Liberty ran into the trees and they tried to find him and kill him. But the kid got away clean. After that, Jake and Della went into a panic and offered anyone who killed the Ute a hundred dollars reward."

Longarm had heard enough. "Are you willing to testify before a court of law this is exactly what happened?"

"Yeah, but I don't know if Nettie will testify against her own daughter."

"I'll bet she will to save her hide," Ochoa said not bothering to hide his contempt.

Casey expelled a deep breath. "Jake is dead so he don't matter now. But Della isn't right in the head and she might get off clean."

"That's for the court to decide," Longarm told the gunman. "Let's go have a talk with Della and Mrs. Hawk."

"I'm worried about how Nettie will take all this," Casey fretted.

"No, you're not," Longarm snapped. "What you're really worried about is that she will turn on you."

"She would never do that."

"Don't count on it," Ochoa said. "After all, the woman you say you love didn't earn her name as the Black Widow because she is good at knitting doilies."

"She would never try to kill me!"

"I'll make sure she doesn't have the chance," Longarm promised the gunman. "We'll all be going to Denver and I won't let her near you."

Casey sighed. "I'll explain to Nettie that I admitted everything in order to protect her from a terrible injustice. She'll understand that I did it for her sake, won't she?"

"I don't know," Longarm answered. "I'm wondering how she's going to react to Jake's death."

"Marshal, to be real honest, she didn't like Jake any better than the senator. Nettie admitted a lot of times that her son was crazy. That's why she believed that Hawk Ranch would be lost if her children inherited it after her death."

"And the next thing you'll tell me is that this is the reason why she was willing to marry an ex-convict like you," Ochoa said.

Longarm had heard more than enough. "Let's ride."

"We gonna just leave Jake's body out here like that?" Casey asked.

"The cowboys will be back soon to retrieve it. When we

meet I'll tell them to take the body into Pagosa for the undertaker to put in a sealed casket. Nobody will want to see Jake Hawk looking that way . . . not even his enemies."

"The whole town hated Jake."

"I bet they weren't real fond of you, either," Ochoa remarked.

"I did what I was told to do and I never hurt anybody. Just scared 'em some. But I'll tell you what . . . they *really* hated Otto Klinger even worse than us. I'm glad you nailed that big bastard."

Longarm mounted Ugly. "Let's ride."

"You gonna tell Nettie about the Navajo blowing half of Jake's head off?"

"I expect that those cowboys will have already told her what happened," Longarm answered.

"Della is the one that you have to watch," Casey warned. "She always carries a derringer."

"What did Jake and Della think about you and their mother getting married?" Ochoa asked as they rode along.

"I'd be lying if I told you they liked the idea of me being their stepfather. At first, I even thought about Della and me . . . well, you know. But then I saw her one night walking out into the woods with Otto."

"She was messing around with Klinger?" Longarm asked to make sure he'd heard correctly.

"They weren't out picking flowers in the meadow every night. Della really liked men and she picked all the Hawk cowboys she wanted. She even picked me, but by then I was thinking of marrying her mother."

"Do you believe that?" Ochoa asked sarcastically.

"I don't know what to believe anymore," Longarm replied. "But I do think that Jake was crazy enough to have lost his temper and killed the senator."

"What about Della?"

"I don't know."

"I'm just telling you the truth about her," Casey argued. "But, Marshal, it doesn't matter to me if you believe me or not. Those two killed their father and that Snyder fella, but don't expect a confession from Della. She'll say or do most anything to save her own neck."

"You could be lying," Longarm reasoned. "Maybe *you're* the real killer."

"Since Nettie and I were talking to an attorney in Durango two days before the murder that would be impossible, because there's no way that we could have gotten back in a buggy fast enough to commit those murders."

"Do you have witnesses to say you were in Durango?"

"Hell, yes! Plenty of 'em."

"Here comes the buckboard for Jake's body," Ochoa said.

When the wagon met them, Longarm gave the still-shaken cowboys instructions to take the body into Pagosa directly to the undertaker's office. "Don't uncover him," were Longarm's final words.

The reason for that order was obvious. Anyone seeing what a shotgun blast had done to a once handsome young man might suffer horrible nightmares. And Longarm especially did not want Milly to see Jake Hawk.

"What we gonna tell the undertaker?" the cowboy driving the buckboard asked.

"Tell him to prepare Jake's body and place it in a sealed casket for burial. Tell him I'll be in later with further instructions."

"Sure thing, Marshal."

The cowboys continued on and when Longarm saw the Hawk mansion, he said, "Big Chief, I want you and Casey to stay back while I speak to Mrs. Hawk and her daughter."

"Okay. You don't want them to hear this man's story until you've heard their own version. Right?"

"Right. And Big Chief?"

"Yeah?"

"Thanks for standing with me when things look fatal for our side."

"No problem. Lawmen need to stick tight together."

Longarm nodded with appreciation. He knew without the slightest doubt that, had Ochoa not been at his side, he might well have been killed. And while he wasn't willing to accept everything the gunfighter had told him, if he really did have witnesses in Durango it would be impossible to call the man a liar.

The two women were standing on the big porch when Longarm rode up to them and tipped his hat. "I guess you heard the news already," he said to the older woman. "Your son is dead."

"Gawdamn you!" Della shouted, her hands clenched into fists.

Longarm did not dismount. "Mrs. Hawk, tell me why you couldn't have killed your husband and Mr. Snyder."

"Because I was coming back from Durango with Mr. Casey, you murdering sonofabitch!"

"Any witnesses to place you in Durango just a few days before the murders?"

"A town full. One of them being the finest attorney in western Colorado. His name is Harry Blake."

"I'll check into that. Della, who can prove that you didn't kill your father and Mr. Snyder?"

"No one can prove . . . or disprove it," she hissed.

"In that case, I'm afraid I have to arrest you for murder."

Della paled, then began to shake her head. "Liberty murdered my father and that other man."

"I don't think so," Longarm told her. He turned to look at the Black Widow. "What do *you* think?"

"She's right. Liberty killed both men down in my husband's study."

174

"I don't believe either one of you. Della, you are under arrest. Pack for a trip to Denver."

"Never!"

Before Longarm could draw his gun, Della whirled and raced back into the house.

"Mrs. Hawk," Longarm said, dismounting and handing his reins to Ochoa, "I strongly suggest you talk to your daughter."

"Prison would kill Della. It would also have killed Jake. Both of them would rather die fighting than be locked in a cell, maybe for life."

"I can't help that."

"And I won't help you."

Longarm couldn't fathom a woman who would calmly stand there and refuse to help her own flesh and blood. So he started into the house.

"Be careful!" Ochoa shouted. "She might be waiting to ambush and kill you!"

Longarm drew his gun, because Ochoa was right about Della being capable of anything.

"Della," he shouted, stepping into the downstairs hallway.

There was no answer.

He looked up the staircase toward the second-floor landing. He thought he could hear the woman. "Della, you can't get away and I'm not going away. So let's do this the easy way. Come down here!"

When she didn't reply, he cautiously started up the stairs with his gun clenched in his fist. He was halfway up the staircase when a loud gunshot froze him in his tracks. "Della!"

She didn't answer so Longarm hurried the rest of the way up to the second-floor landing, shouting the crazy young woman's name over and over and watching to make sure that she wasn't trying to lure him into a deadly trap.

He had to burst into three separate bedrooms before he found the beautiful young woman lying on the floor with a bullet lodged deep in her brain.

Longarm checked her pulse, but he already knew that Della was already dead.

He slowly made his way downstairs to face the Black Widow, who was standing very stiff and straight-backed in the entry hall.

"Your daughter shot herself in the head."

Chapter 16

"Well, Custis," United States Marshal Billy Vail said, "I must say that you did a fine job solving that sensational murder case. The hearing was front-page news and people are still having a hard time accepting Senator John Hawk was murdered by his own children."

"It was a sad affair. I'm not sure that I could have handled the case had it not been for an ex-Navajo Police Chief named Jerome Ochoa."

"Ah, yes! Chief Ochoa. We met one time down in Arizona when I was a deputy marshal like yourself. I'll have to tell you about it someday."

"He's quite a man."

"Yes, he is. What did you think of Della and Jake?"

"Della was beautiful, but rotten inside. Jake was just crazy. He didn't need to die, although I'm sure that he could not have survived a federal penitentiary."

"The world is better off without either one of them. I can't imagine how they both turned out to be killers. I knew they were strange, but I never thought of Jake as being a murderer."

Billy shook his head in amazement. "But what gets me

is the Black Widow and George Casey got married even before the hearing was completed. I've never seen the likes of such cold and callous behavior. That woman has a stone where her heart ought to rest. You'd think she'd have at least waited a few months to give the illusion that she was in mourning."

"The Black Widow was well named."

Billy clucked his tongue and leaned back in his office chair. "And do you know what the worst of it is?"

"It's all bad."

"Sure, but the irony is that the tremendous amount of national publicity caused by those sensational murders has soured the legislature on buying that Ute land."

"That might be bad for Colorado," Longarm said, "but it's good news for the Ute Indians."

"Oh," Billy said a little testily. "I forgot that you've become quite the Indian sympathizer."

"I'm no 'sympathizer'," Longarm replied with annoyance. "But I am sick of watching them getting shafted out of their land."

"They'll never use that timber!"

"That's right, so perhaps it will be there for generations to come."

"Custis, let's not argue the point. I believe in progress and that often comes at the expense of the land and the Indians. You, on the other hand, believe in stopping progress if the land or the Indians suffer."

"I'd agree with that assessment."

"My contention is," Billy said, "that if our founding fathers had that kind of attitude, we'd still be huddled under some tree at Plymouth Rock!"

Longarm dragged a cigar out of his coat pocket. "I'm going on vacation before you find some other awful case to assign me."

"By all means, do take a vacation."

"How long do I have?"

"How about an entire month?"

"Sounds good," Longarm said, pleasantly surprised.

Billy was feeling expansive and Longarm guessed he had probably been congratulated by both the director and the governor of Colorado. "Custis, I suspect that you'll need at least that long to figure out how to handle *two* Denver women. I don't know why you ever allowed Milly to come here when you knew that Miss Lacy would throw an absolute fit."

"I had no choice in the matter."

"If I were you, I'd just go away and hope that things cool down."

"That's exactly what I'm planning." Longarm lit his cheroot, stood up, and said, "So long, Boss."

"Come back rested and ready to go to work!" Billy shouted as Longarm bolted out the door before the man changed his mind about giving him an entire month off.

Two days later, Longarm was relaxing beside a good fishing stream in the southern Rockies thinking of the tragedy that had befallen the Hawk family. He still felt the hairs on the back of his neck stand up when he remembered how the Black Widow had reacted to the deaths of her only children. Or *not* reacted, actually. But at least Liberty had been exonerated. The poor kid had suffered plenty, and the last time that Longarm had seen him, Liberty had vowed never to leave his reservation and live among white people again.

And who could blame the Ute? If Jake and Della had not gotten rattled and missed shooting him from her upstairs bedroom, then—

Longarm's unlit cheroot fell into his lap and he bolted to his feet as something that had been nagging at his mind suddenly sprang into focus. *Oh my gawd! Della's bedroom*

*wasn't facing the horse barn! That meant . . . that meant
that Casey and the Black Widow had lied!*

Longarm took a deep breath and pressed his fingertips to
his temples. *Could it be that the Black Widow and her
lover, George Casey, had managed to return in time to
murder the senator and the dispatcher? Then, when Jake
was killed after proclaiming his innocence, the pair of mur-
derers had set poor Della up to appear as Jake's accom-
plice?*

Of course they had!

"There goes the vacation," Longarm swore, hurrying
along a footpath toward the little town where he'd chosen
to escape all his problems and immerse himself in trout
fishing. "Well, maybe not. Pagosa is only . . . let's see . . .
no more than sixty miles to the west. I can be there the day
after tomorrow, arrest the Black Widow and George Casey,
and be back here fishing by the middle of next week."

Longarm's return to Pagosa Springs did not go unno-
ticed. One of the first to speak to him was a young cowboy
who'd quit the Hawk Ranch. "Welcome back, Marshal!
Didn't expect to see you again. 'Member me? Mort
Seager?"

Longarm vaguely recalled the cowboy's face. "You must
have found a town job?"

"I'm breaking some horses for the freighting company
and making more money than I did cowboying," the young
man said proudly. "What brings you back to Pagosa
Springs?"

Longarm dismounted. "Mort, I'm going to ask you something and I need a straight answer."

The kid's grin slipped and his eyelids dropped a fraction.
"Sure."

"Were Nettie Hawk and George Casey still in Durango
when the senator and that other fella were stabbed to death
in the mansion?"

"No sir. They'd just arrived back to the ranch that afternoon."

Longarm tried to stay calm. "Were they in the mansion when the senator was killed?"

"Now, I wouldn't know about that since me and all the cowboys were out on the range working cattle."

"Was there anyone at the Hawk mansion other than the senator and that other man that was stabbed to death?"

"Nobody except Liberty and Otto."

"Otto Klinger would have been at the ranch?"

"His only job was to repair wagons, corral fences, pumps, and saddles," Mort said. "So yeah, he would have been around the place somewhere."

"Since he's dead, I obviously can't talk to him. Wasn't there a maid or a cook or—"

"Oh yeah, we did have a cook but he quit too. But we both got jobs right here in Pagosa Springs. Luck must have been running with us, don't you think?"

"I do," Longarm said, trying to smother his building excitement. "What is the cook's name?"

"Eli Evers. He's working at that little cafe across the street. Same one that Miss Milly used to work at before you took her away to Denver. Say, how is she doing?"

"Milly is prospering. She started her own cafe and is so busy she's turning customers away in the evenings."

Mort slapped his thigh with glee. "Damn! That woman made the best pies I ever ate. Better'n my own mother's, even."

"Congratulations on your new job. Take care of yourself."

"It was good seein' you!"

Longarm lead his horse over to the cafe, tied the animal, and went inside. The supper crowd hadn't arrived yet and the place was completely empty. Longarm sat down at a table with its checkered linen tablecloth and the place felt

empty without Milly's warm smile and exuberant hello.

A thin man with a long face came out from the kitchen slapping flour from his apron. Longarm said, "Hello, Eli. My name is Marshal Custis Long."

"I know who you are, Marshal. I been expecting you'd come calling on me someday."

"Then you know what I need to ask."

"Yeah, but I'm real scared of both of 'em. If they find out I talked, they'll kill me for damn sure!"

"Who?"

"Why Mrs. Hawk and George Casey. Only I guess it's Mrs. Casey now."

"Did you see them murder the senator and the dispatcher?"

"No sir. Marshal, my life won't be worth—"

"They'll be plotting to kill you, Eli. Their fates rest on the fact that there are no more living witnesses to say what *really* happened that day."

"I didn't see anybody get killed."

"But you heard terrible screams."

Eli took a deep breath and collapsed in the chair opposite Longarm. "Yes, Marshal, I did hear the dying men's screams. I been hearing them ever since they happened and they're slowly driving me insane."

Longarm only had to look into the cook's tortured eyes to see that this was the truth. "So you heard the senator and the other man screaming. Then what?"

"I was out in the root cellar getting some potatoes to boil for supper. When I heard those horrible screams I got a horse and rode off."

"How come you didn't tell me this before?"

"I'd have been a dead man."

Longarm nodded with understanding. "But your silence might have saved Della and Jake. And it almost got Liberty hanged."

"I know and that shames me, Marshal. But I never said I was the bravest of men."

"There's only one way to get rid of the nightmares and that is to be willing to testify in court what you just told me. We'll go to Denver."

Eli's face turned as white as the flour on his apron. "Please, Marshal! I'm so scared of the Black Widow that just the thought of her makes me puke!"

"You should be scared. She hasn't forgotten you. But I'm going to go out there first thing tomorrow morning and arrest both her and her husband for murder. I'll handcuff their wrists and ankles and pass through town to pick you up."

"I can't do it."

"You have to," Longarm told the man in a firm voice that brooked no argument. "Either you come to Denver on your own accord and the government will pay your expenses and make things right, or I'll arrest you. That way you'll still have to testify and you'll be paid nothing."

Eli's hands had begun to shake so violently that he clasped one in the other, squeezing hard. "All right," he whispered.

"Good!" Longarm patted the man on the shoulder. "You got anything to eat here? I'm pretty hungry."

"I got beef hash. I got stew. But I got no pies to match Milly's."

"I'll take the hash and some bread."

Eli got up to prepare the food. "I'm so scared my guts are all tied up in knots, Marshal."

"Look. The only way you're ever going to sleep well at night again is when those two are either serving life sentences in a federal prison where they can't ever hurt anyone again . . . or are hanged. Do you understand me?"

"Yes, sir."

Longarm didn't enjoy his hash, but the bread was satis-

factory. He returned to the Bonner House and slept badly, then got up and had breakfast. Eli was gone but that seemed normal since there was a different breakfast cook. By eight o'clock, Longarm was ready to ride out to the Hawk Ranch and make his arrests. He wished Ochoa were riding at his side but knew he could handle this on his own.

When he rode up to the Hawk mansion, nothing seemed to have changed. A suspicious but respectful cowboy who remembered Longarm came out to greet him. "Can I help you, Marshal?"

"Where is Mr. and Mrs. Casey?"

"Mr. Casey suddenly got sick in the middle of the night and died."

Longarm nearly fell out of the saddle. "No!"

"Yes sir." The cowboy shook his head. "One of the boys saw you in town last night and told Mrs. Casey to expect you this morning. I don't know what happened but Mr. Casey just took ill suddenly and died."

Longarm felt a chill pass the entire length of his body.

"Where is Mrs. Casey?"

"She's in the mansion."

Longarm started that way, but the cowboy followed him a few steps saying, "This place sure is snakebit for people dying! I'm new here but I heard about all the folks that has been killed. Marshal, what's going on?"

"It's a long story."

"I might be drawin' my pay next week. This place must be cursed by the Utes or somebody. I love the country and the higher-than-average wages, but with all the deaths they've had lately, this place gives me the spooks."

"It should."

He was almost to the mansion when the Black Widow emerged to stand on the porch. She was dressed all in black, from the lace shawl over her head to her pointed shoes.

"What do you want?" she demanded. "Can't you see I'm

in mourning again? Haven't I enough to suffer without you adding to my problems?"

"I'd like to see Mr. Casey's body."

"Why?"

"Because I have reason to believe you poisoned him."

The Black Widow gave him a chilling death grin. "Why Marshal Long, you *do* have a wild imagination."

Longarm climbed the porch steps and walked past the woman, yelling over his shoulder, "Where is Casey's body!"

"Upstairs in the bedroom. Don't you dare touch my husband!"

Longarm attacked the stairs two at a time. The last time he'd been up here it had been to discover Della's body just after she'd killed herself. He'd busted into several bedrooms and knew exactly the one where he'd find the gunfighter's body.

George Casey was dressed in an expensive suit and his body was already prepared for burial. Longarm studied the corpse for evidence of poisoning. He had expected that Casey might have died in terrible pain and his face would be contorted with agony and his skin would possess a strange color. Many years earlier Longarm had seen a kid that had swallowed some kind of rat poison, causing his lips to turn a bluish green. But Casey looked absolutely normal.

Then Longarm saw a small, dark stain on the man's coat, just under the corpse's armpit. He pulled back the suit coat and saw it . . . blood. Longarm tore open the corpse's shirt and there it was . . . a bandage tightly pressed over a stab wound located under George Casey's rib cage. At the same instant, he heard a faint creak on the staircase.

Longarm drew his Colt and it came up just as the Black Widow appeared in the doorway with a gun held in both fists. They both fired at the same instant and the Black

185

Widow hit the far wall and slumped to the floor in the sitting position.

"Drop the gun!" he shouted.

"Go to hell," she choked, blood trickling from the corner of her mouth.

The Black Widow struggled to raise the pistol and fire again, but her strength was gone and the gun sagged into her lap. Longarm kept his own pistol trained on her as he knelt by her side. "You killed them all. Two husbands, and you might as well have killed both Jake and Della because you were responsible for their deaths. And now you killed Casey."

"I'd have killed the cook, too," she choked, mouth forming a terrible smile. "But most of all, I wanted to kill *you*!"

Longarm squatted on his haunches. "I've never enjoyed watching a human die. But you're *not* human."

The old woman's face contorted with insane hatred. Her hands grasped the gun in her lap with new determination, and as it came up an instant before, Longarm shot the Black Widow right between the eyes.

Watch for

LONGARM AND THE CHURCH LADIES

260th novel in the exciting LONGARM series
from Jove

Coming in July!

"It's not every da[y] *million dollars." Estelle* [could] *be honest about that. "Nor move to Marbella...."*

"You will love it," Raúl said. "The nightlife is fantastic...."

He just didn't know her at all, Estelle realized.

"How did your parents die?" Raúl asked, watching as her shoulders stiffened. "My family are bound to ask."

"In a car accident," Estelle said, turning then to him. "The same as your mother."

He opened his mouth to speak and then changed his mind.

"I just hope everyone believes us," Estelle said.

"Why wouldn't they? Even when we divorce we maintain the lie. You understand the confidentiality clause," Raúl said, checking. "No one is to ever know that this is a marriage of convenience only."

"No one will ever hear it from me," she assured him. The prospect of being found out was abhorrent to Estelle. "Just a whirlwind romance and marriage that didn't work out."

"Good," Raúl said. "And, Estelle, even if we do get on, even if you do like..."

"Don't worry, Raúl," she interrupted, "I'm not going to be falling in love with you." She gave him a tight smile. "I'll be out of your life as per the contract."

All about the author...
Carol Marinelli

CAROL MARINELLI finds writing a bio rather like writing her New Year's resolutions. Oh, she'd love to say that since she wrote the last one, she now goes to the gym regularly and doesn't stop for coffee and cake and a gossip afterward; that she's incredibly organized and writes for a few productive hours a day after tidying her immaculate house and taking a brisk walk with the dog.

The reality is that Carol spends an inordinate amount of time daydreaming about dark, brooding men and exotic places (research), which doesn't leave too much time for the gym, housework or anything that comes in between, and her most productive writing hours happen to be in the middle of the night, which leaves her in a constant state of bewildered exhaustion.

Originally from England, Carol now lives in Melbourne, Australia. She adores going back to the U.K. for a visit—actually, she adores going anywhere for a visit—and constantly (expensively) strives to overcome her fear of flying. She has three gorgeous children who are growing up so fast (too fast—they've just worked out that she lies about her age!) and keep her busy with a never-ending round of homework, sport and friends coming over.

A nurse and a writer, Carol writes for the Harlequin Presents® and Medical Romance lines and is passionate about both. She loves the fast-paced, busy setting of a modern hospital, but every now and then admits it's bliss to escape to the glamorous, alluring world of her Presents heroes and heroines. A bit like her real life, actually!

Other titles by Carol Marinelli available in ebook format:
PLAYING THE ROYAL GAME (*The Santina Crown*)
BEHOLDEN TO THE THRONE (*Empire of the Sands*)
PLAYING THE DUTIFUL WIFE
A LEGACY OF SECRETS (*Sicily's Corretti Dynasty*)

Carol Marinelli

—

The Playboy of Puerto Banús

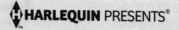

Recycling programs
for this product may
not exist in your area.

ISBN-13: 978-0-373-13185-3

THE PLAYBOY OF PUERTO BANÚS

Copyright © 2013 by Carol Marinelli

HARLEQUIN®
™ www.Harlequin.com

Printed in U.S.A.

The Playboy of Puerto Banús

For Anne and Tony

Thank you for all your love and support.

It means so much.

cxxxx

CHAPTER ONE

'ESTELLE, I PROMISE, you wouldn't have to do anything except hold Gordon's hand and dance....'

'And?' Estelle pushed, pulling down the corner on the page she was reading and closing her book, hardly able to believe she was having this conversation, let alone considering going along with Ginny's plan.

'Maybe a small kiss on the cheek or lips...' As Estelle shook her head Ginny pushed on. 'You just have to look as if you're madly in love.'

'With a sixty-four-year-old?'

'Yes.' Ginny sighed, but before Estelle could argue further broke in, 'Everyone will think you're a gold-digger, that you're only with Gordon for his money. Which you will be...' Ginny stopped talking then, interrupted by a terrible coughing fit.

They were housemates rather than best friends, two students trying to get through university. At twenty-five, Estelle was a few years older than Ginny, and had long wondered how Ginny managed to run a car and dress so well, but now she had found out. Ginny worked for a very exclusive escort agency and had a long-term client—Gordon Edwards, a politician with a secret. Which was why, Ginny had assured her, nothing would happen or be

expected from Estelle if she took Ginny's place as his date
at a very grand wedding being held this evening.

'I'd have to share a room with him.'

Estelle had never shared a room with a man in her life.
She wasn't especially shy or retiring but she certainly had
none of Ginny's confidence or social ease. Ginny thought
the weekends were designed for parties, clubs and pubs,
whereas Estelle's idea of a perfect weekend was looking
around old churches or ruins and then curling up on the
sofa with a book.

Not playing escort!

'Gordon always takes the sofa when we share a room.'

'No.' Estelle pushed up her glasses and returned to her
book. She tried to carry on reading about the mausoleum
of the first Qin Emperor but it was terribly hard to do so
when she was so worried about her brother and he *still*
hadn't rung to let her know if he had got the job.

There was no mistaking the fact that the money would
help.

It was late Saturday morning in London, and the wedding was being held that evening in a castle in Scotland. If
Estelle was going to go then she would have to start getting
ready now, for they would fly to Edinburgh and then take
a helicopter to the castle and time was fast running out.

'Please,' Ginny said. 'The agency are freaking because
they can't get anyone suitable at such short notice. He's
coming to pick me up in an hour.'

'What will people think?' Estelle asked. 'If people are
used to seeing him with you…'

'Gordon will take care of that. He'll say that we had an
argument, that I was pushing for an engagement ring or
something. We were going to be finishing soon anyway,
now that I'm nearly through university. Honestly, Estelle,
Gordon really is the loveliest man. There's so much pres-

sure on him to appear straight—he simply cannot go to this wedding without a date. Just think of the money!'

Estelle couldn't stop thinking about the money.

Attending this wedding would mean that she could pay her brother's mortgage for an entire month, as well as a couple of his bills.

Okay, it wouldn't entirely solve their dilemma, but it would buy Andrew and his young family a little bit more time and, given all they had been through this past year, and all that was still to come, they could certainly use the reprieve.

Andrew had done so much for her—had put his own life on hold to make sure that Estelle's life carried on as normally as possible when their parents had died when Estelle was seventeen.

It was time for Estelle to step up, just as Andrew had.

'Okay.' Estelle took a deep breath and her decision was made. 'Ring and say that I'll come.'

'I've already told him that you've agreed,' Ginny admitted. 'Estelle, don't look at me like that. I know how badly you need the money and I simply couldn't bear to tell Gordon that I didn't have someone else lined up.'

Ginny looked more closely at Estelle. Her long black hair was pulled back in a ponytail, her very pale skin was without a blemish, and there was no last night's make-up smudged under Estelle's green eyes because Estelle rarely wore any. Ginny was trying not to show it but she was actually more than a little nervous as to what a made-up Estelle would look like and whether or not she could carry it off.

'You need to get ready. I'll help with your hair and things.'

'You're not coming near me with that cough,' Estelle said. 'I can manage.' She looked at Ginny's doubtful ex-

pression. 'We can all look like tarts if we have to.' She smiled and Ginny laughed. 'Though I don't actually have anything I can wear…would anyone notice if I wore something of yours?'

'I bought a new dress for the wedding.' Ginny headed to the wardrobe in her bedroom and Estelle followed.

Estelle's jaw dropped when she held the flimsy gold fabric up.

'Does that go under the dress?'

'It looks stunning on.'

'On *you*, perhaps…' Estelle said, because Ginny was a lot slimmer and had a tiny pert bust, whereas, though small, Estelle was curvy. 'I'm going to look like…'

'Which is the whole point.' Ginny grinned. 'Honestly, Estelle, if you just relax you'll have fun.'

'I doubt it,' Estelle said, wrapping her long dark hair in heated rollers at Ginny's dressing table, and setting to work on her face under her housemate's very watchful eye. Gordon was supposed to be a womanizer, and somehow Estelle had to get the balance right between looking as if she adored him while being far, far too young for him too.

'You need more foundation.'

'More?' Estelle already felt as if she had an inch on.

'And lashings of mascara.'

Ginny watched as Estelle took out the heated rollers and her long dark hair tumbled into ringlets. 'Okay, loads of hairspray…' Ginny said. 'Oh, and by the way, Gordon calls me Virginia, just in case anyone mentions me.'

Ginny blinked a few times when Estelle turned around. The smoky grey eyeshadow and layers of mascara brought out the emerald in her green eyes, and the make-up accentuated Estelle's full lips. Seeing the long black curls framing her friend's petite face, Ginny started to believe that Estelle could carry this off.

'You look amazing! Let's see you in the dress.'

'Won't I change there?'

'Gordon's schedule is too busy. Once you land I would imagine you'll be straight into the wedding.'

The dress was beautiful—sheer and gold, it clung everywhere. It was far too revealing but it was delicious too. Ginny gaped when Estelle wobbled on very high shoes.

'I think Gordon might dump me.'

'This,' Estelle said firmly, 'is a one-off.'

'That's what I said when I first started at the agency,' Ginny admitted. 'But if it goes well…'

'Don't even *think* it!' Estelle said as a car tooted in the street.

'You'll be fine,' Ginny said as Estelle nearly jumped out of her skin. 'You look stunning. I know you can do this.'

Estelle clung onto that as she stepped out of her cheap student accommodation home. Teetering on the unfamiliar high heels, she walked out of the drive and towards a sleek silver car, more than a little terrified to meet the politician.

'I have amazing taste!'

Gordon greeted her with a smile as his driver held open the door and Estelle climbed in. He was chubby, dressed in full Scottish regalia, and he made her smile even before she'd properly sat down.

'And you've got far better legs than me! I feel ridiculous in a kilt.'

Instantly he made her relax.

As the car headed for the airport he brought Estelle up to speed. 'We met two weeks ago…'

'Where?' Estelle asked.

'At Dario's…'

'Dario who?'

Gordon laughed. 'You really don't know anything, do you? It's a bar in Soho—sugar daddy heaven.'

'Oh, God…' she groaned.

'Do you work?' Gordon asked.

'Part-time at the library.'

'Maybe don't mention that. Just say you do a little bit of modelling,' Gordon suggested. 'Keep it all very vague, or say that right now keeping Gordon happy is a full-time job.' Estelle blushed and Gordon noticed. 'I know. Awful, isn't it? I seem to have created this terrible persona.'

'I'm worried that I shan't be able to pull it off.'

'You'll be fine,' Gordon said, and he went through everything with her again.

They practised their story over and over on the short flight to Edinburgh. He even asked after her brother and niece, and she was surprised that he knew about their plight.

'Virginia and I have become good friends this past year,' Gordon said. 'She was ever so upset for you when your brother had his accident and when the baby was born so unwell…' He gave her hand a squeeze. 'How is she now?'

'Waiting for surgery.'

'Just remember that you're helping them,' Gordon said as they transferred to the helicopter that would take them to the castle where the very exclusive wedding was being held.

As they walked across the immaculate lawn Gordon took her hand and she was grateful to hold onto it. He really was nice—if they had met under any other circumstances she would be looking forward to this evening.

'I can't wait to get inside the castle,' Estelle admitted. She'd already told Gordon she was studying ancient architecture.

'There won't be much time for exploring,' Gordon said. 'We'll be shown to our room and there will just be time

to freshen up and touch up your hair and make-up before we head down for the wedding.'

'Okay.'

'And just remember,' Gordon said, 'this time tomorrow it will all be over and you'll never have to see any of them again.'

CHAPTER TWO

THE SOUND OF seagulls and the distant throb of music didn't wake Raúl from his slumber; instead they were the sounds that soothed him when he was startled in his sleep. He lay there, heart pounding for a moment, telling himself it was just a dream, while knowing that it was a memory that had jolted him awake.

The gentle motion of his berthed yacht almost tempted him back to sleep, but then he remembered that he was supposed to be meeting with his father.

Raúl forced his eyes open and stared at the tousled blonde hair on his pillow.

'Buenos días,' she purred.

'Buenos días.' Raúl responded, but instead of moving towards her he turned onto his back.

'What time do we leave for the wedding?'

Raúl closed his eyes at her presumption. He had never actually asked Kelly to join him as his guest, but that was the trouble with dating your PA—she knew your diary. The wedding was to be held this evening in the Scottish Highlands. It was nothing for Raúl to fly from Spain to Scotland for a wedding, but Kelly clearly thought that a few weeks out of his office and in his bed meant she was automatically invited.

'I'll speak to you about that later,' Raúl said, glancing at the clock. 'Right now I have to meet with my father.'

'Raúl…' Kelly turned to him in a move that was suggestive.

'Later,' he said, and climbed out of bed. 'I am supposed to be meeting with him in ten minutes.'

'That wouldn't have stopped you before.'

He took the stairs and walked up onto the deck, picking his way through the debris and the evidence of another wild Raúl Sanchez Fuente party. A maid was already starting the mammoth clean up and she gave a cheery wave to Raúl.

'*Gracias,*' she said as he gave her a substantial cash bonus without apologising for the mess. She did not mind his excesses—Raúl paid and treated her well, unlike the owners of some of the yachts, who expected her to work without complaint for very little.

Raúl put on his shades and walked along the Puerto Banús marina, where his yacht was moored. Here, Raúl belonged. Here, despite his decadent ways, he fitted in—because he was not the wildest. Raúl could hear a party continuing on, the music throbbing, the sound of laughter and merriment carrying across the sparkling water, and it reminded Raúl why he loved this place. Rarely was it ever silent. The marina was full of luxurious yachts and had the heady scent of filthy money. Ludicrously expensive cars were casually parked, all the fruits of serious wealth were on display here, and Raúl—dishevelled, unshaven and terribly beautiful—blended in well.

A couple of tourists stumbling home from a club nudged each other as Raúl walked past, trying to place him. For he was as good-looking as any film star and clearly he was *someone*. People-watching was a regular activity in Puerto

Banús, for amongst the tourists and locals were the rich, the famous and the notorious too.

Raúl scored two out of three—though he *was* famous in the business world.

Enrique, his driver, was waiting for him, and Raúl climbed in and gave a brief greeting, and then sat silently as he was driven the short distance to the Marbella branch of De La Fuente Holdings. He had no doubt as to what his father wanted to discuss, but his mind was going over what Kelly had just said.

'That wouldn't have stopped you before.'

Before what? Raúl asked himself.

Before he lost interest?

Before the chase had ended?

Before she assumed that a Saturday night would be shared?

Raúl was an island.

An island with frequent visitors and world-renowned parties, an island of endless sun and unlimited luxury, but one who preferred guests not to outstay their welcome, only allowed the superficial. Yes, Raúl was an island, and he intended to keep it that way. He certainly didn't want permanent boarders and he chose not to let anyone get too close.

He would never be responsible again for another's heart.

'I shan't be long,' Raúl told Enrique as the car door was lifted and he climbed out.

Raúl was not looking forward to this conversation, but his father had insisted they meet this morning and Raúl just wanted it over and done with.

'Buenos días.' He greeted Angela, his father's PA. 'What are you doing here on a Saturday?' he asked, because Angela usually flew home to her family for the weekend.

'I am trying to track down a certain Spaniard who said he would be here at eight a.m.,' Angela scolded mildly. She was the one woman who could get away with telling Raúl how it was. In her late fifties, she had been employed by the company for as long as Raúl could remember. 'I've been trying to call you—don't you ever have your phone on?'

'The battery is flat.'

'Well, before you speak with your father I need to go through your diary.'

'Later.'

'No, Raúl. I'm flying home later this morning. This needs to be done now. We also need to sort out a new PA for you—preferably one you *don't* fancy!' Angela was less than impressed with Raúl's brief eye-roll. 'Raúl, you need to remember that I'm going on long service leave in a few weeks' time. If I'm going to train somebody up for you, then I need to get on to it now.'

'Choose someone, then,' Raúl said. 'And you're right; perhaps it would be better if it was someone that I did not fancy.'

'Finally!' Angela sighed.

Yes, after having it pointed out to him on numerous occasions, Raúl was finally accepting that mixing business with pleasure had consequences, and sleeping with his PA was perhaps not such a good idea.

What was it with women? Raúl wondered. Why, once they'd made it to his bed, did they decide that they could no longer both work *and* sleep with him? Raúl could set his watch by it. After a few weeks they would decide, just as Kelly now had, that frequent dates and sex weren't enough. They wanted exclusivity, wanted inclusion, wanted commitment—which Raúl simply refused to give. Kelly would

be found another position—or paid off handsomely, if that was what she preferred.

'All your flights and transfers are arranged for this afternoon,' Angela said. 'I can't believe that you'll be wearing a kilt.'

'I look good in a kilt.' Raúl smiled. 'Donald has asked that all the male guests wear them. I'm an honorary Scotsman, you know!' He was. He had studied in Scotland for four years, perhaps the best four years of his life, and the friendships he had made there had long continued.

Bar one.

His face hardened as he thought of his ex, who would be there tonight. Perhaps he *should* take Kelly after all, or arrive alone and get off with one of his old flames just to annoy the hell out of Araminta.

'Right, let's get this done…'

He went to walk towards his father's office but Angela called him back. 'It might be an idea to have a coffee before you see him.'

'No need,' Raúl said. 'I will get this over with and then go to Sol's for breakfast.' He loved Saturday mornings at Sol's—a beautiful waterfront café that moved you out quickly if you weren't one of the most beautiful. For people like Raúl they didn't even bother with a bill. They wanted his patronage, wanted the energy he brought to the place. Yes, Raúl decided, he would head there next—except Angela was calling him back again.

'Go and freshen up and I will bring you in coffee and a clean shirt.'

Yes, Angela was the only woman who could get away with speaking to him like that.

Raúl went into his own huge office—which was more like a luxurious hotel suite. As well as the office there was a sumptuous bedroom, and both rooms were put to

good use. Heading towards the bathroom, he glanced at the bed and was briefly tempted to lie down. He had had two, possibly three hours' sleep last night. But he forced himself on to the bathroom, grimacing when he saw himself in the mirror. He could see now why Angela had been so insistent that he freshened up before facing his father.

Raúl's black eyes were bloodshot. He had forgotten to shave yesterday, so now two days' worth of black growth lined his strong jaw. His usually immaculate jet-black hair was tousled and fell over his forehead, and the lipstick on his collar, Raúl was sure, *wasn't* the colour that Kelly had been wearing last night.

Yes, he looked every inch the debauched playboy that his father accused him of being.

Raúl took off his jacket and shirt and splashed water on his face, and then set about changing, calling out his thanks to Angela when he heard her tell him that she had put a coffee on his desk.

'Gracias!' he called, and walked out mid-shave. Angela was possibly the only woman who did not blush at the sight of him without a shirt—she had seen him in nappies, after all. 'And thanks for pointing me in this direction before I meet with my father.'

'No problem.' She smiled. 'There is a fresh shirt hanging on the chair in your office also.'

'Do you know what it is that he wants to see me about?' Raúl was fishing. He knew exactly what his father would want to discuss. 'Am I to be given another lecture about taming my ways and settling down?'

'I'm not sure.' Only now did Angela's cheeks turn pink. 'Raúl, please listen to what your father has to say, though. This is no time for arguments. Your father is sick…'

'Just because he is ill, it does not necessarily make him right.'

'No,' Angela said carefully. 'But he does care for you, Raúl, even if he does not easily show it. Please listen to him… He is worried about you facing things on your own…' Angela saw Raúl's frown and stopped.

'I think you *do* know what this is about.'

'Raúl, I just ask that you listen—I can't bear to hear you two fighting.'

'Stop worrying,' Raúl said kindly. He liked Angela; she was the closest thing to a mum he had. 'I have no intention of fighting. I just think that at thirty years of age I don't have to be told my bedtime, and certainly not who I'm going to bed *with*…'

Raúl got back to shaving. He had no intention of being dictated to, but his hand did pause. Would it be such a big deal to let his father think that maybe he was actually serious about someone? Would it hurt just to hint that maybe he was close to settling down? His father was dying, after all.

'Wish me luck.' Raúl's voice was wry as, clean-shaven and bit clearer in the head, he walked past Angela to face his father. He glanced over, saw the tension and strain on her features. 'It will be fine,' he reassured her. 'Look…' He knew Angela would never keep news from his father. 'I *am* seeing someone, but I don't want him getting carried away.'

'Who?' Angela's eyes were wide.

'Just an old flame. We ran into each other again. She lives in England but I'm seeing her at the wedding tonight…'

'Araminta!'

'Stop there…' Raúl smiled. That was all that was needed. He knew the seed had been sewn.

Raúl knocked on his father's door and stepped in.

There should have been flames, he thought afterwards.

Or the smell of sulphur. Actually, there should have been the smell of car fuel and the sound of thunder followed by silence. There should at least have been some warning, as he was walked through the door, that he was returning to hell.

CHAPTER THREE

ESTELLE FELT AS if everyone knew what a fraud she was.

She closed her heavily made-up eyes and dragged in a deep breath. They were standing in the castle grounds, waiting to be led to their seating, and some pre-wedding drinks and nibbles were being served.

Why they hell had she agreed to this?

You know why, Estelle told herself, her resolve hardening.

'Are you okay, darling?' Gordon asked. 'The wedding should start soon.'

He'd been nothing but kind, just as Ginny had promised he would be.

'I'm fine,' Estelle said, and held a little more tightly onto his arm, just as Gordon had told her to do.

'This is Estelle.'

Gordon introduced her to a couple and Estelle watched the slight rise of the woman's eyebrow.

'Estelle, this is Veronica and James.'

'Estelle.' Veronica gave a curt nod and soon moved James away.

'You're doing wonderfully,' Gordon said, squeezing her hand and drawing her away from the mingling wedding guests so that they could speak without being overheard. 'Maybe you just need to smile a bit more,' he suggested

gently, 'and, I know it calls for brilliant acting, could you try and look just a little more besotted with me? I've got my terrible reputation with women to think of.'

'Of course,' Estelle said through chattering teeth.

'The gay man and the virgin,' Gordon whispered in her ear. 'If only they knew!'

Estelle's eyes widened in horror and Gordon quickly apologised. 'I was just trying to make you smile,' he said.

'I can't believe that she *told* you!'

Estelle was horrified that Ginny would share something as personal and as sensitive as that. Then again, she could believe it—Ginny found it endlessly amusing that Estelle had never slept with anyone. It wasn't by deliberate choice; it wasn't something she'd actively decided. More that she'd been so shell shocked by her parents' death that homework and books had been her escape. By the time she'd emerged from her grief Estelle had felt two steps behind her peers. Clubs and parties had seemed frivolous. It was ancient ruins and buildings that fascinated her, and when she did meet someone there was always a panic that her virgin status must mean she was looking for a husband. More and more it had become an issue.

Now it would seem it was a joke!

She'd be having strong words with Ginny.

'Virginia didn't say it in a malicious way.' Gordon seemed devastated to have upset her. 'We were just talking one night. I really should never have brought it up.'

'It's okay,' Estelle conceded. 'I guess I am a bit of a rarity.'

'We all have our secrets,' Gordon said. 'And for tonight we both have to cover them up.' He smiled at her strained expression. 'Estelle, I know how hard it was for you to agree to this, but I promise you have nothing to feel nervous about. I'm soon to be a happily married man.'

'I know,' Estelle said. Gordon had told her on the plane about his long-term boyfriend, Frank, and the plans they had made. 'I just can't stand the disapproving looks and that everyone thinks of me as a gold-digger,' she admitted. 'Even though that's the whole point of the night.'

'Stop caring what everyone thinks,' Gordon said.

It was the same as she said to Andrew, who was acutely embarrassed to be in a wheelchair. 'You're right.'

Gordon lifted her chin and she smiled into his eyes. 'That's better.' Gordon smiled back. 'We'll get through this together.'

So Estelle held onto his arm and did her best to look suitably besotted, ignoring the occasional disapproving stare from the other guests, and she was just starting to relax and get into things when *he* arrived.

Till that moment Estelle had thought it would be the bride who would make an entrance, and it wasn't the sight of a helicopter landing that had heads turning—helicopters had been landing regularly since Estelle had got there— no, it was the man who stepped out who held everyone's attention.

'Oh, my, the evening just got interesting,' Gordon said as the most stunning man ducked under the blades and then walked towards the gathering.

He was tall, his thick black hair brushed back and gleaming, and his mouth was sulky and unsmiling. His Mediterranean colouring should surely mean that he'd look out of place wearing a kilt, but instead he looked as if he'd been born to wear one. Lean-hipped and long-limbed, but muscular too, he could absolutely carry it off.

He could carry me off right now, Estelle thought wildly—and wild thoughts were rare for Estelle.

She watched as he accepted whisky from a waiter and then stood still. He seemed removed and remote from ev-

eryone else. Even the women who flocked to him were quickly dismissed, as if at any minute he might simply walk off.

Then he met her eyes.

Estelle tried to flick hers away, except she found that she couldn't.

His eyes drifted down over the gold dress, but not in the disapproving way that Veronica's had. Although they weren't approving either. They were merely assessing.

She felt herself burn as his eyes moved then to her sixty-four-year-old date, and she wanted to correct him—wanted to tell him that the rotund, red-faced man who was struggling with the heat in his heavy kilt and jacket was not her lover. Though of course she could not.

She wanted to, though.

'Eyes only for me, darling,' Gordon reminded her, perhaps picking up on the crackle of energy crossing the lawn. His glance followed Estelle's gaze. 'Though frankly no one would blame you a bit for looking. He's completely divine.'

'Who?' Estelle tried to pretend that she hadn't noticed the delicious stranger—Gordon was paying her good money to be here, after all—but she wasn't fooling anyone.

'Raúl Sanchez Fuente,' Gordon said in a low voice. 'Our paths cross now and then at various functions. He owns everything but morals. The bastard even looks good in a kilt. He has my heart—not that he wants it…'

Estelle couldn't help but laugh.

Raúl's eyes lazily worked over the guests. He was questioning now his decision to come alone. He needed distraction tonight, but when he had thought of the old flames that he might run into he had been thinking of the perky breasts and the narrow waists of yesteryear, as if the clock might

have stopped on his university days. Instead the hands of time had moved on.

There was Shona. Her once long red hair was now cut too severely and she stood next to a chinless wonder. She caught his eye and then blushed unbecomingly and shot him a furious look, as if their once torrid times could be erased and forgotten by her wedding ring.

He knew, though, that she was remembering.

'Raúl…'

He frowned when he saw Araminta walking towards him. She was wearing that slightly needy smile that Raúl recognised only too well and it made his early warning system react—because temporary distraction was his requirement tonight, not desperation.

'How are you?'

'Not bad,' she said, and then proceeded to tell him about her hellish divorce, how she was now single, how she'd thought about him often since the break-up, how she'd been looking forward to seeing him tonight, how she regretted the way things had worked out for them…

'I told you that you would at the time.' Raúl did not do sentiment. 'You'll have to excuse me. I have to make a call.'

'We'll catch up later, though?'

He could hear the hope in her voice and it irked him.

Was he good enough for her father now? Rich enough? Established enough?

'There's nothing to catch up on.'

Just like that he dismissed her, his black eyes not even watching her as she gave a small sob and walked off.

What on earth was he doing here? Raúl wondered. He should be getting ready to party on his yacht, or to hit the clubs—should be losing himself instead of getting reacquainted with his past. More to the point, there was hardly a limitless choice of women in this castle in the Scottish

Highlands. And after what Raúl had found out this morning his own company wasn't one he wanted to keep.

His hand tightened on the whisky glass he held. The full impact of what his father had told him was only now starting to hit him.

So black were his thoughts, so sideswiped was he by the revelations, Raúl actually considered leaving—just summoning his pilot and walking out. But then a tumble of dark hair and incredibly pale skin caught his eye and held it. She looked nervous and awkward—which was unusual for Gordon's tarts. They were normally brash and confident. But not this one.

He held her gaze when she caught his and now there was only one woman he wanted to walk towards him—except she was holding tightly to Gordon's arm.

She offered far more than distraction—she offered oblivion. Because for the first time since his conversation with his father he forgot about it.

Perhaps he would stay. At least for the service…

A deep Scottish voice filled the air and the guests were informed that the wedding would soon commence and they were to make their way to their seats.

'Come on.' Gordon took Estelle's hand. 'I love a good wedding.'

'And me.' Estelle smiled.

They walked through the mild night. The grounds were lit by torches and there were chairs set out. With the castle as a backdrop the scene looked completely stunning, and Estelle let go of her guilt, determined to enjoy herself. She'd been on a plane and, for the first time in her life, a helicopter, she was staying the night in a beautiful castle in the Scottish Highlands, and Gordon was an absolute delight. Despite having dreaded it, she was enjoying her-

self, Estelle realised as they took their seats and she made more small talk with Gordon.

'Donald says that Victoria's so nervous,' he told her. 'She's such a perfectionist, apparently, and she's been stressing over the details for months.'

'Well, it all seems to have paid off,' Estelle said. 'I can't wait to see what she's wearing.'

Just as she'd finally started to relax as the music changed and they all stood for the bride, just as she'd decided simply to enjoy herself, she turned to get a first glimpse of the bride—only to realise that Raúl was sitting behind her.

Directly behind her.

It should make no difference, Estelle told herself. It was a simple coincidence. But even coincidence was too big a word—after all, he had to sit *somewhere*. Estelle was just acutely aware that he was there.

She tried to concentrate on the bride as she made her way to Donald. Victoria really did look stunning. She was wearing a very simple white dress and carried a small posy of heather. The smile on Donald's face as his bride walked towards him had Estelle smiling too—but not for long. She could feel Raúl's eyes burning into her shoulder, and a little while later her scalp felt as if it were on fire. She was sure his eyes lingered there.

She did her best to focus on the service. It was incredibly romantic. So much so that when they got to the 'in sickness and in health' part it actually brought tears to her eyes as she remembered her brother Andrew's wedding, just over a year ago.

Who could have known then the hard blows fate had in store for him and his pregnant bride, Amanda?

Ever the gentleman, Gordon pressed a tissue into her hand.

'Thank you.' Estelle gave a watery smile and Gordon gave her hand a squeeze.

* * *

Please! Raúl thought. *Spare me the crocodile tears.* It had been the same with Gordon's previous girlfriend—what was her name? Raúl smiled to himself, as he had the day they were introduced.

Virginia.

This one, though, even if she wasn't to Raúl's usual taste, was stunning. Raven-haired women were far from a rarity where Raúl came from, and for that reason he certainly preferred a blonde—for variety, two blondes!

He wanted raven tonight.

Turn around, Raúl thought, for he wanted to meet those eyes again.

Turn around, he willed her, watching her shoulders stiffen, watching the slight tilt of her neck as if she was aware of but resisting his silent demand.

How she was resisting.

Estelle sat rigid and then stood in the same way after the service was over, when the bride and groom were letting doves fly. They fluttered high into the sky and the crowd murmured and pointed and turned to watch them in flight.

Reluctantly she also turned, and she must look up, Estelle thought helplessly as two black liquid pools invited her to dive in. She should, like everyone else, move her gaze upwards and watch the doves fly off into the distance.

Instead she faced him.

What the hell are you doing with him? Raúl wanted to ask. *What the hell are you doing with a man perhaps three times your age?*

Of course he knew the answer.

Money.

And Raúl knew then what to do—knew the answer to the dilemma that had been force-fed to him at breakfast-time.

His mouth moved into a smile and he watched as her head jerked away—watched as she stared, too late, up into the sky. And he saw her pale throat as her neck arched and he wanted his mouth there.

A piper led them back to the castle. He walked in front of her and Gordon. Estelle's heels kept sinking into the grass, but it was nothing compared to the feeling of drowning in quicksand when she had been caught in Raúl's gaze.

His kilt was greys and lilacs, his jacket a dark purple velvet, his posture and his stride exact and sensual. She wanted to run up to him, to tap him on the shoulder and tell him to please leave her alone. Yet he had done nothing. He wasn't even looking over his shoulder. He was just chatting with a fellow guest as they made their way back to the castle.

Very deliberately Raúl ignored her. He turned his back and chatted with Donald, asked a favour from a friend, and then flirted a little with a couple of old flames—but at all times he knew that her eyes more than occasionally searched out his.

Raúl knew exactly what he was doing and he knew exactly why.

Mixing business with pleasure had caused a few problems for Raúl in the past.

Tonight it was suddenly the solution.

CHAPTER FOUR

'Excuse me, sir.'

A waiter halted Estelle and Gordon as they made their way into the Grand Hall and to their table.

'There's been a change to the seating plan. Donald and Victoria didn't realise that you were seated so far back. It's all been rectified now. Please accept our apologies for the mistake.'

'*Oooh*, we're getting an upgrade,' Gordon said as they were led nearer to the front.

Estelle flushed when she saw that the rather teary woman she had seen earlier speaking with Raúl was being quietly shuffled back to the bowels of the hall. Estelle knew even before they arrived at the new table which one it would be.

Raúl did not look up as they made their way over. Not until they were being shown into their seats.

She smiled a greeting to Veronica and James, but could not even attempt one for Raúl—both seats either side of him were empty.

He had done this.

Estelle tried to tell herself she was imagining things, or overreacting, but somehow she knew she was right. Knew that those long, lingering stares had led to this.

The chair next to him was being held out. She wanted

to turn to Gordon, to ask if they could swap seats but she knew that would look ridiculous.

It was a simple change of seating, Estelle told herself.

She acknowledged to herself that she lied.

'Gordon.' Raúl shook his hand.

'Raúl.'

Gordon smiled as he took the seat next to Estelle, so she was sandwiched between them, and she leant back a little as they chatted.

'I haven't seen you since…' Gordon laughed. 'Since last wedding season. This is Estelle.'

'Estelle.' He raised one eyebrow as she took her seat beside him. 'In Spain you would be Estela.'

'We're in England.' She was aware of her brittle response, but her defences were up—though she did try to soften it with a brief smile.

'Of course.' Raúl shrugged. 'Though I must speak with my pilot. He was most insistent, when we landed, that this was *Scotland*.'

She tried so hard not to, but Estelle twitched her lips into a slight smile.

'This is Shona and Henry…' Raúl introduced them as a waiter poured some wine.

Estelle took a sip and then asked for water—for a draughty castle, it felt terribly warm.

There was brief conversation and more introductions taking place, and all would have been fine if Raúl were not there. But Estelle was aware, despite his nonchalant appearance, that he was carefully listening to her responses.

She laughed just a little too loudly at one of Gordon's jokes.

As she'd been told to do.

Gordon was busy speaking with James, and for something to do Estelle looked through the menu, squinting

because Ginny had suggested that she leave her glasses at home.

Raúl misconstrued it as a frown.

'Vichyssoise,' came his low, deep voice. 'It is a soup. It's delicious.'

'I don't need hand-holding for the menu.' Estelle stopped herself, aware she was coming across as terribly rude, but her nerves were prickling in defensiveness. 'And you failed to mention it's served cold.'

'No.' He smiled. 'I was just about to tell you that.'

Soup was a terribly hard ask with Raúl sitting next to her, but she worked her way through it, even though her conversation with Gordon kept getting interrupted by his phone.

'I can't even get a night off.' He sighed.

'Important?' Estelle checked.

'It could be soon. I'll have to keep it on silent.'

The main course was served and it was the most gorgeous beef Estelle had ever tasted. Yet it stuck in her throat—especially when Veronica asked her a question.

'Do you work, Estelle?'

She took a drink of water before answering. 'I do a bit of modeling.' Estelle gave a small smile, remembering how Gordon had told her to respond to such a question. She just hadn't expected to be inhaling testosterone when she answered. 'Though, of course, taking care of Gordon is a full-time job...'

Estelle saw the pausing of Raúl's fork and then heard Gordon's stab of laughter. She was locked in a lie and there was no way out. It was an act, Estelle told herself. Just one night and she would never have to see these people again—and what did she care if Raúl thought her cheap?

'Could you pass me the pepper?' came the silk of his voice.

Was it the fact that it had been asked with a Spanish accent that made the question sound sexy, or was it that she was going mad?

She passed it, holding the heavy silver pot and releasing it to him, feeling the brief warmth of his fingertips as he took it. He immediately noticed her error. 'That's the salt,' Raúl said, and she had to go through it again.

It was bizarre. He had said hardly two words to her, had made no suggestions. There were no knees pressing into hers under the table and his hands had not lingered when she'd passed him the pepper, yet the air between them was thick with tension.

He declined dessert and spread cheese onto Scottish oatcakes. 'I'd forgotten how good these taste.'

She turned and watched as he took a bite and then ran his tongue over his lip, capturing a small sliver of quince paste.

'Now I remember.'

There was no implication. He was only making small talk.

It was Estelle's mind that searched every word.

She spread cheese on an oatcake herself and added quince.

'Fantastic?' Raúl asked.

'Yes.'

She knew he meant sex.

'Now the speeches.' Gordon sighed.

They were long. Terribly long. Especially when you had no idea who the couple were. Especially when you were supposed to be paying attention to the man on your right but your mind was on the one to your left.

First it was Victoria's father, who rambled on just a touch too long. Then it was the groom Donald's turn, and he was thankfully a bit quicker—and funnier too. He

moved through the formalities and, on behalf of himself and his new wife, especially thanked all who had travelled from afar.

'I was hoping Raúl wouldn't make it, of course,' Donald said, looking over to Raúl, as did the whole room. 'I'm just thankful Victoria didn't see him in a kilt until *after* my ring was on her finger. Trust a Spaniard to wear a kilt so well.'

The whole room laughed. Raúl's shoulders moved in a light, good-natured laugh too. He wasn't remotely embarrassed—no doubt more than used to the attention and to having his beauty confirmed.

Then it was the best man's turn.

'In Spain there are no speeches at a wedding,' Raúl said, leaning across her a little to speak to Gordon.

She could smell his expensive cologne, and his arm was leaning slightly on her. Estelle watched her fingers around the stem of her glass tighten.

'We just have the wedding, a party, and then bed,' Raúl said.

It was the first hint of suggestion, but even so she could merely be reading into things too much. Except as he leant over her to hear Gordon's response Estelle wanted to put her hand up, wanted to ask for the lights to come on, for this assault on her senses to stop, to tell the room the inappropriateness of the man sitting beside her. Only not a single thing had he done—not a word or hand had he put wrong.

So why was her left breast aching, so close to where his arm was? Why were her two front teeth biting down on her lip at the sight of his cheek, inches away?

'Really?' Gordon checked. 'I might just have to move to Spain! In actual fact I was—'

Gordon was interrupted by the buzz of his phone and

Raúl moved back in his seat. Estelle sat watching the newly wed couple dancing.

'Darling, I am so sorry,' Gordon said as he read a message on his phone. 'I am going to have to find somewhere I can make some calls and use a computer.'

'Good luck getting internet access,' drawled Raúl. 'I have to go outside just to make a call.'

'I might be some time.'

'Trouble?' Estelle asked

'Always.' Gordon rolled his eyes. 'Though this is unexpected. But I'll deal with it as quickly as I can. I hate to leave you on your own.'

'She won't be on her own,' Raúl said. 'I can keep an eye.'

She rather wished that he wouldn't.

'Thanks so much,' Gordon said. 'In that dress she deserves to dance.' He turned to Estelle. 'I really am sorry to leave you...' For appearances' sake, he kissed her on the cheek.

What a waste of her mouth, Raúl thought.

Once Gordon had gone she turned to James and Veronica, on her right, desperately trying to feed into their conversation. But they were certainly not interested in Gordon's new date. Over and over they politely dismissed her, and then followed the other couples at their table and got up to dance—leaving her alone with Raúl.

'From the back you could be Spanish...'

She turned to the sound of his voice.

'But from the front...'

His eyes ran over her creamy complexion and she felt heat sear her face as his eyes bored into hers. And though they did not wander—he was far too suave for that—somehow he undressed her. Somehow she sat there on her seat beside him at the wedding as if they were a

couple. And when he looked at her, she felt, for a bizarre second, as if she was completely naked.

He was as potent as that.

CHAPTER FIVE

'IRISH?' HE CHECKED, and Estelle hesitated for a moment before nodding.

She did not want to give any information to this man—did not even want to partake in conversation.

'Yet your accent is English?'

'My parents moved to England before I was born.' She gave a tight swallow and hoped her stilted response would halt the conversation. It did not.

'Where in England are they?'

'They're not,' Estelle answered, terribly reluctant to reveal *anything* of herself.

Raúl did not push. Instead he moved the conversation on.

'So, where did you and Gordon meet?'

'We met at Dario's.' Estelle answered the question as Gordon had told her to, trying to tell herself he was just being polite, but every sense in her body seemed set to high alert. 'It's a bar—'

'In Soho,' Raúl broke in. 'I have heard a lot about Dario's.'

Beneath her make-up her cheeks were scalding.

'Not that I have been,' Raúl said. 'As a male, I would perhaps be too young to get in there.' His lips rose in a slight smile and he watched the colour flood darker in her neck and to her ears. 'Maybe I should give it a try...'

He looked more closely at Estelle. She had eyes that were a very dark green and rounded cheeks—she really was astonishingly attractive. There was something rather sweet about her despite the clothes, despite the make-up, and there was an awkwardness that was as rare as it was refreshing. Raúl was not used to awkwardness in the women he dated.

'So, we both find ourselves alone at a wedding...'

'I'm not alone,' Estelle said. 'Gordon will be back soon.' She did not want to ask, but she found herself doing just that as she glanced to the empty chair beside him. 'How come...?' Her voice faded out. There was no polite way to address it.

'We broke up this morning.'

'I'm sorry.'

'Please don't be.' He thought for a moment before continuing. 'Really to say we broke up is perhaps an exaggeration. To break something would mean you had to have something, and we were only going out for a few weeks.'

'Even so...' Still she attempted to be polite. 'Break-ups are hard.'

'I've never found them to be,' Raúl said. 'It's the bit before that I struggle with.'

'When it starts to go wrong?'

'No,' Raúl said. 'When it starts to go right.'

His eyes were looking right into hers, his voice was deep and low, and his words interesting—because despite herself she *did* want to know more about this fascinating man. So much so that she found herself leaning in a little to hear.

'When she starts asking what we are doing next weekend. When you hear her saying "Raúl said..." or "Raúl thinks..."' He paused for a second. 'I don't like to be told what I'm thinking.'

'I'm sure you don't.'

'Do you know what I'm thinking now?'

'I wouldn't presume to.' She could hardly breathe, because she was surely thinking the same.

'Would you like to dance?'

'No, thank you,' Estelle said, because it was far safer to stay seated than to self-combust in his arms. He was sinfully good-looking and, more worryingly, she had a sinking feeling as she realised he was pulling her in deeper with each measured word. 'I'll just wait here for Gordon.'

'Of course,' Raúl said. 'Have you met the bride or groom?'

'No.' Estelle felt as if she were being interviewed. 'You're friends with the groom?'

'I went to university with him.'

'In Spain?'

'No, here in Scotland.'

'Oh!' She wasn't sure why, but that surprised her.

'I was here for four years,' Raúl said. 'Then I moved back to Marbella. I still like to come here. Scotland is a very beautiful country.'

'It is,' Estelle said. 'Well, from the little I've seen.'

'It's your first time?'

She nodded.

'Have you ever been to Spain?'

'Last year,' Estelle said. 'Though only for a few days. Then there was a family emergency and I had to go home.'

'Raúl?'

He barely looked up as a woman came over. It was the same woman who had been moved from the table earlier.

'I thought we could dance.'

'I'm busy.'

'Raúl…'

'Araminta.' Now he turned and looked at her. 'If I wanted to dance with you then I would have asked.'

Estelle blinked, because despite the velvet of his voice his words were brutal.

'That was a bit harsh,' Estelle said as Araminta stumbled off.

'Far better to be harsh than to give mixed messages.'

'Perhaps.'

'So…' Raúl chose his words carefully. 'If taking care of Gordon is a full-time job, what do you do in your time off?'

'My time off?'

'When you're not *working*.'

She didn't frown this time. There was no mistake as to what he meant. Her green eyes flashed as she turned to him. 'I don't appreciate the implication.'

He was surprised by her challenge, liked that she met him head-on—it was rare that anyone did.

'Excuse me,' he said. 'Sometimes my English is not so good…'

When it suited him.

Estelle took a deep breath, her hand still toying with the stem of her glass as she wondered how to play this, deciding she would do her best to be polite.

'What work do you do?' She looked at him. She had absolutely no idea about this man. 'Are you in politics too?'

'Please!'

He watched the slight reluctant smile on her lips.

'I am a director for De La Fuente Holdings, which means I buy, improve or build, and then maybe I sell.' Still he watched her. 'Take this castle; if I owned it I would not have it exclusively as a wedding venue but also as a hotel. It is under-utilised. Mind you, it would need a lot of refurbishment. I have not shared a bathroom since my university days.'

She was far from impressed and tried not to show it. Raúl, of course, could not know that she was studying ancient architecture and that buildings were a passion of hers. The castle renovations she had seen were modest, the rooms cold and the bathrooms sparse—as it should be. The thought of this place being modernised and filled to capacity, no matter how tastefully, left her cold.

Unfortunately *he* didn't.

Not once in her twenty-five years had Estelle even come close to the reaction she was having to Raúl.

If they were anywhere else she would get up and leave.

Or, she conceded, if they were anywhere else she would lean forward and accept his mouth.

'So it's your father's business?' Estelle asked, trying to find a fault in him—trying to tell herself that it was his father's money that had eased his luxurious path to perfection.

'No, it was my mother's family business. My father bought into it when he married.' He saw her tiny frown.

'Sorry, you said De La Fuente, and I thought Fuente was *your* surname…'

For an occasional model who picked up men at Dario's she was rather perceptive, Raúl thought. 'In Spain it is different. You take your father's surname first and then your mother's…'

'I didn't know that.' She tried to fathom it. 'How does it work?'

'My father is Antonio Sanchez. My mother was Gabriella De La Fuente.'

'Was?'

'She passed away in a car accident…'

Normally he could just say it. Every other time he revealed it he just glossed over it, moved swiftly on—tonight, with all he had learnt this morning, suddenly he could not.

Every man except Raúl had struggled in the summer heat with full Scottish regalia. Supremely fit, and used to the sun, Raúl had not even broken a sweat. But now, when the castle was cool, when a draught swirled around the floor, he broke into one—except his face drained of colour.

He tried to right himself, reached for water; he had trained his mind not to linger. Of course he had not quite mastered his mind at night, but even then he had trained himself to wake up before he shouted out.

'Was it recent?' Estelle saw him struggle briefly, knew surely better than anyone how he must feel—for she had lost her parents the same way. She watched as he drained a glass of water and then blinked when he turned and the suave Raúl returned.

'Years ago,' he dismissed. 'When I was a child.' He got back to their discussion, refusing to linger on a deeply buried past. 'My actual name is Raúl Sanchez De La Fuente, but it gets a bit long during introductions.'

He smiled, and so too did Estelle.

'I can imagine.'

'But I don't want to lose my mother's name, and of course my father expects me to keep his.'

'It's nice that the woman's name passes on.'

'It doesn't, though,' Raúl said. 'Well, it does for one generation—it is still weighted to the man.' He saw her frown.

'So, if you had a baby…?'

'That's never going to happen.'

'But if you did?'

'God forbid.' He let out a small sigh. 'I will try to explain.'

He was very patient.

He took the salt and pepper she had so nervously passed to him and, heads together, they sat at the table while he made her a small family tree.

'What is your surname?'

'Connolly.'

'Okay, we have a baby and call her Jane…'

How he made her burn. Not at the baby part, but at the thought of the part to get to that.

'Her name would be Jane Sanchez Connolly.'

'I see.'

'And when Jane marries…' he lifted a hand and grabbed a fork as he plucked a name from the ether '…Harry Potter, her daughter…' he added a spoon '…who shall also be called Jane, would be Jane Sanchez Potter. Connolly would be gone!' He looked at her as she worked it out. 'It is simple. At least the name part is simple. It is the fifty years of marriage that might prove hard.' He glanced over to today's happy couple. 'I can't imagine being tied down to another, and I certainly don't believe in love.'

He always made that clear up-front.

'How can you sit at a wedding and say that?' Estelle challenged. 'Did you not see the smile on Donald's face when he saw his bride?'

'Of course I did,' Raúl said. 'I recognised it well—it was the same smile he gave at the last wedding of his I attended.'

She laughed. There was no choice but to. 'Are you serious?'

'Completely,' Raúl said.

Yet he was smiling, and when he did that she felt as if she should scrabble in her bag for sunglasses, because the force of his smile blinded her to all faults—and she was quite positive a man like Raúl had many.

'You're wrong, Raúl.' She refused to play his cynical game. 'My brother got married last year and he and his wife are deeply in love.'

'A year.' He gave a light shrug. 'It is still the honey-moon phase.'

'They've been through more in this year than most have been through in a lifetime.' And she'd never meant to but she found herself opening up to him. 'Andrew, my brother, was in an accident on their honeymoon—a jet ski…'

'Serious?'

Estelle nodded. 'He's now in a wheelchair.'

'That must take a lot of getting used to.' He thought for a moment. 'Is that the family emergency you had to fly home from your own holiday for?'

Estelle nodded. She didn't tell him it had been a trip around churches. No doubt he assumed she'd been hauled out of a club to hear the news. 'I raced home, and, really, since then things have been tough on them. Amanda was already pregnant when they got married…'

She didn't know why she was telling him. Perhaps it was safer to talk than to dance. Maybe it was easier to talk about her brother and the truth than make up stories about Dario's and seedy clubs in Soho. Or perhaps it was the black liquid eyes that invited conversation, the way he moved his chair a little closer so that he could hear.

'Their daughter was born four months ago. The prospect of being a dad was the main thing that kept Andrew motivated during his rehabilitation. Just when we thought things were turning around…'

Raúl watched her green eyes fill with tears, saw her rapid blink as she tried to stem them.

'She has a heart condition. They're waiting till she's a little bit bigger so they can operate.'

He watched pale hands go to her bag and Estelle took out a photo. He looked at her brother, Andrew, and his wife, and a small frail baby with a slight blue tinge to her skin, and he realised that they hadn't been crocodile tears

he had witnessed during the wedding ceremony. He looked
back to Estelle.

'What's her name?'

'Cecelia.'

Raúl looked at her as she gazed at the photo and he
knew then the reason she was here with Gordon. 'Your
brother?' Raúl asked, just to confirm things in his mind.
'Does he work?'

'No.' Estelle shook her head. 'He was self-employed.
He…' She put away the photo, dragged in a breath, could
not stand to think of all the problems her brother faced.

Exactly at that moment Raúl lightened things.

'My legs are cold.'

Estelle laughed, and as she did she blinked as a photographer's camera flashed in her face.

'Nice natural shot,' the photographer said.

'We're not…' Oh, what did it matter?

'I need to move.' He stood. 'And Gordon asked that I
take care of you.' Raúl held out his hand to her. This dance
was more important than she could ever know. This dance
must ensure that tonight she was thinking only of *him*—
that by the time he approached her with his suggestion it
would not seem so unthinkable. But first he had to set the
tone. First he had to make her aware that he knew the sort
of business she was in. 'Would you like to dance?'

Estelle didn't really have a choice. Walking towards the
dance floor, she had the futile hope that the band would
break into something more frivolous than sensuous, but
all hope was gone as his arms wrapped loosely around her.

'You are nervous?'

'No.'

'I would have thought you would enjoy dancing, given
that you two met at Dario's.'

'I do love to dance.' Estelle forced a bright smile, re-

membered who she was supposed to be. 'It's just a bit early for me.'

'And me,' Raul said as he took her in his arms. 'About now I would only just be getting ready to go out.'

She couldn't read this man. Not in the least. He held her, he was skilled and graceful, but the eyes that looked down at her were not smiling.

'Relax.'

She tried to—except he'd said it into her ear, causing the sensitive skin there to tingle.

'Can I ask something?'

'Of course,' Estelle said, though she would rather he didn't. She just wanted this duty dance to end.

'What are you doing with Gordon?'

'Excuse me?' She could not believe he would ask that— could not think of anyone else who would be so direct. It was as if all pretence had gone—all tiny implications, all conversation left behind—and the truth was being revealed in his arms.

'There is a huge age difference...'

'That's none of your business.' She felt as if she was being attacked in broad daylight and everyone else was just carrying on, oblivious.

'You are twenty, yes?'

'Twenty-five.'

'He was ten years older than I am now when you were born.'

'They're just numbers.'

'We both work in numbers.'

Estelle went to walk off mid-dance, but his grip merely tightened. 'Of course...' He held her so she could feel the lean outline of his body, inhale the terribly masculine scent of him. 'You want him only for his money.'

'You're incredibly rude.'

'I'm incredibly honest,' Raúl corrected. 'I am not criti-
cizing—there is nothing wrong with that.'

'Vete al infierno!' Estelle said, grateful for a Spanish
schoolfriend and lunchtimes being taught by her how to
curse. She watched his mouth curve as she told him in
his own language to go to hell. 'Excuse me,' Estelle said.
'Sometimes my Spanish is not so good. What I mean to
say is…'

He pressed a finger to her lips before she could tell
him, in her own language and rather more crudely, exactly where he could go.

The contact with her mouth, the sensual pressure, the
intimacy of the gesture, had the desired effect and silenced
her.

'One more dance,' Raúl said. 'Then I return you to Gordon.' He removed his finger. 'I'm sorry if you thought I
was being rude—believe me, that was not my intention.
Accept my apology, please.'

Estelle's eyes narrowed in suspicious assessment. She
was aware of the pulse in her lips from his mere touch.
Logic told her to remove herself from this situation, yet
the stir of first arousal won.

The music slowed and, ignoring brief resistance, he
pulled her in tighter. If she thought he was judging her,
she was right—only it was not harshly. Raúl admired a
woman who could separate emotion from sex.

Raúl needed exactly such a woman if he were to see
this through.

He did not think her cheap: on the contrary, he intended
to pay her very well.

She should have gone then—back to the table, to be ignored by the other guests. Should have left this man at a
safer point. But her naïve body was refusing to walk away;
instead it was awakening in his arms.

He held her so that her head was resting on his chest. She could feel the soft velvet of his jacket on her cheek. But she was more aware of his hand resting lightly on the base of her spine.

A couple dancing, each in a world of their own.

Raúl's motives were temporarily suspended. He enjoyed the soft weight that leant against him, the quiet of his mind as he focused only on her. The hand on her shoulder crept beneath her hair, his fingers lightly stroking the back of her neck, and again he wanted his mouth there, wanted to lift the raven curtain and taste her.

His fingers told her so—they stroked in a soft probing and they circled and teased as she swayed in time to the music. Estelle felt the stirring between them, and though her head denied what was happening her body shifted a little to allow for him. Her nipples hurt against his chest. His hand pressed her in just a little tighter as again he broke all boundaries. Again he voiced what perhaps others would not.

'I always thought a sporran was for decorative purposes only…'

She could feel the heat of its fur against her stomach.

'Yet it is the only thing keeping me decent.'

'You're *so* far from decent,' Estelle rasped.

'I know.'

They danced—not much, just swaying in time. Except she was on fire.

He could feel the heat of her skin on his fingers, could feel her breath so shallow that he wanted to lower his head and breathe into her mouth for her. He thought of her dark hair on his pillow, of her pink nipples in his mouth at the same time. He wanted her more than he had wanted any other, though Raúl was not comfortable with that thought.

This was business, Raúl reminded himself as motive re-

turned. Tonight she would think of *his* lean, aroused body. When she was bedded by Gordon it would be *his* lithe body she ached for. He must now make sure of that. It was a business decision, and he made business decisions well.

His hand slid from beneath her hair down to the side of her ribs, to the bare skin there.

She ached. She ached for his hand to move, to cup her breast. And again he confirmed what was happening.

'Soon I return you to Gordon,' Raúl said, 'but first you come to *me*.'

It was foreplay. So much so she felt that as if his fingers were inside her. So much so that she could feel, despite the sporran, the thick outline beneath his kilt. It was the most dangerous dance of her life. She wanted to turn. She wanted to run. Except her body wanted the feel of his arms. Her burning cheeks rested against purple velvet and she could hear the steady thud of his heart as hers tripped and galloped. No one around them had a clue about the fire in his arms.

He smelt exquisite, and his cheek near hers had her head wanting to turn, to seek the relief of his mouth. She did not know the range of *la petit mort* or that he was giving her a mere taste. Estelle was far too innocent to know that she was building up to doing exactly as instructed and coming to him.

Raúl knew exactly when he felt the tension in his arms slowly abate, felt her slip a little down his chest as for a brief moment she relaxed against him.

'Thank you for the dance.' Breathless, stunned, she went to step back.

But still he held her as he lifted her chin and offered his verdict. 'You know, I would like to see you *really* cuss in Spanish.'

He let her go then, and Estelle headed to the safety of the ladies' room and ran her wrists under the tap to cool them.

Careful, she told herself. *Be careful here, Estelle.*

There was a blaze of attraction more intense than any she had known. What Estelle *did* know, though, was that a man like Raúl would crush her in the palm of his hand.

She looked up into the mirror and took out her lipstick; she could not fathom what had just taken place—nor that she had allowed it.

That she had partaken in it.

And willingly at that.

'There you are.'

Gordon smiled as she headed back to the table and she could not feel more guilty: she'd even failed as an escort.

'I'm so sorry to have left you—some foreign minister wanted to speak urgently with me, but we couldn't get him on the line and when we did…' Gordon gave a weary smile. 'He had no idea what he wanted to speak to me about. I've been going around in circles.' Gordon drained his drink. 'Let's dance.'

It felt very different dancing with Gordon. They laughed and chatted as she tried not to think about the dance with Raúl.

Yes, she danced with Gordon—but it was the black eyes still on her that held her mind. Raúl sat at the table drinking whisky.

'I think you've made quite an impression. Raúl can't keep his eyes off you.'

She started in his arms. 'It's okay, Estelle.' Gordon smiled. 'I'm flattered—or rather my persona is. To have Raúl as competition is a compliment indeed.'

He kissed her cheek and she rested her head on his shoulder, and then her eyes fell to Raúl's black eyes that still watched and there was heat in her body, and she tried

to look away but she could not. She watched his mouth move in a slow smile till Gordon danced her so that Raúl was out of her line of vision. Then, a moment later, her eyes scanned the room for him and prayed that the dangerous part of her night was now over.

Raúl was gone.

CHAPTER SIX

'SORRY!'

Gordon apologised profusely for scaring her, after Estelle had walked into the guest room much later that night to find a monster!

He whipped the mask off. 'It's for my breathing. I have sleep apnoea.'

Estelle had changed in a tiny bathroom along the draughty hall and was now wearing some very old, very tatty pale pink pyjamas that she only put on when she was sick or reading for an entire weekend. It was all she'd had at short notice, but Estelle was quite sure Gordon wasn't expecting cleavage and sexy nightdresses.

She offered to take the sofa bed—he was paying her, after all—but true to his word he insisted that she have the bed.

'Thank you so much for tonight, Estelle.'

'It's been fine,' Estelle said as she rubbed cold cream into her face and took her make-up off. 'It must be so hard on you, though,' she mused, trying to get off the last of her mascara. 'Having to hide your real life.'

'It certainly hasn't been easy, but six months from now I'll be able to be myself.'

'Can't you now?'

'If it was just about me then I probably would have by

now,' Gordon explained. 'Frank is so private, though—it would be awful for him to have our relationship discussed on the news, which it would be. Still, six months from now we'll be sunning it in Spain.'

'Is that where you're going to live?'

'And marry,' Gordon said. 'Gay marriage is legal there.'

Estelle was really tired now; she slipped into bed and they chatted a little while more.

'You know that Virginia has nearly finished her studies…?'

'I know.' Estelle sighed—not only because she would miss her housemate, but also because she would need to find someone else to share if she continued with *her* course. But then she realised what Gordon was referring to.

'She's starting work next month. I don't want to offend you by suggesting anything, but if you did want to accompany me to things for a few months…'

He didn't push, and for that Estelle was grateful.

'Have a think about it,' Gordon said, and wished her goodnight.

Estelle was soon drifting off, thinking not about Gordon's offer but about Raúl and his pursuit.

And it *had* been a pursuit.

From the moment their eyes had locked he had barely left her thoughts or her side, whether standing behind her at the wedding or sitting beside her at dinner. She still could not comprehend what had taken place on the dance floor; she had been searching for the bells and whistles and sirens of an orgasm, but how delicious and gentle that had been—how much more was there to know?

She didn't dare think too much about it now. Exhausted from a long and tiring day, Estelle was just about to drift off to sleep when Gordon turned on his ventilation machine.

Ginny hadn't told her about this part.

She lay there, head under pillow, at two a.m., still listening to the CPAP machine whirring and hissing. In the end she gave in.

She padded through the castle, her bare feet making not a sound on the stone floor. She headed to the small bathroom and took a drink from the tap, willing the night to be over.

Then she looked at her surroundings and regretted willing it over.

She stepped out onto a huge stone balcony, stared out to the loch. It was incredibly light for this time of the morning. She breathed in the warm summer night air and now her thoughts *did* turn to Gordon and his offer.

Estelle had already been coming to a reluctant decision to defer her studies and work full-time. It was all so big and scary—a future that was unknown.

She turned as the door opened, her eyes widening as Raúl stepped out.

He was wearing only his kilt.

Estelle would have preferred him with clothes on. Not because there was anything to disappoint—far from it— but the sight of olive skin, the light fan of hair on his chest and the way the kilt hung gave her eyes just one place to linger. There was nothing safe about meeting his gaze.

It was only then that she realised he had not followed her out here—that instead he was speaking on the phone.

He must have come out to get better reception. She gave him a brief smile and went to brush past, to get away from him without incident, but his hand caught her wrist and she stood there as he spoke into the phone.

'You don't need to know what room I am in…' He rolled his eyes. 'Araminta, I suggest that you go to bed.' He let out an irritated hiss. 'Alone!'

He ended the call and only then dropped Estelle's wrist. She stood as he examined her face.

'You know, without all the make-up you slather on...' His eyes searched her unmade-up skin. Her hair was tied in a low ponytail and she was dressed in a way he would not expect Gordon to find pleasing.

Raúl did.

She looked young—so much younger without all the make-up—and her baggy pyjamas left it all to Raúl's imagination. Which he was using now.

And then came his verdict.

'You look stunning,' Raúl said. 'I'm surprised Gordon has let you out of his sight.'

'I just needed some air.'

'I am hiding,' Raúl admitted.

'From Araminta?'

'Someone must have given her my phone number. I am going to have to change it.'

'She'll give in soon.' Estelle smiled, feeling a little sorry for the other woman. If Araminta had had a fling with him a few years ago and had known he would be here to-night—well, Estelle could see why her hopes might have been raised.

His phone rang again and he rolled his eyes and chose not to answer. 'So, what are you doing out here at this time of morning?'

'Just thinking.'

'About what?'

'Things.' She gave a wry smile, didn't add that far too many of her thoughts had been about him.

'And me,' Raúl admitted. 'It has been an interesting day.'

He looked out to the still, silent loch and felt a world away from where he had woken this morning. He didn't

even know how he was feeling. He looked over to Estelle, who was gazing out into the night too, a woman who was comfortable with silence.

It was Raúl who was not—Raúl who made sure his days and nights were always filled to capacity so that exhaustion could claim him each night.

Here, for the first time in the longest time, he found himself alone with his thoughts—and that was not pleasant. But he refused to pick up to Araminta, knowing the chaos that might create.

It was Raúl who broke the silence. He wanted to hear her voice.

'When do you go back?'

'Late morning.' Estelle stared out ahead. 'You?'

'I will leave early.'

He walked to lean over the balcony, gazed into the night, and Estelle saw the huge scar that ran from his shoulder to his waist. He glanced around and saw the slight shock on her face. Usually he refused to offer an explanation for the scar—he did not need sympathy. Tonight he chose to explain it.

'It's from the car accident...'

'That killed your mother?'

He gave a curt nod and turned back to look into the night, breathing in the cool air. He was glad that she was here. For no other reason, Raúl realised, than he was glad. It was two a.m. in the second longest night of his life, and for the first one he had been alone.

'Can I ask again?' He had to know. 'What are you doing with Gordon?'

'He's nice.'

'So are many people. It doesn't mean we go around...' He did not complete his sentence yet he'd made his rather crude point. 'Are you here tonight for your brother?'

Estelle could not answer. She had agreed to be here for Gordon, yet she knew they both knew the truth.

'Do you have siblings?' Estelle asked.

There was a long stretch of silence. His father had asked that he not reveal anything just yet, but it would all be out in the open soon. Estelle came and stood beside him as she awaited his answer. Perhaps she would go straight to the press in the morning. Raúl actually did not care right now. He could not think about tomorrow. It was taking all his control to get through the night.

'Had you asked me that yesterday the answer would have been no.' He turned his head, saw her frown at his answer and was grateful that she did not push for more detail. Instead she stayed silent as Raúl admitted a little of the truth. 'This morning my father told me that I have a brother—Luka.' It felt strange to say his name. 'Luka Sanchez Garcia.'

From their little lesson earlier, Estelle knew they did not share the same mother. 'Have you met him?'

'Unwittingly.'

'How old is he?'

She asked the same question that he had asked his father, though the relevance of the answer she could not know.

'Twenty-five,' Raúl said. 'I walked into my father's office this morning, expecting my usual lecture—he insists it is time for me to settle down.' He gave a small mirthless laugh. 'I had no idea what was coming. My father is dying and he wants his affairs put in order. My affairs too. And so he told me he has another son...'

'It must have been the most terrible shock.'

'Skeletons in the closet are not unique,' Raúl said. 'But this was not some long-ago affair that has suddenly come to light. My father has kept another life. He sees his mis-

tress in the north of Spain. I thought he went there so regularly for work. We have a hotel in San Sebastian. It is his main interest. Now I know why.'

Estelle tried to imagine what it was like, finding out something like this, and Raúl stood trying to comprehend that he had actually told another—how readily he had opened up to her. Then he reminded himself why. For his solution to come to fruition of *course* Estelle had to be told.

Some of it, at least.

He would never reveal all.

'His PA—Angela—she has always been…'

He gave a tight shrug. Angela had not been so much like a mother, but she had been a constant—a woman he trusted. Raúl closed his eyes, remembered walking out of his father's office and the words he had hurled to the one woman he had believed did not have an agenda.

'We have always got on. It turns out the son she speaks of often is in fact my half-brother.' He gave a wry smile. 'A lot of my childhood was spent with my aunt or uncle. I assumed my father was working at the hotel in San Sebastian. It turns out he was with his mistress and his son.' Black was the hiss that came from his mouth. 'It's all sorry and excuses now. I always prided myself on knowing what goes on, on being astute. It turns out I knew nothing.'

He had said enough. More than enough for one night.

'So, in answer to your question—yes. I have a brother.'

He shrugged naked shoulders and her fingers balled into her palms in an effort not to rest her hand on them.

'Unlike you, I care nothing for mine.'

'You might if you knew him.'

'That's not going to happen.'

She felt a small shiver, put it down to the night air. But his voice was so black with loathing it could have been that. 'I'm going to go in.'

'Please don't.'

Estelle had to get back—back to the safety of Gordon—yet she did not want to walk away from him.

She had to.

'Goodnight, Raúl…'

'Stay.'

She shook her head, grateful for the ringing of his phone—for the diversion it offered. But as she went to open the door she heard a woman's frantic voice coming down the corridor.

'Pick up Raúl. Where the hell are you?'

He had lightning reflexes. Quickly Raúl turned his phone off and pulled Estelle into the shadows.

'I need a favour.'

Before she knew what was happening she was in his arms, his tongue prising her lips open, his hand at her pyjama top. Estelle struggled against him before realising what was happening. She could hear Araminta calling out to Raúl, and if she saw the balcony any moment now she would come out.

But Araminta didn't. She stumbled past the balcony, the couple on it unseen.

He could stop now, Estelle thought. Except her pyjama top was completely open, her breasts splayed against his naked chest.

We *should* stop now, she thought as his tongue chased hers.

He made a low moan into her mouth; it was the sexiest thing she had ever heard or felt. He slid one hand over her bottom and his tongue was hot and moist.

Suddenly sending a message to Araminta was the last thing on Raúl's mind.

Estelle wanted his kiss to end, and yet she yearned for it to go on—like a forbidden path she was running down,

wanting to get to the end, to glimpse again the woman he made her. It was a kiss that should not be happening, but it was one she did not want to end.

'Don't go back to him…' Raúl's mouth barely left hers as he voiced his command.

He had intended to speak with her at a later point, perhaps get her phone number, but having tasted her, having kissed her, he could not stand the thought of her in Gordon's bed. He would reveal his plan right now.

He peeled his mouth off hers, his breath coming hard on her lips. 'Come now with me.'

It was then that she fully realised her predicament. Raúl assumed this was the norm for her, that she readily gave her body.

As he moved in to kiss her again she slapped him. It was the only way she knew how to end this.

'You pay more, do you?' She was disgusted with his thought processes.

'I did not mean it like that.' Raúl felt the sting on his cheek and knew that it was merited—knew how his suggestion must have come across. But business had been the last thing on his mind. He had simply not wanted her going back to another man. 'I meant—'

'I know exactly what you meant.'

'Bastard!'

They both turned at the sight of a tear-streaked Araminta. 'You said you were tired, that you were in bed.'

'Can I suggest that you go back to your bed?' Raúl snapped to Araminta, clearly not welcoming the intrusion.

Estelle saw again just how brutal this man could be when he chose.

'How much clearer can I make it that I have absolutely no interest in you?'

He turned and came to help a mortified Estelle with her buttons, but her hand slapped him off.

'Don't touch me!'

She flew from the balcony and back to her room, stepped quietly in and slipped into bed, listened to the whirring of Gordon's machine, trying to forget the feel of Raúl's hands, his mouth.

Trying to deny that she lay there for the first time truly wanting.

CHAPTER SEVEN

'ESTELLE...'

Gordon was lovely when she told him what had happened. Well, not all of it. She didn't tell him about her conversation with Raúl, just that he had been trying to avoid a woman and had kissed her...

It was a terribly awkward conversation, but Gordon was writing her a cheque, so as not to embarrass her in front of his driver, and Estelle simply couldn't accept it and had to tell him why.

'Frank and I have three free passes.'

Estelle blinked as Gordon smiled and held out the cheque.

'We have three people each who, should something happen, wouldn't be construed as cheating with.' He gave her a smile. 'It's just a game, of course, and it's mainly movie stars, but Raúl could very easily make it to my list. No one can resist him when he sets his sights on them—especially someone as darling and innocent as you.'

'I feel awful.'

'Don't.' Gordon closed her hand around the cheque. 'My being in competition with Raúl Sanchez Fuente could only do wonders for my reputation, if word were ever to get out. It might even be the reason for our breaking up and me realising just how much I care for Virginia.'

'I'm sorry.'

'Don't be,' Gordon said, and gave her a kiss on the cheek. 'Just be careful.'

'I'll never see him again,' Estelle said. 'He doesn't know anything about me.'

'Mere details to a man like Raúl—and he takes care of them easily.'

Estelle felt the hairs on her arms stand up as she remembered that she had given him her name.

'Just do your hair and put on a ton of make-up and we'll head down for breakfast,' Gordon told her. 'If anyone says anything about last night just laugh and shrug it off.'

It was a relief to hide her blushes behind thick make-up. Estelle put on a skirt that was too short and some high wedges, and tied her hair in a high ponytail and then teased it with a comb and sprayed it.

'I feel like a clown,' she said to Gordon as she checked her reflection in the mirror.

'Well, you make *me* smile.'

Raúl had gone, and all Estelle had to endure were some daggers being thrown in her direction by Araminta as they ate a full Scottish breakfast. She was relieved not to see him, yet there was a curious disappointment at his absence which Estelle chose not to examine.

Finally they were on their way, but it was late afternoon before Gordon dropped her at her home.

'Think about what I said,' Gordon reminded Estelle as she climbed out.

'I think I've had my excitement for the year,' Estelle admitted as she farewelled him.

She let herself step into familiar surrounds and released a breath before calling out to Ginny that she was home.

'How are you feeling?' Estelle asked as she walked into the lounge.

'Awful!'

Ginny certainly looked it.

'I'm going to go home for a couple of days. My dad's coming to pick me up—I need Mum, soup and sympathy.'

'Sounds good.'

'How was it?

'It was fine,' Estelle said, really not in the mood to tell Ginny all that had happened.

Ginny would no doubt find out from Gordon, given how much the two of them discussed. Estelle was still irritated that Ginny told Gordon about her virginity but, seeing how sick Ginny was, Estelle chose to save that for later.

'Gordon was lovely.'

'I told you there was nothing to worry about.'

'I'm exhausted,' Estelle admitted. 'You didn't tell me about Gordon's sleep apnoea. I got the fright of my life when I walked in and he was strapped to a machine.'

Ginny laughed. 'I honestly forgot. Your brother's been calling you. A few times, actually.'

The phone rang then, and Estelle's heart lurched in hope when she saw that it was her brother. 'Maybe he's got that job.'

He hadn't.

'I found out on Friday,' Andrew said. 'I just couldn't face telling you.'

'Something will come up.'

'I'm not qualified for anything.'

Estelle could hear the hopelessness in his voice.

'I don't know what to do, Estelle. I've asked Amanda's parents if they can help—'

His voice broke then. Estelle knew the hell that would have paid with his pride.

'They can't.'

She could feel his mounting despair.

'Something will come up,' Estelle said, but she was finding it harder and harder to sound convincing. 'You've just got to keep applying for work.'

'I know.' He blew out a long breath in an effort to compose himself. 'Anyway, enough about me,' Andrew said, 'Ginny said you were in Scotland. How come?'

'I was at a wedding.'

'Whose?'

'I'll tell you all about it tomorrow.'

'Tomorrow?'

'I want to speak to you about something.' As a car tooted outside, Ginny stood. 'Andrew, I've got to go,' Estelle said. 'I'll call in tomorrow.'

Estelle didn't know how to tell Andrew she had some money for him, but anyway she knew that one month's mortgage payment would only be a Band-Aid solution. She was relieved that Ginny would be out for a few days because she really wanted some time to go over what she was considering.

The library was offering her more hours. Perhaps she could defer her studies and move in with Andrew and Amanda for a year, pay them rent, help out with little Cecelia, maybe even take Gordon up on his offer... Yes, she was glad Ginny would be away, because she needed to think properly.

'Your dad's here,' Estelle said.

'Thanks so much for last night, Estelle,' Ginny said, grabbing her bag and heading out of the door, waving to her father, who had climbed back into the car when he saw her.

Ginny was too dosed up on flu medication even to notice the expensive car a little further down the road.

Raúl noticed *her*, though—and a frown appeared on his face as he saw Virginia, Gordon's regular date, disappear-

ing into a car driven by another older male. After Raúl's father's revelations he was past being surprised by anything, but there was a curious feeling of disappointment as he thought of Estelle and Virginia together with Gordon.

No.

He did not like the images that conjured, so he settled for the slightly more palatable version—that Estelle hadn't picked him up at Dario's; instead Estelle and Virginia must both work for the same escort agency.

He needed someone tough, Raúl told himself. He needed a woman who could separate sex from emotion, who could see what he was about to propose as a financial opportunity rather than a romantic proposition.

Except his knuckles were white as he clutched the steering wheel. Since last night there had been an incessant gnawing in his stomach when he thought of Estelle with Gordon. Now that gnawing had upgraded to a burn in the lining of his gut.

Estelle would be far better with him.

Was he arrogant to think so? Raúl pondered briefly as he walked up her garden path.

Perhaps, he conceded, but he was also assured enough to know that he was right.

'What did you forget...?' Estelle's voice trailed off when she saw that it wasn't Ginny.

Raúl preferred the way she'd looked last night on the balcony, but her appearance now—the short skirt, the heavy make-up, the lacquered hair—actually made things easier.

'What do you want?'

'I wanted to apologise for what I said last night. I think it was misconstrued.'

'I think you made things perfectly clear.' She drew in

a breath and then gave a small nod. 'Apology accepted. Now, if you'll excuse me?'

Her hand was ready to close the door on him. There was just a moment and Raúl knew he had to use it wisely. There was no time for mixed messages. He knew he had better reveal the truth up-front.

'You were right—I didn't want you to go back to Gordon, but not just because…' The door was closing on him so Raúl told her exactly what he was here for. 'I wanted to ask you to marry me.'

Estelle laughed.

After the tension of the last twenty-four hours, then her brother's tears on the phone, and now Raúl, standing absolutely immaculate in black jeans and a shirt at her door with his ridiculous proposal, all she could do was throw her head back and laugh.

'I'm serious.'

'Of course you are,' Estelle answered. 'Just as you were serious last night when you told me just how much you don't want to marry—ever.'

'I don't want to marry for love,' Raúl said, 'but I do need a bride. One with a level head. One who knows what she wants and goes for it.'

There was that implication again, Estelle realised. She was about to close the door, but then she looked down to the cheque Raul was holding—one with her name on it—and she saw the ridiculous amount he was offering. He surely wasn't serious. She looked up at him and realised that possibly he was—that he could pay for her services. As Gordon had.

Estelle gave a nervous swallow, reminding herself that whatever happened, whatever Raúl thought, she must not betray Gordon's confidence.

'Look—whatever you think, Gordon and I…'

'Should that be, Gordon, *Virginia* and I?' He watched her flaming cheeks pale. 'I just saw her leave. Are you both dating him?'

'I don't have to explain anything to you.'

'You're right,' Raúl conceded.

'How did you know where I lived?'

'I checked your bag when you were dancing with Gordon.'

Estelle blinked. He was honest, brutally honest—and, yes, she couldn't help herself. She was curious.

'Are you going to ask me in or do I stand and speak here?'

'I don't think so.' Common sense told her to close the door on him, but as she stared into black eyes curiosity was starting to win. Things like this—conversations like this—simply didn't happen to Estelle. But, more than that, she wanted to find out more about this man who had been on her mind from the second their eyes had locked.

'I ask for ten minutes,' Raúl said. 'If you want me to leave then, I shall, and I will never bother you again.'

He spoke in such a matter-of-fact voice. This was business to him, Estelle realised, and he assumed it was the same for her. She chose to keep it that way.

'Ten minutes,' Estelle said, and opened the door.

He looked around the small house. It was typical student accommodation, yet she was not your typical student.

'You are studying?'

'Yes.'

'Can I ask what?'

Estelle hesitated, not keen on revealing anything to him, but surely it could do no harm. 'Ancient architecture.'

'Really?' Raul frowned. Her response was not the one he'd been expecting.

She offered him a seat and Raúl took it. Estelle chose a

chair on the opposite side of the room to him. He wasted
no time getting to the point.

'I have told you that my father is sick?' Raúl said, and
Estelle nodded. 'And that for a long time he has wanted
to see me settled? Now, with his death nearing, more and
more he wishes to see his wish fulfilled—he has convinced
himself that a wife will tame my ways.'

Estelle said nothing. She just looked at this man she
doubted would ever be tamed; she had tasted his passion,
had heard about his appalling reputation. A ring on his
finger certainly wouldn't have stopped what had taken
place last night.

'You might remember I told you my father revealed he
has another son?'

Again Estelle nodded.

'He has said that if I do not comply, if I do not settle
down, then he will leave his share of the business to my…'
He could not bring himself to call Luka his brother. 'I refuse to allow that to happen.'

She could see the determination in his eyes.

'Which is why I have come this evening to speak with
you.'

'Why aren't you having this conversation with Araminta? I'm sure she'd be delighted to marry you.'

'I did briefly consider it,' Raúl admitted, 'but there are
several reasons. The main one being she would not be able
to reconcile the fact that this is a business transaction. She
would agree, I think, but it would be with hope that love
would grow, that perhaps a baby might change my mind.
It will not,' Raúl said. His voice was definite. 'Which is
why I come to speak with you. A woman who understands
a certain business.'

'I really think you have the wrong idea about me.'

'I am not here to judge you. On the contrary, I admire a woman who can separate love from sex.'

He did not understand the wry smile on her face. If only he knew. It faded as he continued.

'We are attracted to each other.' Raúl said it as a fact. 'Surely for you that can only be a bonus?'

Estelle blew out a breath; he was practically calling her a hooker and yet she was in a poor position to deny it.

'We both like to party,' Raúl said. 'And we like to live life in the fast lane—even if we know how to take things seriously at times.'

He was wrong about the fast lane, and Estelle knew if she admitted the truth he'd be gone. But, yes, she *was* undeniably attracted to him. Her skin was tingling just from his presence. Her mind was still begging for a moment of peace just to process the dance and the kiss they had shared last night.

He interrupted her wandering thoughts.

'Estelle. I have spoken with my father's doctor; it is a matter of weeks rather than months. You would only be away for a short while.'

'Away?'

'I live in Marbella.'

Now she definitely shook her head. 'Raúl, I have a life here. My niece is sick. I am studying…'

'You can return to your studies a wealthy woman—and naturally you will have regular trips home.'

He looked at her, with her gaudy make-up and teased hair. He chose to remember her fresh-faced on the balcony, recalled the comfort she had given even before they had kissed. He should not care, but he did not like the life she was leading. Suddenly it was imperative for reasons other than appeasing his father that she take this chance.

'I do not judge you, Estelle, but you could come back

and start over. You can live the life you want to without ever having to worry about the rent.'

Estelle stood and walked to the window, not wanting him to see the tears that sprang in her eyes because for a moment there he had sounded as if he actually cared.

'You certainly won't have to host dinner parties or cook for me. I work hard all day. You can shop. We'll eat out every night. And there are many clubs to choose from, parties to attend. You would never be bored.'

He had no idea about her at all.

'After my father's death, after a suitable pause, we will admit our whirlwind marriage cannot deal with the grief—that with regret we are to part. No one will ever know you married for money. That would be written into the contract.'

'Contract?'

'Of course,' Raúl said. 'One that will protect both of us, that will lay down all the rules. I have asked my lawyer to fly in for a meeting at midday tomorrow. Naturally it will be a lengthy meeting. We will have to go over terms.'

'I won't be there.'

He didn't look in the least deterred.

'Raúl, my brother would never believe me.'

'I will come with you and speak to him.'

'Oh, and he'll believe *you*? He'll believe we met yesterday and fell madly in love? He'll have me certified insane before he lets me fly off with a stranger—'

'We met last year.' Raúl interrupted her tirade. It was clear he had thought it all through. 'When you were in Spain. It was then that we fell madly in love, but of course with your brother's accident it was not the time to say so, or to make plans to move, so we put it down to a holiday romance. We met again a few weeks ago and this time around I had no intention of letting you go.'

'I don't want to lie to him.'

'You are always truthful?' Raúl checked. 'Does he know about Gordon, then? Does he know—?'

'Okay,' she interrupted. Because of course there were things her brother didn't know. She was actually considering it—so much so that she turned to him with a question. 'Would *your* family believe it?'

'Before I found out about my father's other life I chose to let him think I was serious about someone I used to date. It was not you I had in mind, but they do not know that.'

It could work.

The frown that was on her brow was smoothed, the impossibility of it all was fading, and Raúl knew it was time to leave.

'Sleep on it,' Raúl said. 'Naturally there is more that I have to tell you, but I am not prepared to discuss certain things until after the marriage.'

'What sort of things?'

'Nothing that impacts on you now—just things that a loving wife would know all about. It is something I would not reveal to anyone I did not trust or love.'

'Or pay for?'

'Yes.' He placed the cheque on the coffee table and handed her two business cards.

'That is the hotel my lawyer will be staying at. I have booked an office there. The other card contains my contact details—for now.'

'For now?'

'I am changing my phone number tomorrow,' Raúl said. 'One other thing…' He ran a finger along her cheek, looked at the full mouth he had so enjoyed kissing last night. 'There will be no one else for the duration of our contract…'

'It's not going to happen.'

'Well, in case you change your mind—' he handed her an envelope '—you might need this.'

She opened it, stared at the photo that had been taken last night. His arm was on the chair behind her, she was laughing, and there was Raúl—smiling, absolutely beautiful, his eyes on her, staring at her as if he was entranced.

He must have known the photographer was on his way, Estelle realised. He had been considering this even last night.

Raúl *had* rearranged the seating—she was certain of it now.

She realised then the lengths he would go to to get his way.

'Did you arrange for Gordon to be called away?'

'Of course.'

'You don't even try to deny it?'

He heard her anger.

'You'd prefer that I lie?' Raúl checked.

She looked to the mantelpiece, to the photo of her brother and Amanda holding a tiny, frail Cecelia. She was so tired of struggling. But she could not believe that she was considering his offer. She had considered Gordon's, though, Estelle told herself. Tomorrow she had been going to tell her brother she was deferring her studies and moving in with them.

She had already made the decision to up-end her life.

This would certainly up-end it—but in a rather more spectacular way.

She went into the kitchen with the excuse of making coffee, but really it was to gather her thoughts.

Bought by Raúl.

Estelle closed her eyes. It was against everything she believed in, yet it wasn't just the money that tempted her. It was something more base than that.

A man as beautiful as Raúl, for her first lover. The thought of sharing his bed, his life—even for a little while—was as tempting as the cheque he had written. Estelle blew out a breath, her skin on fire, aroused just at the thought of lying beside him. Yet she knew that if Raúl knew she was a virgin the deal would be off.

'Not for me.'

He was standing at the kitchen door, watching as she spooned instant coffee into two mugs.

'I'll leave you to think about it. If you do not arrive at the appointment then I will accept your decision and stop the cheque. As I said, tomorrow my phone number will be changing. It will be too late to change your mind.'

It really was, Estelle knew, a once-in-a-lifetime offer.

CHAPTER EIGHT

'I WILL FLY your family out for the wedding…'

They were sitting in Raúl's lawyer's office, going over details that made Estelle burn, but it was all being dealt with in a cool, precise manner.

'I will speak with your parents and brother.'

'My parents are both deceased.' Estelle said it in a matter-of-fact way. She was not after sympathy from Raúl and this was not a tender conversation. 'And my brother and his wife won't be able to attend—Cecelia is too sick to travel.'

'You should have *someone* there for you.'

'Won't your family believe us otherwise?' There was a slight sneer to her voice, which she fought to check. She had chosen to be here, after all. It was just the mention of her parents, of Cecelia, that had her throat tightening—the realisation that everything in this marriage bar love would be real and she would be going through it all alone.

'It has nothing to do with that,' Raúl said. 'It is your wedding day. You might find it overwhelming to be alone.'

'Oh, please,' Estelle responded, determined not to let him see her fear. 'I'll be fine.'

'Very well.' Raúl nodded. 'It will be a small wedding, but traditional. The press will go wild—they have been

waiting a long time for me to marry—but we will not let them know we are married till after.'

They had been talking for hours; every detail from wardrobe allowance to hair and make-up had been discussed.

Estelle had insisted she could choose her own clothes.

'I have a reputation to think of,' had been Raúl's tart response.

Estelle was entitled to one week every month to come back to the UK and visit her family for the duration of the contract.

'I am sure we will both need the space,' had been Raúl's explanation. 'I am not used to having someone permanently around.'

There was now an extremely uncomfortable conversation—for Estelle, in any case—about the regularity of sex, and also about birth control and health checks. Raúl didn't appear in the least bit fazed.

'In the event of a pregnancy—' the lawyer started.

Raúl was quick to interrupt. Only now did he seem concerned by the subject matter being discussed. 'There is to be no pregnancy.' There was a low menace to his voice. 'I don't think my bride-to-be would be foolish enough to try and trap me in *that* way.'

'It still needs to be addressed.' The lawyer was very calm.

'I have no intention of getting pregnant.' Estelle gave a small nervous laugh, truly horrified at the prospect. She had seen the stress Cecelia had placed on Andrew and Amanda, and they were head over heels in love.

'You might change your mind,' Raúl said, for he trusted no one. 'You might decide that you like the lifestyle and don't want to give it up.' He looked to his lawyer. 'We need to make contingency plans.'

'Absolutely,' the lawyer said.

It could not be made clearer that this was all business.

Estelle sat as with clinical detachment he ensured that he would provide for any child they might have on the condition that the child resided in Spain.

If she moved back to England, Estelle would have to fight against his might just to make the rent.

'I think that covers it,' the lawyer said.

'Not quite.' Estelle cleared her throat. 'I'd like us to agree that we won't sleep with each other till after the wedding.'

'There's no need for quaint.'

'I've agreed to all your terms.' She looked coolly at him. It was the only way for this to work. If he knew she was a virgin this meeting would close now. 'You can surely agree to one of mine? I'd like some time off before I start *working*.' She watched his jaw tighten slightly as she made it clear that this *was* work.

'Very well.' Raúl did not like to be told that sleeping with him would be a chore. 'You may well change your mind.'

'I shan't.'

'You will be flown in a couple of days before the wedding. I will be on my yacht, partying as grooms do before their marriage. You shall have the apartment to yourself.' He had no intention of holding hands and playing coy for a week. He waited for her nod and then turned to his lawyer. 'Draft it.'

They waited in a sumptuous lounge as the lawyer got to work, but Estelle couldn't relax.

'You are tense.'

'It's not every day you get offered a million dollars.' She could at least be honest about that. 'Nor move to Marbella…'

'You will love it,' Raúl said. 'The night-life is fantastic…'

He just didn't know her at all, Estelle realised yet again.

'How did your parents die?' Raúl asked, watching as her shoulders stiffened. 'My family are bound to ask.'

'In a car accident,' Estelle said, turning to him. 'The same as your mother.'

He opened his mouth to speak and then changed his mind.

'I just hope everyone believes us,' Estelle said.

'Why wouldn't they? Even when we divorce we'll maintain the lie. You understand the confidentiality clause?' Raúl checked. 'No one is ever to know that this is a marriage of convenience only.'

'No one will ever hear it from me,' she assured him. The prospect of being found out was abhorrent to Estelle. 'Just a whirlwind romance and a marriage that didn't work out.'

'Good,' Raúl said. 'And, Estelle—even if we do get on…even if you do like—'

'Don't worry, Raúl,' she interrupted. 'I'm not going to be falling in love with you.' She gave him a tight smile. 'I'll be out of your life, as per the contract.'

CHAPTER NINE

RAÚL HAD BEEN RIGHT.

Estelle stood on the balcony of his luxurious apartment, looking out at the marina, on the morning of her wedding day, and was, as Raúl had predicted, utterly and completely overwhelmed.

She had arrived in Marbella two days ago and had barely stopped for air since. Stepping into this vast apartment, she had fully glimpsed his wealth. Every room bar the movie screening room was angled to take in the stunning view of the Mediterranean, and every whim was catered for from Jacuzzi to sauna. There was a whole new wardrobe waiting for her too. The only thing lacking was that the kitchen cupboards and fridge were empty.

'Call Sol's if you don't want to go out,' Raúl had said. 'They will bring whatever you want straight over.'

The only vaguely familiar thing had been the photo of them both, taken at Donald's wedding, beautifully framed and on a wall. But even that had been dealt with by Raúl. It had been manipulated so that her make-up was softer, her cleavage less revealing.

It had been a sharp reminder that he thought her a tart.

Raúl knew the woman he wanted to marry, and it wasn't the woman he had met, so there had been trips to a beauty salon for hair treatments and make-up lessons.

'I don't *need* make-up lessons,' Estelle had said.

'Oh, baby, you do,' had been his response. 'Subtle is best.'

Constantly she had to remind herself to be the woman he thought he had met. A woman who acted as if delighted by her new designer wardrobe, who didn't mind at all when he told her to wear factor fifty-plus because he liked her pale skin.

But it wasn't that which concerned Estelle this morning as she looked out at the glittering sea and the luxurious yachts, wondering which one was Raúl's.

Tonight she would be on his yacht.

This night they would be sharing a bed.

Estelle wasn't sure if she was more terrified of losing her virginity, or of him finding out that she had never slept with anyone before.

Maybe he wouldn't notice, she thought helplessly. But she knew she didn't have a hope of delivering to his bed the sexually experienced woman that Raúl was expecting. Last night, before heading off with his sponsors for his final night as a single man, Raúl had kissed her slowly and deeply. The message his tongue had delivered had been an explicit one.

'Why do you make me wait?'

Tonight he would find out why.

'You have a phone call.' Rosa, his housekeeper, brought the phone up to the balcony. It was Amanda on the line.

'How are you doing?' Amanda asked.

'I'm petrified.' It was nice to be honest.

'All brides are,' Amanda said. 'But Raúl will take good care of you.'

He had utterly and completely charmed Amanda, but had not quite won over Andrew.

'I am not letting her go again.' He had looked Andrew

straight in the eye as he said it. 'If I move Estelle to Spain I want to make a proper commitment. That is why she will come to be my wife.'

So easily he had lied.

Estelle knew she must remember that fact.

'How did the dress turn out?' Amanda asked.

'It's beautiful,' Estelle said. 'Even better than I imagined it would be.'

It was the only thing Estelle had been allowed to organise. It had all be done online and by phone, and the final adjustments made when she had arrived.

'How is Cecelia?' Estelle asked, desperate for news of her niece.

'She's still asleep.'

It was nine a.m. in Spain, which meant it was eight a.m. in the UK. Cecelia had always been an early riser. More and more she slept these days, though Amanda always did her best to be upbeat.

'I'm going to dress her up for the wedding and take a photo and send it. Even if we can't be there today, know that we're thinking of you.'

'I know.'

'And I'm not your sister, but I do think of you as one.'

'Thank you,' Estelle said, her eyes welling up. 'I think of you as a sister too.'

They weren't idle words; many hours had been spent in hospital waiting rooms this past year.

'Is that the door?' Amanda asked.

'Yes. Don't worry, someone else will get it.'

'Do you have a butler?'

'No!' Estelle laughed, swallowing down her tears. 'Just Raúl's housekeeper. Though it's going to start to get busy soon, with the hairdresser...' She turned around as she

heard her name being called, and Estelle's jaw dropped as she saw her brother coming through the door.

'Andrew!'

'Is that where he's got to?' Amanda laughed, and then she was serious. 'I'm so sorry that I couldn't be with you today—I'd have given anything. But with Cecelia…'

'Thank you,' Estelle said, and promptly burst into tears, all her pent-up nerves released.

'I think she's pleased to see me,' Andrew said, taking the phone and chatting to Amanda briefly before hanging up.

'I can't believe you're here,' Estelle admitted.

'Raúl said he thought you might need someone today, and of course I wanted to give you away. If anything happens with Cecelia he's assured me I'll be able to get straight back.'

She couldn't believe that Raúl would do this for her. Until now she hadn't fully realised how terrifying today was, how real it felt.

Raúl had.

'When did you get in?'

'Last night,' Andrew said. 'We went to Sol's.'

'You were out with Raúl?'

'He certainly knows how to party.' Andrew smiled. 'I'd forgotten how.'

Even if she was doing all this for her brother and his wife, of the many benefits of marrying Raúl, this was one Estelle had not even considered—that her brother, who was still having trouble accepting the diagnosis that he would never walk again, who had, apart from job interviews and hospital appointments, become almost reclusive, would fly not just to Spain but so far out of his comfort zone.

It was a huge and important step, and it was thanks to Raúl that he was here.

'I've got something for you.'

Estelle bit her lip, hoping they hadn't spent money they didn't have on a gift for a wedding that wasn't real.

'Remember these?' Andrew said as she opened the box. 'These' were small diamond studs that had belonged to her mother. 'Dad bought them for her for their wedding day.'

She had never felt more of a fraud.

'Enough tears,' Andrew said. 'Let's get this wedding underway.'

Raúl was rarely nervous, but as he stood at the altar and waited for Estelle, to his own surprise, he was.

His father had almost bought their story, and Raul's future with the company was secure, but instead of a gloating satisfaction that his plans were falling into place today he thought only of the reasons he had had to go to these lengths.

His head turned briefly and he caught a glimpse of Angela in the middle of the church. She was seated with his father, as ever-present PA. His mother's family were still unaware of the real role she played in his father's life—and the role she had played in his mother's death.

He stared ahead, anger churning in his gut that Angela had the gall to be here. He wouldn't put it past her to bring her bastard son.

Then he heard the murmur of the congregation and Raúl turned around. The churning faded. Just one thought was now in his mind.

She looked beautiful.

He had wondered how Estelle might look—had worried that, left to her own devices, a powder-puff ball would be wobbling towards him on glittery platform shoes, smiling from ruby-red lips.

He had not—could not have—imagined this.

Her dress was cream and made of intricate Spanish lace. It was fitted, and showing her curves, but in the most elegant of ways. The neckline was a simple halter neck. She carried orange blossom, as was the tradition for Spanish brides, and her lipstick was a pale coral.

'Te ves bella.' He told her that she looked beautiful as she joined him, and he meant every word. Not one thing would he change, from her black hair, piled high up on her head, to the simple diamond earrings and elegant cream shoes. She was visibly shaking, and he made a small joke to relax her. 'Your sewing is terrible.'

She glanced at his shirt and they shared a smile. With so little history, still they found a piece now, at the altar—as per tradition, the bride-to-be must embroider her groom's shirt.

'I'm not marrying a billionaire to sit sewing!' she had said teasingly, and Raúl had laughed, explaining that most women did not embroider all of the front of the shirt these days. Only a small area would be left for her, and Estelle could put on it whatever she wanted.

He had half expected a € but had frowned this morning when he had put on his shirt to find a small pineapple. Raúl still couldn't work out what it meant, but it was nice to see her relax and smile as the service started.

They knelt together, and as the service moved along he explained things in his low, deep voice, heard only by her.

'El lazo,' he said as a loop of satin decorated with orange blossom was placed over his shoulders and then another loop from the same piece was placed over hers. The priest spoke then for a moment, in broken English, and Estelle's cheeks burnt red as he told them that the rope that bound them showed that they shared the responsibility for this marriage. It would remain for the rest of the ceremony.

But not for life.

She felt like a fraud. She *was* a fraud, Estelle thought, panic starting to build. But Raúl took her hand and she looked into his black eyes. He seemed to sense that she was suddenly struggling.

'He asks now that you hand him the Arras,' Raúl said and she handed over the small purse he had given her on arrival. It contained thirteen coins, he had explained, and it showed his financial commitment to her.

It was the only honest part of the service, Estelle thought as the priest blessed them and handed it back to her.

Except it felt real.

'It's okay,' he said to her. 'We are here in this together.'

It felt far safer than being in it alone.

The service ended and an attendant removed the satin rope and presented it to Estelle; then they walked out to cheers and petals and rice being thrown at them. Raúl's hand was hot on her waist, and he gripped her tighter when she nearly shot out of her dress at the sound of an explosion.

'It's firecrackers,' Raúl said. 'Sorry I forgot to warn you.'

And there would be firecrackers later too, Estelle thought, when they got to bed and she told him the truth! But it was far too late now to warn him.

It really was a wonderful wedding.

As Raúl had told her on the night they had met, there were no speeches; instead it was an endless feast, with dancing and celebration and congratulations from all.

She met Paola and Carlos, Raúl's aunt and uncle, and they spoke of Raúl's mother, Gabriella.

'She would be so proud to be here today,' Paola said. 'Wouldn't she, Antonio?'

Estelle saw how friendly they were with Raúl's father,

and also with Angela, who was naturally seated with them. No longer were they names, but faces, and a shiver went down her arms as she imagined their reaction when the truth came out.

'My son has excellent taste.' Antonio kissed her on the cheek.

Estelle had met him very briefly the day before, and Raúl had handled most of the questions—though both had seen the doubt in his eyes as to whether this union was real.

It was slowly fading.

'It is good to see my son looking so happy.'

He *did* look happy.

Raúl smiled at her as they danced their first dance as husband and wife, with the room watching on.

'Remember our first dance?' Raúl smiled.

'Well, we shan't be repeating *that* tonight.'

'Not till later.' Raúl gazed down, saw her burning cheeks, and mistook it for arousal.

He could never have guessed her fear.

'I ache to be inside you.'

Other couples had joined them. The music was low and sensual and it seemed to beat low in her stomach. His hand dusted her bare arm and she shivered at the thought of what was to come, wondered if those eyes, soft now with lust and affection, would darken in anger.

'Raúl…' Surely here was not the place to tell him, but it felt better with people around them rather than being alone. 'I'm nervous about tonight.'

'Why would you be nervous?' he asked. 'I will take good care of you.'

He would, Raúl decided. He was rarely excited at the thought of monogamy but he actually wanted to take care of her, could not stand to think of what she might have put her body through. There was a surge of protectiveness that

shot through him then, and his arms tightened around her. He could feel her tension and nervousness and again he wanted to make her smile.

'Can I ask why,' he whispered into her ear as they danced, 'you embroidered a pineapple on my shirt?'

'It's a thistle!'

A smile spread on her lips and he felt her relax a little in his arms.

'For Scotland.'

Raúl found himself smiling too. 'All day I have been trying to work out the significance of a pineapple.'

She started to laugh and Raúl found himself laughing a little too.

He lowered his head and kissed her lightly.

It was expected, of course. What groom would *not* kiss his bride?

Many times since he had put his proposition to her Estelle had had doubts—the morality of it, the feasibility of it, the logistics—but as he kissed her, as she felt his warm lips and the soft caress of his hand near the base of her spine, true doubt as to her ability to go through with the deal surfaced. For once it had nothing to do with her hymen. She was suddenly more worried about her heart.

It was the music. It was the moment. It was having her brother here. It was Raúl's kiss. All these things, she told herself, were the reasons she felt as she did—as if this were real…as if this were love.

Estelle excused herself a little while later and went to the bathroom, just so she might collect herself, but brides could not easily hide on their wedding day.

'Estelle?' She turned at the sound of a woman's voice. 'I am Angela—Raúl's father's PA.'

'Raúl has spoken about you,' Estelle responded carefully.

'I'm sure what he had to say was not very flattering.' There were tears in the older woman's eyes. 'Estelle, I don't know what to believe…'

'Excuse me?'

'About this sudden marriage.' Angela was being as upfront with Estelle as she was with Raúl. 'I do know, though, that Raúl seems the happiest I have seen him. If you *do* love your husband…'

'If?'

'I apologise,' Angela said. 'Given that you surely love your husband, I ask this not for me, and not even for Antonio's sake. Whatever Raúl thinks of me, I care for him. I want him to come and visit us. I want us to be a family, even for a little while.'

'You could have had that years ago.' Estelle answered as she hoped Raúl would expect his loyal wife to.

'I want him to make peace with his father while there is still time. I don't want him to have any guilt when his father passes. I know how much guilt he has over his mother.'

Estelle blinked, unsure how to respond because there was so much she didn't know about Raúl. What did he have to feel guilty about? Raúl had been a child, after all. He had agreed to tell her more on their honeymoon—had said that he would be the one to deal with any questions tonight.

'I have always loved Raúl. I have always thought of him as a son.'

'So why did you leave it so late to tell him?' Perhaps it was the emotion of the day, but the tears that flashed in Estelle's eyes were real. 'If you cared so much for him—'

Estelle halted. It wasn't her place to ask, and Raúl certainly wouldn't thank her for delving. She was here to ensure his father left his share of the business to him, that was all. She would do well to remember that.

'I *do* care,' Angela responded. 'Whatever Raúl thinks of me, from a distance I have loved him as a son.'

'From a distance?' Estelle repeated, making the bitter point.

Turning on her heel, she walked out and straight into Raúl's arms.

'She wanted to speak about you,' Estelle told him. 'I don't know how well I handled it.'

'We'll discuss it later,' Raúl said, for he had seen Angela follow her in. 'Now we have to hand out the favours.'

It really was an amazing party, and for reasons of her own Estelle didn't particularly want it to end.

As per tradition, the bride and groom had to see off all their guests and be the last to leave. Antonio tired first, and she felt the grip of Raúl's hand tighten on hers as his father left with his loyal PA.

'It's been great,' Andrew said as he prepared to head back to the hotel he was staying in. 'Once Cecelia is well, and I'm working, I'm going to bring Amanda and Cecelia here for a holiday, to visit you.'

'You do that,' Estelle said, and bent down and gave her brother a cuddle, then stood as Raúl shook his hand.

'Look after my sister.'

'You do not have to worry about that.'

'Have a great honeymoon.'

A driver sorted out the wheelchair and they waved Andrew off and then headed back inside.

Apart from the staff it was just Raúl and Estelle now, and still the music went on as they danced their last dance of the night.

'It really helped having Andrew here.' Her hands were round the back of his neck, he held her hips, and she would give anything not to disappoint him tonight—anything to be the experienced lover he assumed she was.

'I thought it might.'

'It didn't just help me,' Estelle admitted, and started to tell him about how Andrew's confidence had been lacking.

But he dropped a kiss on her shoulder. 'Enough about others.'

Estelle swallowed. She could feel his fingers exploring the halter neck, his other hand running down the row of tiny buttons that ran to the base of her spine, and she knew he was planning his movements, undressing her slowly in his mind as they danced.

'Raúl…' His mouth was working over her bare shoulder, kissing it deeply; she could feel the soft suction, feel the heat of his tongue and his ardour building. 'I've never slept with anyone before.'

He moaned into her shoulder and pulled her tighter into him, so she could feel every inch of the turn-on he thought she was giving him.

'I mean it.' Her voice was shaking. 'You'll be my first.'

'Come on, then.' His mouth was now at her ear. 'Let's go and play virgins.'

CHAPTER TEN

THEY WERE DRIVEN the short distance to the marina, but for Estelle it just passed in a blur.

It was almost morning, yet despite the hour the celebrations continued.

Alberto, the skipper, welcomed them, and briefly introduced the staff—but Estelle barely took in the names, let alone her surroundings. All she could think of was what was soon to come as the crew toasted them and then Raúl dismissed them.

'Tomorrow I will show you around properly,' Raúl said, taking her champagne glass. 'But for now…'

There was no escaping. He pulled her towards him, his tongue back on her neck, at the crease between her neck and shoulder. He *had* been mentally undressing her before, for now his hands moved straight to the halter neck and expertly unravelled the carefully tied bow.

He had been expecting a basque, had anticipated another contraption to disable, but the dress had an inbuilt bra and he gave a low growl of approval as one of the breasts that had filled his private visions in recent days fell heavy and ripe into his palm.

'Raúl, someone might come…'

'That would be *you*,' he said, but she did not relax. 'No one will disturb us.'

Raúl lowered his head and licked around the pale are-
ola, flicked a nipple that had been crushed all day by fabric back into rapid life, surprised that she was concerned
that someone might come in. The staff on his yacht had
seen many a decadent party—a husband and wife on their
wedding night paled in comparison with what usually took
place. He took the breast he craved in his mouth again, felt
her hand try to push him back. He was at first surprised
by her reticence—but then he remembered their game.

'Of course.' He smiled. 'You are nervous.'

He lifted her up and carried her down to the master
stateroom, kissing her the entire way. He lowered her to
the ground, turning her around so he could work on the
tiny buttons from behind. It did not halt his mouth; his
tongue kissed every inch of newly exposed flesh till her
spine felt as if it were on fire.

He peeled off her dress, then her shoes and stockings.
As his tongue licked and nibbled her sex through her silk
panties the sensations his mouth delivered drove her wild.
He only removed her panties when the moisture his mouth
had made matched the dampening silk.

'Raúl…' Her hands were on his head—contrary hands
that tried to halt him, while her moans of mounting desire urged him on.

'I want you so bad.' He peeled off her panties and,
kneeling, parted her lips, his tongue darting to the swelling bud over and over as her hands knotted in his hair.

'Raúl…' she whimpered, lost between bliss and fear.
'I'm serious. I really haven't slept with anyone before.'

He simply didn't believe her. As she came under his
mouth she had a hopeless thought that maybe he wouldn't
guess, maybe he wouldn't know. Because despite her
naïveté her body responded with ease. She throbbed

against his mouth, more aroused than sated as he softly kissed the lingering orgasm.

He relished her taste, was assured she was moist. He was desperate now to take her.

He rose to his full height then, and shrugged his jacket off.

Breathless, aroused, moving on instinct, her hands shaking with want, she undid the buttons of his shirt. He was so dark and sultry, and he wore it well. His lips parted as her hands roamed his chest and she licked at his nipples as she undid his belt.

Raúl wanted her fingers at his zipper, and he wished she would hurry, but she lingered instead, feeling his thick heat through the fabric, her fingers lightly exploring. His already aching erection hardened further beneath her fingers. 'Estelle…' He could barely get the word out, but thankfully she read the urgency and slid the zipper down, and he let out a breath as she freed him.

He was delicious to her hands. She ran her fingers along his length, felt the soft skin that belied the strength beneath. She was petrified at the thought of him inside her, but wanting him just the same. She could see a trickle of silver and caught it with her finger, then swirled it around the head, entranced by its beauty.

Raúl closed his eyes in a mixture of frustration and bliss, for he wanted her hand to grip him tight, yet conversely he liked the tentative tease and exploration, liked the feel of her other hand gently weighing him.

Deeply they kissed, his tongue urging her to move faster, his erection twitching at the pleasure of her teasing, till he could take it no more.

'Te quiero.'

He told her he wanted her in Spanish as he pushed her

onto the bed. *'Tengo que usted tiene.'* He told her he had to have her as he parted her legs.

'Be gentle.' She was writhing and hot beneath him, her words contrary to the wanton woman in his arms. Her sex was slippery and warm and engorged as his hand stroked her there. She was as close to coming as Raúl, and his answer to her final plea was delivered as he nudged her entrance.

'It's way too late for gentle, baby.'

How he regretted those words as he seared and tore into her.

Raúl heard her sob, heard her bite back a scream.

Estelle knew then she had been a fool to think he might somehow not notice. He tore through her barrier but the pain did not end there. His fierce erection drove through tight muscles full of resistance. Too late to halt, too late to be tender, he froze—just not quickly enough. He leant on his elbows above her as she tried to work out how to breathe with Raúl inside her.

He attempted slow withdrawal. She begged that he did not. She lay there, trying to accommodate him, waiting for the heat and pain to subside, her muscles clamped around him.

'I take it out slowly,' Raúl said. He felt sick—appalled by his own brutality—and guilty too at the pleasure of her, hot and tight around him. He was so close to coming and trying to hold on. 'I'll just—'

'Don't.'

Her eyes were screwed tight as he moved a fraction backwards, but when he halted, when he stilled, her body relaxed a little. Estelle tried to release herself. She moved to slide away from him. Yet the pain was subsiding to a throbbing heat so she moved again, warming to the sensation of him inside her.

It was a different type of command she gave next. 'Don't stop.'

'Estelle?' He did not want to stop, and yet he did not want to hurt her; he moved slowly a little within her, his breath shallow, panting as if he had already come.

Her hands moved to his buttocks and she felt them tauten beneath her fingers. It was Estelle who pressed and dictated the tempo and, rarely for Raúl, he let her. Rarely for Raúl, he was humbled. He did not think of the questions he must ask her, just focused on the tight grip and the heat of her on his unsheathed skin, and all he could do was kiss her. Every inch of him held back, resisting the beckoning of oiled muscles that gripped as he slid past them, that urged him now to move faster, to take her deeper.

Estelle's breath was quickening. He felt the somewhat impatient rise of her groin, the press of her hands in his buttocks, and he could hold back no more.

Still he had not taken her fully, but now he thrust in. Estelle's neck arched as he probed and located fresh virgin flesh with each deepening thrust, and when he had filled her, when every part of her was consumed, he moved out and did it again, angling his hips, hitting her deep inside till she was moaning.

He was moving fast now, and she wrapped her legs around him, could not believe how her body had just taken over. For she lifted to him, was building to him, working with him, both heading to the same mutual goal.

No longer naïve, her body shattered in an orgasm like nothing she had ever given herself—for there she could stop, there she could halt. And it was nothing like the teasing he had given her either, for here in Raúl's bed he urged her on further, broke all limits, ensured that she screamed.

She pulsed around the head of him. He was stroking her deep inside—one spot that had her sobbing, one tender

spot that he hit over and over—till she sobbed, and then he released himself into her. Her thighs were in spasm as a fresh wave of orgasm crashed through her body—and, yes, just as he had warned her, she cussed him in Spanish till he kissed her, till she was lying beneath him no longer a virgin.

She looked up at him, expecting a barrage of questions, a demand for an explanation, but instead he moved onto his side and put his arm around her, pulling her into him.

'I should have known' was his reprimand.

'I tried to tell you.'

'Estelle…' he warned.

She gave a small nod, conceding that tonight might have been rather too late.

'We will speak about it in the morning.'

For now, they held each other, lay in each other's arms, tired and sated and both in a place they had never thought they might be.

Estelle a bought bride; Raúl a man who had married and made love to a virgin.

CHAPTER ELEVEN

ESTELLE WOKE AND had no idea where she was for a moment.

Her body was bruised and sore. She could hear a shower.

She rolled over in bed and saw the evidence of their union, and moved the top sheet to cover it.

'Hiding the evidence?'

Estelle turned and was shocked at the sight of him. There was a towel round his hips, but his chest was covered in the bruises she now remembered her mouth making. He turned and took a drink from the breakfast table that had presumably been delivered and she saw the scratches on his back, remembered the wanton place he had taken her to.

'I need to have a shower.'

'We need to talk.' But then he conceded, 'Have some lunch and a shower. Then we will talk.'

'Lunch?'

'Late lunch,' Raúl said. 'It is nearly two.'

Estelle quickly gulped down some grapefruit juice and then headed to the bathroom. When she had found out they would be honeymooning on a yacht she had expected basic bathroom facilities; instead it was like a five-star hotel. The bathroom was marble, the taps and lighting incredible, yet she barely noticed. Her only thought was getting to her make-up bag.

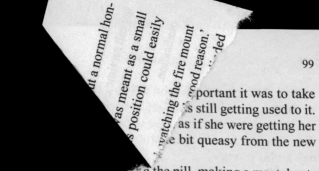

...t a normal hon-
...as meant as a small
...s position could easily
...watching the fire mount
...ood reason.'
...ded

...portant it was to take
...s still getting used to it.
...as if she were getting her
...e bit queasy from the new

...n the pill, making a mental note
...alarm on her phone to two p.m.—or should
...take it at seven tomorrow?

Her mind felt dizzy. She had seen that Raúl was less than impressed with her this morning and no doubt he would want a thorough explanation. She still hadn't worked out what to say.

Estelle showered and put on the factor fifty he insisted on, then sorted out her hair and make-up, relieved when she headed back into the bedroom and Raúl wasn't there. She selected a bikini from the many he had bought her, and also a pale lilac sarong. Her head was splitting from too much champagne and too much Raúl. She sat on the bed and put on espadrilles. Then, dressed—or rather barely dressed, as Raúl would want her to be—she stood. But her eyes did not go to the mirror—instead they went to the bed.

Mortified at the thought of a maid seeing the stained sheets, Estelle started to strip the bed.

'What are you doing?'

'I'm just making up the bed.'

'If I had a thing for maids then it would have been stipulated in the contract,' Raúl said. 'And if I had a thing for virgins,' he added, 'that would have been stipulated too.'

Estelle said nothing.

'Just leave it.' His voice was dark. 'The crew will take care of that. I will show you around.'

'I'll just wander…' She went to walk past.

'You can't hide from me here,' he warned, taking her wrist. 'But we will discuss it later. I don't want the staff

getting even a hint that this is anything b
eymoon.'

'Don't you trust your staff?' It
dig—because surely a man in hi
pay for his privacy?

'I don't trust anyone,' Raúl said, w
on her cheeks as his words sank in. 'And wit g

She followed him up onto the deck. The sun blin
her for a moment.

'Where are your sunglasses?'

'I forgot to bring them.' She turned to head back down,
but Raúl halted her, calling out to one of the crew. 'I can
get them myself.'

'Why would you?'

Sometimes she forgot just how rich and spoilt he was.
This was not one of those times. Despite the fact there were
some of the crew around, he pulled her into his arms and
very slowly kissed her.

'Raúl....' She was embarrassed by his passion. She
looked into his black eyes and knew he was making a
point.

'We are here for two days, darling. The plan is for us
to fully enjoy them.'

His words were soft, the message not.

'I'll show you around now.'

A maid handed her her sunglasses and then Raúl
showed her their abode for the next few days. The lounge
that she had barely noticed last night was huge, littered
with low sofas; another maid was plumping the cushions.
There was a huge screen and, though nervous around him,
Estelle did her best to be enthusiastic. 'This will be lovely
for watching a movie.'

Raúl swallowed and caught the maid's eyes, and as Es-

telle went over to look at his DVD collection he quickly led her away.

'Here is the gym.' He opened a door and they stepped in. 'Not that you'll need it. I will ensure that you get plenty of exercise.'

Only there, with the door safely closed, did he let his true frustration slip out. He closed the door and gave her a glimpse of what was to come.

'If you think we are going to be sitting around watching movies and holding hands—'

'I know what I'm here for.'

'Make sure that you do.'

Raúl had woken at lunchtime from his first decent sleep in days, from his first night without nightmares. For a moment he had glimpsed peace—but then she had stirred in his arms and he had looked down to a curtain of raven hair and felt the weight of her breast on his chest. The sheet had tumbled from them; he'd seen her soft pale stomach and the evidence of their coupling on her inner thigh.

He had gone to move the sheet to cover them, but the movement had disturbed her a little and he had lain still, willing her back to sleep, fighting the urge to roll over and kiss her awake, make love to her again. He had felt the heat from her palm on his stomach and had physically ached for that hand to move down. His erection had been uncomfortable.

He'd fought the bliss of the memories of last night as his hand had moved down—and then halted when he'd realised his own thought-processes.

Sex Raúl could manage—and often.

Making love—no.

Last night had been but one concession, and he reminded himself she had lied.

He had removed her hand from him then and spent a

full ten minutes examining her face—from the freckles dusting her nose to the full lips that had deceived him.

He stood in the well-equipped gym and looked at them now. Absolutely he would make things clear.

'We have several weeks of this,' Raúl said. 'I wanted a woman who could handle my life, who knew how to have fun.' He did not mince words. 'Who was good in bed.'

He watched her cheeks burn.

'I'm sure I'll soon learn. I'll keep up my end of the deal—I don't need hand-holding.'

'There will be no holding hands.' He took her hand and placed it exactly where it had been agreed it would visit regularly. 'You knew what you were signing up for…'

He had to hold her back; he had to be at his poisonous worst. He could not simply dump her, as he usually did when a woman fell too hard. They had weeks of this and he could not risk her heart.

Instead he would put her to work.

'Let's have a spa.'

She saw the challenge in his eyes, knew that he was testing her, and smiled sweetly. 'Let's!'

She followed him up onto the deck, trying to ignore the fact that he had fully stripped off as she took off her espadrilles and dropped her sarong.

'Take off your top.'

'In a moment…'

He could sense rather than see that she was upset, and it made him furious. He was actually wishing his father dead, just so this might end.

'Take off your top,' he said again. Because if she thought she was here to discuss the passing scenery, or for them to get to know each other better, then she was about to find out she was wrong.

Estelle might have taken him for a fool.

...race was one burning blush as her shaking hands undid the clasp, and she sank beneath the water as she removed it and placed the bikini top on the edge.

'Good morning!' The skipper made his way over. Naked breasts were commonplace on the Costa Del Sol—and especially on Raúl Sanchez Fuante's boat. He had no trouble at all looking Estelle in the eye as he greeted her. She, though, Raúl noted, was close to tears as she attempted to smile back.

'We are heading towards Acantilados de Maro-Cerro Gordo,' Alberto said, and then turned to Raúl. 'Would you like us to stop there tonight? The chef is looking forward to preparing your dinner and he wondered if you would like us to set up for you to eat on the bay?'

'We'll eat on the boat,' Raúl said. 'We might take a couple of jet skis out a little later and take a walk.'

'Of course,' Alberto said, then turned to Estelle.

'Do you have any preferences for dinner? Any food choices you would like the chef to know about?'

'Anything.'

Raul heard her try to squeeze the word out through breathless lips.

'It's a beautiful bay we are stopping at.' Albert happily chatted on. 'It's not far at all from the more built-up areas, but soon we will start to come into the most stunning virgin terrain.'

He wished them a pleasant afternoon and headed off.

'I've already explored the virgin terrain...' Raúl drawled, once he was out of earshot.

Estelle said nothing.

'Here.' Annoyed with himself for giving in, but hating her discomfort, he threw her the bikini top. 'Put it on ...ou want.'

She really was shaken, Raúl thought as he watched her trembling hands trying to put the garment on. Going topless was nothing here—nothing at all—but then he remembered last night: her shaking, her asking him to be gentle. Pleas he had ignored.

He strode through the water and turned her around, helping her with the clasp of her bikini top. Then, and he didn't know why, he pulled her into his arms and held her till she had stopped shaking—held her till the blush had seeped from her skin.

And then he made her burn again as he dropped a kiss on her shoulder and admitted a truth to her about that virgin terrain.

'…and it was stunning.'

CHAPTER TWELVE

NORMALLY RAÚL'S YACHT sailed into the busiest port, often
with a party underway.

This early evening, though, they sailed slowly into
Acantilados de Maro-Cerro Gordo. The sky was an amazing pink, the cliffs sparkling as they dropped anchor near
a secluded bay.

'The beaches are stunning here,' Alberto said, 'and
the tourists know it. But this one has no road access.' He
turned to Raúl. 'The jet skis are ready for you both.'

Only as they were about to be launched did Raúl remember. He turned and saw her pale face, saw that she
was biting on her lip as she went to climb on the machine,
and his apology was genuine.

'Estelle, I'm sorry. I forgot about your brother's accident.'

'It's fine,' she said through chattering teeth. 'He was
showing off…mucking around…' She was trying to pretend that the machine she was about to climb on *didn't*
petrify her. 'I know we'll be sensible.'

Raúl had had no intention of being sensible. He loved
the exhilaration of being on a jet ski and had wanted to
share it with her—had wanted to race and to chase.

Instead he was taking her hand. 'It's not fine. You don't
have to pretend.'

Oh, but she did. At every turn she had to pretend, if she was to be the temporary woman he wanted.

'Come on this one with me,' Raúl said. 'Alberto, take her hand and help her on.'

They rode towards the bay in a rather more subdued fashion than Raúl was used to.

The maid who was setting up the dinner table caught Alberto's eye when he came to check on her progress and they shared a brief smile.

His bride and the effect she was having on Raúl was certainly not one they had been expecting.

'I think I might go and reorganise his DVD collection,' the maid suggested and Alberto nodded.

'I think that might be wise.'

Estelle held tightly onto Raul's waist as the jet ski chopped through the waves, and because her head kept knocking into his back in the end she gave in and rested it there, not sure if her rapid heart-rate was because she was scared by the vehicle, by the questions she would no doubt soon be facing, or just by the exhilaration.

Making love with Raúl had been amazing. She was sore and tender but now, feeling his skin beneath her cheek, feeling the ocean water sting her and the wind whip her hair, she could not regret a moment. Even her lie. Feeling his passion as he had seared into her was a memory she would be frequently revisiting. For now, though, Estelle knew she had to play it tough—had to convince him better than she had so far that she was up to the job he had paid her for.

He skidded into the shallows and she unpeeled herself from him and stepped down.

'It's amazing…' She looked up at the cliffs, shielding her eyes. 'Look how high it is.'

He did, but only briefly. Estelle was too busy admiring the stunning view to notice his pallor.

'What did Angela say to you at the wedding?' Raúl asked.

She had been expecting a barrage of questions about her lack of experience, and was momentarily sideswiped at his choice of topic for conversation, but then she reminded herself his interest in her was limited.

'She wasn't sure whether or not we were a true couple,' Estelle said.

'You corrected her?'

'Of course,' Estelle said. 'She seems to think that *if* I love my husband, then I should encourage you to make peace with your father while there is still time.' She glanced over to him as they walked. 'She wants us to go there and visit.'

'It is too late to play happy families.'

'Angela said that she doesn't want you to suffer any guilt, as you did over your mother's death…'

'Misplaced guilt,' Raúl said, but didn't elaborate any more.

He stopped and they sat on the beach, looking out to the yacht. She could see the lights were on, the staff on deck were preparing their meal. It was hard to believe such luxury even existed, let alone that for now it was hers to experience. It was the luxury of *him* she wanted, though; there was more about Raúl that she needed to know.

'I didn't know how to answer her,' Estelle admitted. 'You said there was more you would tell me. I have no real idea about your family, nor about you.'

'So I will tell you what you need to know.' He pondered for a moment on how best to explain it. 'My grandfather—my mother's father—ran a small hotel. It did well

and he built another, and then he purchased some land in the north,' Raúl explained.

'In San Sebastian?' Estelle asked.

He nodded. 'On his death the business was left to his three children—De La Fuente Holdings. My father and mother married, and my father started to work in the family business. But he was always an outsider—or felt that he was, even though he oversaw the building of the San Sebastian hotel. When I was born my mother became unwell. In hindsight I would say she was depressed. It was then he started to sleep with Angela. Apparently Angela felt too much guilt and left work, moved back to her family, but they started seeing each other again...'

'How do you know all this?'

'My father told me the morning I met you.'

It was only then that Estelle fully realised this was almost as new to him as it was to her.

'Angela got pregnant, the guilt ate away at him, and he told my mother the truth. He wanted to know if she could forgive him. She cried and wailed and screamed. She told him to get out and he went to Angela—the baby was almost due. He assumed my mother would tell her family, that she would turn to them. Except she did not. When she had the car accident and died my father returned and soon realised no one knew he had another son. Instead they welcomed him back into the company.' He was silent for a moment. 'Soon they will find out the truth.'

'Angela said that you blamed yourself for your mother's death?'

'That is all you need to know.' He looked over to her. 'Your turn.'

'I don't know what to tell you.'

'Why you lied?'

'I didn't lie.'

'The same way my father didn't lie when he didn't tell me had another son? The same way Angela didn't lie when she failed to tell mention her son, Luka, was my brother?' He did not want to think about that. 'Okay, if you didn't outright lie, you *did* deceive.'

He watched her swallow, watched as her face jerked away to look out to the ocean.

'I wanted an experienced woman.'

'Sorry I don't know enough tricks—'

'I wasn't talking about *sex*!' Raúl hurled. 'I wanted a woman who could handle things. Who could keep to a deal. Who wasn't going to fall in love...'

'Again you assume!' Estelle flared. 'Why would I fall in love with some cold bastard who thinks only in money—who has no desire for true affection? A man who tells me what to wear and whether or not I can tan.'

Her eyes flashed as she let out some of the anger she had suppressed over the past few days while every decision apart from her wedding dress had been made by him.

'Raúl, I would not have a man choose my clothes or dictate to the hairdresser the style of my hair, or the beautician the colour of my nails. You're getting what you paid for—what you wanted—what you demanded. Consider my virginity a bonus!'

She dug her heels deep into the sand and almost believed her own words. Tried to ignore that last night, as she'd been falling asleep in his arms, foolish thoughts had invaded. Raúl's doubts about her ability to see this through perhaps had merit, for he would be terribly easy to love...

She turned around and faced him.

'I'm here for the money, Raúl.' And not for a single second more would she allow herself to forget it. 'I'm here with you for the same reason I was with Gordon.'

He could not stand the thought of her in bed with him—

could not bear to think about it. But when he did, Raúl frowned.

'If you were with Gordon for money, how come you were trying to change the sheets before the maid got in.'

'I was never with Gordon in that way. I just stood in for Ginny.'

'You shared his bed,' Raúl said. 'And we all know his reputation…'

'Unlike you, Gordon didn't feel comfortable going to a wedding alone,' Estelle said carefully.

'So he paid you to look like his tart?' Raúl checked. 'What about Dario's…?' His voice trailed off and he frowned as he realised the lengths Gordon had gone to, then frowned a little more as realisation hit. 'Is Gordon…?' He didn't finish the question—knew it was none of his business. 'You needed the money to help out your brother?'

She conceded with a nod.

'Estelle, it is not for me to question your reasons—'

'Then don't.'

Her warning did not stop him.

'Andrew would not want it.'

'Which is why he will never find out.'

'I know that if I had a sister I would not want her—'

'Don't compare yourself to my brother. You don't even have a sister, and the brother you *do* have you don't want to know.'

'What's that got to do with it?'

'We're two very different people, Raúl. If I discovered that I had a brother or sister somewhere I'd be doing everything I could to find out about them, to meet them—not plotting to bring them down.'

'I'm not plotting anything. I just don't want him taking what is rightfully mine. Neither do I want to end up working alongside him.'

She looked at the seductive eyes that invited you only to bed, at the mouth that kissed so easily but insisted you did not get close.

'You miss out on so much, Raúl.'

'I miss out on nothing,' Raúl said. 'I have everything I want.'

'You have everything money can buy,' Estelle said, remembering the reason she was here. 'Including me.'

When he kissed her it tasted of nothing. It tasted empty. It was a pale comparison to the kiss he had been the recipient of last night. And when he took her top off he knew she was faking it, knew she was thinking of the boat and of people watching, knew she was trying not to cry.

'Not here,' Raúl said for her.

'Please, Raúl…'

Her mouth sought his. She was still playing the part, too inexperienced to understand that he knew her body lied.

He wanted it back, the intimacy of last night, which meant taking care of her.

For now.

Surely for a couple of days he could take care of her. They could just enjoy each other and break her in properly. The last thing he wanted was her tense and teary, feeling exposed.

He had glimpsed her toughness, admired the lengths she would go to for her family, and he believed her now—she did not want his love

'Later.' Raúl pulled his head back from her mouth. 'I'm starving.'

He helped her with her bikini, used his chest as a shield as he did up the clasp, just in case any passing fish were having a peek, or telescopes were trained on them. But rather than making him feel irritated, her coyness now made him smile.

Especially when he thought of her unleashed.

'Come on,' Raúl said, despite the ache in his groin. 'Let's head back.'

CHAPTER THIRTEEN

'WE WILL GO and shower and get dressed for dinner,' Raúl said as they boarded and Alberto took the jet ski. 'Do you want me to ask Rita to come down and do your hair?'

'Rita?'

'She is a masseuse and a beautician. If you want her to come and help just ask Alberto,' Raúl said, heading off to the stateroom.

Estelle called him back. She could smell the food and was honestly starving. 'Why do we have to get dressed for dinner?' Estelle did not notice the twitch of his lips, though Alberto did. 'It's only us.'

'On a yacht such as this one, when the chef…' Raúl began. But he was torn, because etiquette often had no place on board and it seemed petty to put her right. 'Very well.' He turned to Alberto, who was already on to it.

'I'll let the chef know.'

They rinsed off under the shower on deck and then took their seats.

Raúl was rather more used to a well-made-up blonde in a revealing dress sitting opposite him, but there was something incredibly appealing about sitting for dinner half-naked and scooping up the delicacies the waiters were bringing.

'I could get far too used to this,' Estelle started, and

then stopped herself, remembering his words at the lawyer's. 'I meant…'

'I know what you meant.'

She was relieved to see he was smiling.

'The food really is amazing,' Raúl agreed. 'They chef is marvellous. Chefs on yachts generally are—that is why we keep coming back for more.'

They chatted as they ate, far more naturally than they had before, and it wasn't just for the benefit of the staff.

It was simply a blissful night.

They danced.

On the deck of his yacht they danced when the music came on.

'I understand now why we should have changed for dinner,' Estelle admitted. 'Do you think I've offended anyone?'

'I don't think you could if you tried.'

The sky was darkening and Raúl looked out to the cliffs, and rather than remembering hell he buried his face in her hair. It took only the smell of the ocean in her hair for him to escape.

'And for the record,' Raúl said, 'although you accuse me being a controlling bastard, I was worried about you burning. I have never seen paler skin.'

'I think I *am* a bit sunburnt.'

'I know.'

They moved down to the lounge room. Estelle was starting to relax—so much so that she didn't spring from his arms when some dessert wine was brought through to them.

'Let's go to bed…' His hand was in her bikini top, trying to free her breast.

'Not yet,' she breathed into his mouth. 'I'll never sleep.'

'I have no intention of letting you sleep.'

'Let's watch a movie,' Estelle said, unwrapping herself from him and heading over to his collection.

'Estelle—no!'

'Oh, sorry.' She'd forgotten what he'd told her in the gym, about no hand-holding and movies, and she turned and attempted a smile. 'Sure—let's go to bed.'

'I didn't mean that,' Raúl said through gritted teeth, wondering how he'd ended up with the one hooker to whom he'd have to apologise for his DVDs. 'I just don't think there will be anything there to your taste.'

He braced himself for the rapid demise of a pleasant night as Estelle flicked through his collection.

'I love this one.'

'Really?' Raúl was very pleasantly surprised.

'Actually...' She skimmed through a couple more. 'This one's my favourite.' She held up the cover to him and didn't understand his smile.

'Of course it is,' Raúl said, pulling her down beside him, smiling into her hair. One day he would tell her how funny that was—one day when it wouldn't offend, when she knew him better. He would laugh about it with her.

But there would not *be* that day, he reminded himself.

This was just for now.

He had not lain on a sofa and watched a movie—not one with a plot, anyway—since he couldn't remember when.

Estelle shivered. The doors were open and the air was cooling. He pulled down a rug from the back of the sofa and covered them, felt her bottom curving into him.

'Sore?' He kissed her pink shoulders as he made light work of her bikini top.

'A bit.'

Estelle concentrated on the movie as Raúl concentrated on Estelle. He kissed her neck and shoulders for ages, then played with her breasts, massaging them with

his palms, taking her nipples between thumb and fingers. Then slowly, when he knew there would be no qualms from Estelle, moved one hand down and untied her bikini bottoms.

His question, when repeated, was a far more personal one as his fingers crept in.

'Sore?'

'A bit,' she said again, but he was so gentle, and it felt so sublime.

She could feel the motion of the boat, and him huge and hard behind her; she could feel the urging of his mouth to turn to him and growing insistence from behind.

'Turn around, Estelle.' His breathing was ragged.

'In a minute.' She wasn't even watching the film. Her eyes were closed. She was just loving the feel of him playing with her and longing for it to go on. 'It's coming to the best bit.'

He pulled her up a little further, so that her naked bum was against his stomach, and he angled her perfectly. She felt the long, slow slide of him where he had stabbed into her last night. She was still bruised and swollen and hot down below, and yet she closed around him in relief.

'*This* is the best bit,' Raúl's low voice corrected her.

He pressed slowly into her, his fingers playing with her clitoris, slid slowly and deeply, with none of the haste of last night, and it was Estelle who was fighting to hold back.

'I'm going to come.'

'Not yet,' he told her, teasing her harder with his fingers, thrusting himself deeper inside.

'I am.' She was trembling and trying to hold on.

'Not yet.'

He stroked her somewhere so deep, the feeling so intense that she let out a small squeal.

'There?' he asked.

Estelle didn't know what he meant, but then he stroked her there again and she sobbed. 'There!' She was begging as over and over he massaged her deep, hitting her somewhere she hadn't even known existed. 'There…'

She was starting to cry, but with intense pleasure, and then she could no longer hold it. There was no point even trying.

There was a flood of release as she pulsed around him, and Raúl moaned as she tightened over and over around his thick length. He felt the rush of her orgasm flowing into him and he shot back in instant response, spilling deep into her, loving her abandon, loving the Estelle his body revealed.

Loving too the tinge of embarrassment that crept in as she struggled to get her breath back.

'What was that?'

'Us,' he said, still inside her. And it was not the cliffs he feared now, but the perfume of the ocean in her hair as he inhaled it—a fear that was almost overwhelming as he realised how much he had enjoyed this night.

Not just the sex, not just the talking, not just dinner.

But *now*.

'We should head back.'

They had been snorkelling. It had all started off innocently, but had turned into a slightly more grown-up activity. Raúl did not know if it was her laughter, or the feel of her legs wrapped around him, or just that he was simply enjoying her too much, but he kissed her cheek and unwrapped her legs from his waist.

'Is it dinner-time?'

'I meant we should head back for Marbella…'

It had been two nights and two amazing days, and more of a honeymoon than Raúl had ever intended for it to be.

They *were* dressing for dinner tonight, because they wouldn't be dawdling on their return. Which meant this would be their last night on the yacht.

She missed it already.

Even as Rita did her hair and make-up she missed the yacht, because it had been the most magical time. As if they had suspended the rules of the contract, their time had been spent talking, laughing, eating, making love— but Raúl had made it clear that things would be different when they returned to Marbella.

She felt as if they were approaching that already as Rita pushed the last pin into Estelle's hair. Raúl's expression was tense as he picked up his ringing phone.

'I will tell the chef you will be up soon,' Rita said, and Estelle thanked her and started to put on her dress.

She didn't understand what was being said on the phone, but given the terse words, she guessed it wasn't pleasant.

'They are getting married.' Raúl hung up and was silent.

By the time he told her what the call had been about he was doing up his tie, but kept getting the knot wrong.

'Oh.' She didn't know what else to say, just went on struggling with her zip.

'Come here.' He found the side zipper. 'It's stuck.'

She stood still as he tried to undo it.

'My father says he wants to do the right thing by Angela—wants to give her the dignity of being his wife and his widow. He wants her to have a say in decisions by the medical staff.'

'What did you say?'

'That it was the first decent thing I had heard on the subject.'

'Are you going to attend?'

He didn't answer her question; instead he hurried her

along. 'Come on. They will be serving up soon. It is not fair to keep the chef waiting.'

Since when was Raúl thoughtful about his staff? Estelle thought, but said nothing.

It was an amazing dinner. The chef had made his own paella, and even Raúl agreed, it was the best he had tasted.

Yet he barely touched it.

He looked at Estelle; she looked exquisite. Her hair was up, as it had been on their wedding day, her black dress looked stunning, and he told himself he could do it—that it wasn't a problem after all.

'What would you think if we did not turn around for Marbella?'

Estelle swallowed the food she was relishing and took a drink of water, nervous for the same reasons as Raúl.

'We could head to the islands, extend our trip…'

'So that you miss your father's wedding?'

'He has chosen to marry when I am on my honeymoon. He doesn't know we were to be on our way back.'

'You'll have to face him at some point.'

'You don't tell me what I have to do!' he snapped, and then righted himself, trying to explain things a little better. 'He wants a wedding—one happy memory with his wife. I doubt that will be manageable with me there. Especially if Luka attends.' He took a breath. 'So how about a few more days?' He made it sound so simple. 'I have not had a proper holiday in years…'

'I thought your life was one big holiday?'

'No,' Raúl said. 'My life is one big party. We will return to that in a few days.' He issued it as a warning, telling her without saying as much that what happened at sea stayed at sea.

He was waiting for her decision. But then Raúl remem-

bered the decision was entirely his. He was paying for her company—not her say in their location.

'I will let the staff know.'

'Now?'

'They have to plot the route, inform…'

He didn't finish, just headed off to let the crew know, and Estelle sat there, suddenly nervous.

She wanted to be back on safe water—because living with Raúl like this, seeing this side of him, she was struggling to remember the rules.

Their 'couple of days' turned into two weeks.

They sailed around Menorca and took their time exploring its many bays. Estelle's skin turned from pale to pink, from freckles to brown. He watched her get bolder, loved seeing her stretch out on a lounger wearing only bikini bottoms, not even a little embarrassed now. Her sexuality was blossoming to his touch, before his eyes.

Finally they sailed back into Marbella. Normally the sight of it was the one he loved best in the world, yet there was a moment when he wanted to tell the skipper to keep sailing, to bypass Marbella and head to Gibraltar, take the yacht to Morocco, just to prolong their time. Except he was growing far too fond of her.

She put a hand on his shoulder, joined him to watch the splendid sight, but she felt his shoulder tense beneath her touch.

Raúl turned. She was wearing espadrilles and bikini bottoms, his own wedding shirt knotted beneath her now rosy bust, her cheeks flushed and her lips still swollen from their recent lovemaking.

'You'd better get dressed.'

Usually Raúl was telling her she was *over*dressed.

'The press may be there. The cream dress,' he told her. 'And have Rita do your make-up.'

As easily at that he demoted her, reminded her of her place.

Back on dry land he took her hand. But it was just for the cameras that he put his shoulders around his new wife.

It was in case of a long lens that he picked up her and carried her into his apartment, back to the reality of his life.

CHAPTER FOURTEEN

IT WAS A life she could never have imagined.

Raúl worked harder than anyone she knew.

His punishing day started at six, but rather than coming in drained at the end of it he would have a quick swim in the pool, or they'd make love—or rather they'd have sex. Because the Raúl from the yacht was gone now. A quick shower after that and then they'd get changed for dinner. Meals were always eaten out, and then they would hit the pulsing nightlife, dancing and partying into the early hours.

Estelle couldn't believe this was the toned-down version of Raúl.

'I can cook,' Estelle said, and smiled one night as they sat at Sol's and waited for their dishes to be served. 'It might be a novelty…'

'Why would you cook when a few steps away you can have whatever you choose?'

It was how he lived: life was a smorgasbord of pleasure. But six weeks married to Raúl, even with a week off to visit her family, was proving exhausting for Estelle—and she wasn't the one working. Or rather, she corrected herself as the waiter brought her a drink, she *was* working, twenty-four-seven, because no way would she be dining out every night, no way would she be wandering along

streets that still pumped with music well after midnight on a Tuesday.

It had been Cecelia's cardiology appointment today, and Estelle was worried sick and doing her best not to show it. But she kept glancing at her phone, willing it to ring, wondering when she'd hear.

'How's your new PA?' Estelle asked as she bit into the most gorgeous braised beef, which had been cooked over an open fire.

'Okay.' Raúl shrugged. 'Angela trained her well...'

He looked down at her plate, stabbed a piece of beef with a fork and helped himself. Estelle was getting used to the way they shared their meals; it was the norm here.

'It *is* much more difficult without Angela,' Raúl admitted. 'Only now she is gone are we seeing how much she did around the place.'

'When will she be back?'

'She won't,' Raúl said. 'She is taking long service leave to nurse my father. Once he dies and it gets out about her she won't be welcome there.'

'Oh, well, you'll only have to see her at the funeral, then.'

Raúl glanced up. He could never be sure if she was being flip or serious. 'When are you going to see your father?' she asked him.

She was being serious, Raúl quickly found out.

'He chose to live in the north—he chose to end his days with his other family. Why should I....?' He closed his tense lips. 'I do not want to discuss it.'

'Angela called again today.'

'I told you not answer to her.'

'I was waiting for my brother to ring,' Estelle said. 'It was Cecelia's cardiology appointment today. I didn't think

to look when I picked up.' Estelle could not finish her dinner and pushed the plate away.

'You're not hungry?'

'Just full.'

'I was thinking…' Raúl said. 'There is a show premiering in Barcelona at the weekend. I think it might be something we would enjoy.'

'Raúl…' She just could not sit and say nothing—could not lie beside him at night and sleep with him without caring even a bit, without having an opinion. Surely he could understand that? 'I was riddled with guilt when my parents died.'

'Why?'

'For every row, for every argument—for all the things we beat ourselves up about when someone dies. Guilt happens whatever you do. Why not make it about something you couldn't have changed, instead of something you can?' On instinct she went to take his hand, but he pulled it back.

'You're starting to sound like a wife.'

She looked at him.

'Believe me, I don't feel like one.'

Estelle pounced on her phone when it rang.

'I need to take this.'

'Of course.'

It was Amanda, doing her best, as always, to sound upbeat. 'They're going to keep Cecelia in for a few nights. She's a bit dehydrated…'

'Any idea when she's going to have surgery?'

'She's too small,' Amanda said. 'They've put a tube in, and we're going to be feeding her through that. She might come home on oxygen…'

Raúl watched Estelle's eyes filling with tears but she turned her shoulders and hunched into the phone in an effort to hide them. He heard her attempt to be positive

even while she was twisting her hair around and around her finger.

'She's a fighter,' Estelle said, but as she did so she closed her eyes.

'How is your niece?' Raúl asked as she rang off.

'Much the same.' She didn't want to discuss it for fear she might break down—Raúl would be horrified! Seeing that he'd finished eating, Estelle gave him a bright smile. 'Where do you want to go next?'

'Where do *you* want to go?' Raúl offered.

Home, her body begged as they walked along the crowded street. But that wasn't what she was here for. She'd been transferring money over to Andrew since he'd gone back to England. The first time she'd told Andrew it was money she'd been saving to get a car. The second time she'd said it was a loan. Now she'd just given him a decent sum that would see them through the next few months, telling Andrew that she and Raúl simply wanted to help.

It was time to earn her keep.

They passed a club that was incredibly loud and very difficult to get into. It was a particular favourite of Raúl's. 'How about here?'

Estelle woke to silence. It was ten past ten and Raúl would long since have gone to work.

She sat up in bed and then, feeling dizzy, lay back down.

How the hell he lived like this on a permanent basis, Estelle had no idea. All she knew was she was not going out tonight.

He could, she decided, dressing and heading out not for the trendy boutiques but for the markets. She just wanted a night at home—or rather a night in Raúl's home— and something simple for dinner. There must be some

subclause in the contract that allowed for the occasional night off?

Marbella was rarely humid, the mountains usually shielded it, but it struggled today. The air was thick and oppressive and the markets were very busy. Estelle had bought the ripest, plumpest vine tomatoes, and was deciding between lamb and steak when she passed a fish stall and gave a small retch. She tried to carry on, to continue walking, tried to focus on a flower stall ahead instead of the appalling thought she had just had.

She couldn't be pregnant.

Estelle took her pill at the same time every day.

Or she had tried to.

All too often Raúl would come home at lunchtime, or they'd be in a helicopter flying anywhere rather than to his father's—the one place he needed to be.

She couldn't be pregnant.

'Watch where you're going!' someone scolded in Spanish as she bumped into them.

'Lo sierto,' Estelle said, changing direction and heading for the *Pfarmacia*, doing the maths in her head and praying she was wrong.

Less that half an hour later she found out she was right.

Raúl didn't get home from work till seven, and when he did it was to the scent of bread baking and the sight of Estelle in his underutilised kitchen, actually cooking.

'Are we taking the wife thing a bit far?' Raúl checked tentatively. 'You don't have to cook.'

'I want to,' Estelle said. She was chopping up a salad. 'I just want to have a night in, Raúl.'

'Why?'

'Because.' She frowned at him. 'Do you ever stop?'

'No,' he admitted, then came over and give her a kiss. 'Are you okay?'

'I'm fine. Why?'

'You didn't wake up when I left this morning. You seem tense.'

'I'm worried about my niece,' Estelle said, removing herself from him and adding two steaks to the grill.

She was curiously numb. Since she'd done the test Estelle had been operating on autopilot and baking bread, which she sometimes did when she didn't want to think.

She just couldn't play the part tonight.

They carried their food out to the balcony and ate steak and tomato salad, with the herb bread she had made, watching a dark storm rolling in.

Estelle wanted to go home, wanted this over. Though she knew there was no getting out of their deal. But she needed a timeframe more than ever now. She wanted to be far away from him before the pregnancy started showing.

She could never tell him.

Not face to face, anyway.

Estelle could not bear to watch his face twist, to hear the accusations he would hurl, for him to find another reason not to trust.

'I spoke with my father today.'

She tore her eyes from the storm to Raúl. 'How is he?'

'Not good,' Raúl said. 'He asks that I go and see him soon.'

'Surely you can manage to be civil for a couple of days?' She was through worrying about saying the wrong thing. 'Yes, your father had an affair, but clearly it meant something. They're together all this time later…'

'An affair that led to my mother's death.' He stabbed at his steak. 'Their lies left the guilt with *me*.' He pushed his plate away.

The eyes that lifted to hers swirled with grief and confusion and now, when all she wanted was to be away from him, when she must guard her heart properly, when she needed it least, Raúl confided in her.

'I had an argument with my mother the night she died. She had missed my performance at the Christmas play—as she missed many things. When I came home she was crying and she said sorry. My response? *Te odio.* I told her I hated her. That night she lifted me from my sleep and put me in a car. The mountains are a different place in a storm,' Raúl explained. 'I had no idea what was happening; I thought I had upset her by shouting. I told her I was sorry. I told her to slow down...'

Estelle could not imagine the terror.

'The car skidded and came off the mountain, went down the cliffside. My father returned from his so-called work trip to be told his wife was dead and his son was in hospital. He chose not to tell anyone the reason he'd been gone.'

'Did they never suspect he and Angela?'

'Not for a moment. He just seemed to be devoting more and more time to the hotel in San Sebastian. Angela was from the north and she resumed working for him again. Over the years, clearly when Luka was older, she started to come to Marbella more often with my father. We had a flat for her, which she stayed in during the working week.'

'He had two sons to support,' Estelle said. 'Maybe it was the only way he could see how.'

'Please!' Raúl scoffed. 'He was with Angela every chance he could get, leaving me with my aunt and uncle. Had he wanted one family he could have had it. Perhaps it would have been a struggle, but his family would have been together. He chose this life, and those choices caused my mother's death.'

'Instead of you?'

'I blamed myself for years for her death. I thought the terrible things I said…'

'You were a child.'

'Yes,' he said. 'I see that now. The night she died was two days after Luka's birth. I realise now that she was on her way to confront them.'

'In a storm, with a five-year-old in the back of her car,' Estelle pointed out.

'I thought she was trying to kill me.'

'She was ill, Raúl.'

He nodded. 'It would have been nice to know that she was,' Raúl said. 'It would have been nice to know that it was not my words that had her fleeing into the night.'

'It sounds as though she was sick for a long time, and I would imagine it was a very tough time for your father…' Estelle did not want involvement. She wanted to remove herself as much as she could before she told him. Yet she could not sit back and watch his pain. 'He just wants to know you're happy, that you're settled. He just wants peace.'

'We all want peace.' He was a moment away from telling her the rest, but instead he stood and headed through the balcony door. 'I'm going out.'

Estelle sat still.

'Don't wait up.'

'I won't.'

She didn't want him going out in this mood, and she followed him into the lounge while knowing he wouldn't welcome her advice. 'Raúl, I don't think—'

'I don't pay you to think.'

'You're upset.'

'Now she tells me what I'm *feeling*!'

'Now *she* reminds you that she read that contract before she signed it. If you think you're going to go out clubbing

and carrying on in your usual way I'll be on the next plane home…' she watched his shoulders stiffen '…with every last cent you agreed to pay me.'

He headed for the door.

'Hope the music's loud enough for you, Raúl!' she called out to him.

'It could never be loud enough.'

There was a crack from the storm and the balcony doors flew wide open. He turned then, and she glimpsed hell in his eyes. There was more than he was telling her, she knew that, and yet she did not need to know at this moment.

He was striding towards her and she understood for a moment his need for constant distraction, for *she* was craving distraction now. She was pregnant by the man she loved, who was incapable of loving her. How badly she didn't want to think about it. How nice it would be for a moment to forget.

His mouth was, perhaps for the last time, welcome. The crush of his lips was so fierce he might have drawn blood. Yet it was still not enough. He wrestled her to the floor and it was still too slow.

Here beneath him there were no problems—just the weight of him on her.

He was pulling at his zipper and pressing up her skirt. She was kissing him as if his lips could save them both. The balcony doors were still wide open. It was raining on the inside, raining on them, yet it did not douse them.

He had taught her so much about her body, but she learned something new now—how fast her arousal could be.

He was coming even before he was inside her; she could feel the hot splash on her sex. Estelle was sobbing as he thrust inside her, holding onto him for dear life. Each thrust of his hips met with her own desperation. It

was fast and it was brutal, and yet it was the closest they had ever been.

He was at her ear and breathing hard when he lifted his face. She opened her eyes to a different man.

'Come with me to see them?'

He was asking, not telling.

'Yes.'

'Tomorrow?'

'Yes.'

It felt terribly close to love.

CHAPTER FIFTEEN

THEY FLEW EARLY the next morning, over the lush hills of Spain to the north, and even as his jet made light work of the miles there was a mounting tension. Had they run out of time?

Far from anger from Raúl, there was relief when Angela came out of the door to greet them, a wary smile on her face.

'Come in,' she said. 'Welcome.'

She gave Estelle a kiss on the cheek, and gave one too to Raúl. 'We can do this,' she said to him, even as he pulled back. 'For your father. For one day…'

Raúl nodded and they headed through to the lounge.

If Estelle was shocked at the change in his father, it must be hell for Raúl.

'Hey,' he greeted his son. 'You took your time.'

'I'm here now,' Raúl said. 'Congratulations on your wedding.' He handed Antonio a bottle of champagne as he kissed him on the cheek. 'I thought we could have a toast to you both later.'

'I finally make an honest woman of her,' Antonio said.

Estelle watched as Raúl bit back a smart response. There really was no time for barbs.

'Your brother is flying in from Bilbao tonight. Will you stay for dinner?' Antonio's eyes held a challenge.

'I'm not sure that we can stay…'

'A meeting between the two of you is inevitable,' Antonio said. 'Unless you boycott my funeral. I am to be buried here,' he added.

She watched Raúl's jaw tighten as he told his son that this was the home he loved. Yet he had denied his first son the chance of having a real home.

'I will make a drink,' Angela said to Estelle. 'Perhaps you could help me?'

Estelle went into the kitchen with her. It was large and homely, and even though she was hoping to keep things calm for Raúl, Estelle was angry on his behalf.

'We will leave them to it,' Angela said as Estelle sat at the table. 'You look tired.'

'Raúl doesn't live a very quiet life.'

'I know.' Angela smiled and handed her a cup of hot chocolate and a plate of croissants.

Estelle took a sip of her chocolate, but it was far too sickly and she put the cup back down.

'I can make you honey tea,' Angela offered. 'That is what I had when…' Her voice trailed off as she saw the panic in Estelle's eyes and realised she must not want anyone to know yet. To Angela it was obvious—she hadn't seen Estelle since her wedding day, and despite the suntan her face was pale, and there were subtle changes that only a woman might notice. 'Perhaps your stomach is upset from flying.'

'I'm fine,' Estelle said, deliberately taking another sip.

'I am worried that when Antonio dies I will see no more of Raúl…'

Estelle bit her lip. Frankly she wouldn't blame him. Because being here, seeing first-hand evidence of years of lies and deceit, she understood a little better the darkness of his pain.

'He is like a son to me.'

Estelle simply couldn't stay quiet. 'From a distance?' She repeated Angela's own words from the wedding day and then looked around. There were pictures of Luka, who looked like a younger Raúl.

'Raúl is here too.' Angela pointed to a photo.

'He wasn't, though.' Estelle could not stand the pretence. 'You had a home here—whereas Raúl was being shuffled between his aunt and uncle, occasionally seeing his dad.'

'It was more complicated than that.'

'Not really.' Estelle simply could not see it. 'You say you think of him as a son, and yet…'

'We did everything the doctor said,' Angela wrung her hands. 'I need to tell you this—because if Raúl refuses to speak with me ever again, then this much I would like you to know. The first two years of Luka's life Antonio hardly saw him. He did everything to help Raúl get well, and that included keeping Luka a secret. The doctor said Raul needed his home, needed familiarity. How could we rip him away from his family and his house? How could we move him to a new town when the doctor insisted on keeping things as close to normal as possible?'

Estelle gave a small shrug. 'It would have been hard on him, but surely no harder than losing his mother. He thought it was because of something he had said to her.'

'How could we have known that?'

'You could have spoken to him. You could have asked him about what happened. Instead you were up here, with his dad.'

There was a long stretch of silence, finally broken by Angela. 'Raúl hasn't told you, has he?'

'He's told me everything.'

'Did Raúl tell you that he was silent for a year?' She

watched as Estelle's already pale face drained of colour. 'We did not know what happened that day, for Raúl could not tell us. The trauma of being trapped with his dead mother…'

'How long were they trapped for?'

'For the night,' Angela said. 'They went over a cliff. It would seem Gabriella died on impact. When the *médicos* got there he was still begging her to wake up. He kept telling her he was sorry. Once they released him he said nothing for more than a year. How could we take him from his home, from his bed? How could we tell him there was a brother?'

'Excuse me—'

Estelle retched and cried into the toilet, and then tried to hold it together. Raúl did not need her drama today. So she rinsed her mouth and combed her hair, then headed back just as Raúl was coming out from the lounge.

'Are you okay?'

'Of course.'

'My father is going to have a rest. As you heard, my brother is coming for dinner tonight. I have agreed that we will stay.'

Estelle nodded.

'Somehow we will get through dinner without killing each other, and then,' Raúl said, 'as my reward for behaving…' He smiled and pulled her in, whispered something crude in her ear.

Far from being offended, Estelle smiled and then whispered into *his* ear. 'I can do it now if you want.'

She felt him smile on her cheek, a little shocked by her response.

'It can wait.' He kissed her cheek. 'Thank you for today. Without you I would not be here.'

'How is he?'

'Frail…sick…'

'He loves you.'

'I know,' Raúl said. 'And because I love him also, we will get through tonight.'

She wasn't so sure they'd get through it when she met Luka. He was clearly going through the motions just for the sake of his parents. Angela was setting up dinner in the garden and Antonio was sitting in the lounge. It was Estelle who got there first, and opened the door as Raúl walked down the hall.

The camera did not lie: he was a younger version of Raúl—and an angrier one too.

Luka barely offered a greeting, just walked into his family home where it seemed there were now two bulls in the same paddock. He refused Raúl's hand when he held it out to him and cussed and then spoke in rapid Spanish.

'What did he say?' Estelle asked as Luka strode through.

'Something about the prodigal son's homecoming and to save the acting for in front of his father.'

'Come on,' Estelle said. There would be time for dwelling on it later.

He caught her wrist. 'You're earning your keep tonight.'

He saw the grit of her teeth and the flash of her eyes.

'Do you do it deliberately, Raúl?' she asked 'Does it help to remind me of my place on a night like tonight?'

'I am sorry. What I meant was that things are particularly strained. When I asked you I never anticipated bringing you here. Certainly I never thought I would set foot in this house.'

They could not discuss it properly here, so for now she gave him the benefit of the doubt. They went out to the garden, where Luka was talking with his father, and they all sat at the table for what should have been a most diffi-

cult dinner. Instead, for the most part, it was nice. It was little uncomfortable at first, but soon conversation was flowing as Estelle helped Angela to bring out the food.

'I never thought I would see this day,' Antonio said. 'My family all at the same table...'

Antonio would never see it again.

He was so frail and weak it was clear this would be the last time. It was for that reason, perhaps, that Luka and Raúl attempted to be amicable.

'You work in Bilbao?' Raúl asked.

'I do,' Luka said. 'Investment banking.'

'I had heard of you even before this,' Raúl said. 'You are making a name for yourself.'

'And you.' Luka smiled but it did not meet his eyes. 'I hear about your many acquisitions...'

Thank God for morphine, Estelle thought, because Antonio just smiled and did not pick up on the tension.

The food was amazing—a mixture of dishes from the north and south of Spain. There was *pringá*, an Andalusian dish that was a slow-cooked mixture of meats and had been Raúl's favourite as a child. And there was *marmitako* too, a dish from the Basque Country, which was full of potatoes and pimientos and, Antonio said, had kept him going for so long.

'So you study?' Antonio said to Estelle.

'Ancient architecture.' Estelle nodded. 'Although, I haven't been doing much lately.'

'Yes, what happened to your online studies?' Raúl teased.

'Sol's happened.' Estelle smiled.

Raúl laughed. 'Being married to me is a full-time job...'

Raúl used the words she had used about Gordon. It was a gentle tease, a joke that caused a ripple of laughter—

except their eyes met for a brief moment and it hurt her
that he was speaking the truth.

It *was* a job, Estelle reminded herself. A job that would
soon be over. But then she thought of the life that grew inside her, the baby that must have the two most mismatched
parents in the world.

Not that Raúl knew it.

He thought she loved the clubs and the parties, whereas
sitting and eating with his family, as difficult as it was,
was where she would rather be. This night, for Estelle,
was one of the best.

'You would love San Sebastian.' Antonio carried on
speaking to her. 'The architecture is amazing. Raúl, you
should take Estelle and explore with her. Take her to the
Basilica of Santa Maria—there is so much she would love
to see…'

'Estelle would prefer to go out dancing at night. Anyway,' Raúl quipped, 'I haven't been inside a church for
years.'

'You will be inside one soon,' his father warned. 'And
you should share in your wife's interests.'

Estelle watched thankfully as Raúl took a drink rather
than delivering a smart response to his father's marital
advice.

And, as much as she'd love to explore the amazing city,
she and Raúl were simply too different. And the most bizarre thing was Raúl didn't even know that they were.

She tried to imagine a future: Raúl coming home from
a night out to a crying baby, or to nannies, or having access weekends. And she tried to picture the life she would
have to live in Spain if she wanted his support.

Estelle remembered the menace in his voice when he
had warned that he didn't want children and decided then
that she would never tell him while this contract was be-

tween them. When she was back home in England and there was distance, when she could tell him without breaking down, or hang up on him if she was about to, *then* she would confess.

And there would be no apology either. Estelle surged in sudden defensiveness for her child—she wasn't going to start its life by apologising for its existence. However Raúl dealt with the news was up to him.

'So…' Still Antonio was focused on Estelle. 'You met last year?'

'We did.' Estelle smiled.

'When he said he was seeing an ex, I thought it was that…' Antonio snapped his fingers. 'The one with the strange name. The one he really liked.'

'Antonio.' Angela chided, but he was too doped up on morphine for inhibition.

'Araminta!' Antonio said suddenly.

'Ah, yes, Araminta.' Estelle smiled sweetly to her husband. 'Was that the one making a play for you at Donald's wedding?'

'That's the one.' Raúl actually looked uncomfortable.

'You were serious for a long time,' Antonio commented.

Estelle glanced up, saw a black smile on Luka's face.

'Weren't you engaged to her?' he asked. 'I remember my mother saying that she thought there might soon be a wedding.'

'Luka,' Angela warned. 'Raúl's wife is here.'

'It's fine,' Estelle attempted—except her cheeks were on fire. She was as jealous as if she had just found out about a bit of her husband's past she'd neither known of nor particularly liked. 'If I'd needed to know about all of Raúl's past before I married him we'd barely have got to his twenties by now.'

She should have left it there, but there was a white-hot

feeling tearing up her throat when she thought of how he'd so cruelly dismissed Araminta—and that was someone he'd once cared about.

It was for that reason her words were tart when she shot Raúl a look. 'Though you failed to mention you'd ever been engaged.'

'We were never engaged.'

'Please!'

Antonio's crack of laughter caught them all by surprise and he raised a glass to Estelle. 'Finally you have met your match.'

It wasn't a long night. Antonio soon tired, and as they headed inside Luka farewelled his father fondly. But the look he gave to Estelle and Raúl told them both he didn't need them to see him to the door in *his* home.

They headed for bed. Estelle was a bit embarrassed by her earlier outburst, especially as everyone else seemed to have managed to behave well tonight.

'I'm sorry about earlier,' she said as she undressed and climbed into bed. 'I shouldn't have said anything about Araminta.'

'You did well,' Raúl said. 'My father actually believes us now.'

He thought she had been acting, Estelle realised. But she hadn't been.

It felt very different sleeping in his father's home from sleeping in Raúl's apartment or on his yacht. Even Raúl's ardour was tempered, and for the first time since she had married him Estelle put on her glasses and pulled out a book. It was the same book she had been reading the day she had met him, about the mausoleum of the First Qin Emperor.

She was still on the same page.

As soon as this was over she was going to focus on

her studies. It had been impossible even to attempt online learning with Raúl around.

'Read me the dirty bits,' Raúl said, and when she didn't comment he took the book from her and looked at the title. 'Well, that will keep it down.'

For his effort he got a half smile.

'You really like all that stuff?'

'I do.'

His hand was on her hip, stroking slowly down. 'They should hear us arguing now,' he teased lightly. 'You demanding details about my past.'

'I don't need to know.'

'My time in Scotland was amazing.' Raúl spoke on regardless. 'I shared a house with Donald and a couple of others. For the first time since my mother died I had one bedroom, one home, a group of friends. We had wild times but it was all good. Then I met Araminta, we started going out, and I guess it was as close to love as I have ever come. But, no, we were never engaged.'

'I really don't need to hear about it.' She turned to him angrily. 'Do you remember the way you spoke to her?' She struggled to keep her voice down. 'The way you treated her?' She looked at his black eyes, imagined running into him a few years from now and being flicked away like an annoying fly. She wasn't hurting for Araminta, Estelle realised. She was hurting for herself—for a time in her future without him.

'So, should I have slept with her as she requested?'

'No!'

'Should I have danced with her when she asked?'

Estelle hated that he was right.

'Anyway, we were never engaged. Her father looked down on me because I didn't come with some inherited title, so I ended things.'

'You dumped her for that?'

'She was lucky I gave a reason,' Raúl said.

Estelle let out a tense breath—he could be so arrogant and cold at times.

'Normally I don't.'

She returned to her book, tried to pick up where she had left off. Just as she would try to pick up her life in a few weeks' time. Except now everything had changed.

'Put down the book,' Raúl said.

'I'm reading.'

'You are the slowest reader I have ever met,' Raúl teased. 'If we ever watch a movie with subtitles we will have to pause every frame.'

She gave up pretending to read, and as she took off her glasses and put down the book he was suddenly serious.

'Not that we will be watching many more movies.'

She lay on her pillow and faced him.

'I could not have done this without you,' Raúl said. 'I nearly didn't come here in time.' He brushed her hair back from his face with her hand.

'You made it, though.'

'It will be over soon.' He looked into her eyes and didn't know if he was dreading his father dying or that soon she would be gone. 'You'll be back to your studies...'

'And you'll be back on your yacht, partying along the coastline.'

'We could maybe go out on the yacht this weekend?' Was he starting to think of her in ways that he had sworn not to? Or was he simply not thinking straight, given that he was here? 'We had a good time.'

'We did have a good time,' Estelle said, but then she shook her head, because she was tired of running away from the world with Raúl. 'But can we just leave it at that?'

She did not want to taint the memory—didn't want to

return to the yacht with hope, only to find out that what they had found there no longer existed.

But for one more night it did.

He held her face and kissed her—a very slow kiss that tasted tender. She felt as if they were back on the boat, could almost hear the lap of the water as he pulled her closer to him and wrapped her in his arms, urged her to join him in one final escape.

Estelle did.

She kissed him as though she were his wife in more than name. She kissed him as though they were really the family they were pretending to be, sharing and loving each other through difficult times.

He had never known a kiss like it; her hands were in his hair, her mouth was one with his, their bodies were meshing, so familiar with each other now. And he wanted her in his bed for ever.

'Estelle....' He was on the edge of saying something he must not, so he made love to her instead.

His hands roamed her body; he kissed her hard as he slid inside her. Side on, they faced each other as he moved and neither closed their eyes.

'Estelle?'

He said it again. It was a question now—a demand to know how she felt. She could feel him building inside her but she was holding back—not on her orgasm. She was holding back on telling him how she felt. They were making love and they both knew it, though neither dared to admit it.

She stared at this man who had her heart. She didn't even need to kiss him to feel his mouth, because deep inside he consumed her. She was pressing her hips into him, her orgasm so low and intense that he moaned as she gripped him. He closed his eyes as he joined her, then

forced them open just to watch the blush on her cheeks, the grimace on her face, just to see the face he loved come to him.

She knew he would turn away from her afterwards. Knew they had taken things too far, that there had been true tenderness.

She looked at the scar on his back and waited till dawn for his breathing to quicken, for Raúl to awake abruptly and take her as he did most mornings.

It never happened.

CHAPTER SIXTEEN

HE WOKE AND he waited for reason.

For relief to flood in because he had held back his words last night.

It never came.

He turned and watched her awaken. He should be bored by now. She should annoy him by now.

'What am I thinking?' he asked when she opened her eyes and smiled at him.

'I wouldn't presume to know.'

'I *did* meet you that night,' he said. 'Despite the dress and the make-up, it *was* Estelle.'

He was getting too close for comfort. Raúl had never been anything other than himself. She, on the other hand, changed at every turn—he didn't actually know her at all. Sex was their only true form of communication.

Estelle could hear noises from the kitchen and was relieved to have a reason to leave. 'I'll go and give Angela a hand.' She went to climb out of bed, wondering if she should say anything about what Angela had told her last night. 'I spoke to her yesterday…'

'Later,' Raúl said, and she nodded.

Today was already going to be painful enough.

* * *

'Buenos días,' Raúl greeted Angela.

'Buenos días.' Angela smiled. 'I was just making your father his breakfast. What would you like?'

'Don't worry about us,' Raúl said. 'We'll have some coffee and then Estelle and I might go for a walk.'

'What time are you going back?'

'I'm not sure,' Raúl said. 'Maybe we might stay a bit longer?'

'That would be good,' Angela said. 'Why don't you take your father's tray in and tell him?'

He was in there for ages, and Angela and Estelle shared a look when at one point they heard laughter.

'I am so glad that they have had this time,' Angela said, and then Raúl came out, and he and Estelle headed off for a walk along the sweeping hillsides on his father's property.

'Have you been here before?' Estelle asked. 'To San Sebastian, I mean?'

'A couple of times,' Raúl said. 'Would you like to explore?'

'We're here to spend time with your father,' Estelle said, nervous about letting her façade down, admitting just how much she would like to.

'I guess,' Raúl said. 'But, depending on how long we stay, I am sure the newlyweds would like some private time too.'

'Wouldn't you be bored?'

'If I am I can wait in the gift shop.' Raúl smiled, and so did she, and then he told her some of what he had been talking about with his father. 'He has told my aunt and uncle about Angela and Luka.'

'When?'

'Yesterday. When he knew I was on my way,' Raúl said. 'He didn't want to leave it to me to tell them.'

'How did they take it?'

'He asked if we heard any shouting while we were flying up.' Raúl gave a small mirthless laugh. 'They want him dead, of course. He told them they wouldn't have long to wait.'

They walked for ages, hardly talking, and Raúl was comfortable with silence, because he was trying to think— trying to work out if she even wanted to hear what he was about to ask her.

'You miss England?'

'I do,' Estelle said. 'Well, I miss my family.'

'Will you miss me?' He stopped walking.

She turned to him and didn't know how to respond. 'I won't miss the clubs and the restaurants...'

'Will you miss *us*?'

'I can't give the right answer here.'

'You can.' He took her in his arms. 'You were right. I miss out on so much...'

It was a fragile admission, she could feel that, and she was scared to grasp it in case somehow it dispersed. But she could not deny her feelings any longer. 'You don't have to.'

His mouth was on hers and they were kissing as if for the first time—a teenage kiss as they paused in the hills, a kiss that had nothing to do with business; a kiss that had nothing to do with sex. His fingers were moving into her hair, touching her face as if he were blind, and she was a whisper away from telling him, from confessing the truth. Just so they could tell his father—just so there might be one less regret.

'Raúl...'

He looked into her eyes and she thought she could tell him anything when he looked at her like that. But for the moment she held back. Because a child was something

far bigger than this relationship they were almost exploring. She remembered her vow to do this well away from their contract.

'Let's get back.'

They walked down the hill hand in hand, talking about nothing in particular—about France, so close, and the drive they could maybe take tomorrow, or the next day. They were just a couple walking, heading back home to their family—and then she felt his hand tighten on hers.

'It's the *médico*.'

They ran the remaining distance, though he paused for just a moment to collect himself before they pushed open the front door. Because even from there they could hear the sound of Angela sobbing.

'Your father…' Angela stumbled down the hall and Raúl held her as she wept into his arms. 'He has passed away.'

CHAPTER SEVENTEEN

ESTELLE COULDN'T BELIEVE how quickly things happened.

Luka arrived soon after, and spent time with his father. But it was clear he did not appreciate having Raúl and Estelle in his home.

'Stay,' Angela said.

'We'll go to a hotel.'

'Please, Raúl…'

Estelle's heart went out to her, but it was clear that Luka did not want them there and so they spent the night in a small hotel. Raúl was pensive and silent.

The next morning they stood in the small church to say farewell. The two brothers stood side by side, but they were not united in their grief.

'I used to think Luka was the chosen one,' Raúl said as they flew late that afternoon back to Marbella for the will to be read, as per his father's wishes. 'When I found out—when my father said he wanted to die there—I felt his other family were the real ones.' His eyes met hers. 'Luka sees things differently. He was a secret—his father's shame. I got to work alongside him. I was the reason he did not see much of his father when he was small. His hatred runs deep.'

'Does yours?'

'I don't know,' Raúl admitted. 'I don't know how I feel. I just want to get the reading of the will over with.'

It wasn't a pleasant gathering. Paola and Carlos were there, and the look they gave Angela as she walked in was pure filth.

'She doesn't need this—' Estelle started, but Raúl shot her a look.

'It was never going to be nice,' he said.

Estelle bit her lip, and tried to remember her opinion on his family was not what she was here for. But she kept remembering the night they had made love, their walk on the hill the next morning, and tried to hold on to a love that had almost been there—she was sure of it.

She sat silent beside him as the will was read, heard the low murmurs as the lawyer spoke with Angela. From her limited Spanish, Estelle could make out that she was keeping the home in San Sebastian and there were also some investments that had been made in her name.

And then he addressed Luka.

Estelle heard a shocked gasp from Paola and Carlos and then a furious protest started. But Raúl sat still and silent and said nothing.

'What's happening?'

He didn't answer her.

As the room finally settled the lawyer addressed Raúl. He gave a curt nod, then stood.

'Come on.'

He took her by the arm and they walked out.

Angela followed, calling to him. 'Raúl…'

'Don't.' He shrugged her off. 'You got what you wanted.'

Estelle had to run to keep up with his long strides, but finally he told her what was happening.

'His share of the business goes to Luka.' His face was grey when he turned and faced her. 'Even dying still he

plays games, still he lies.' He shook his head. 'I get a vine-yard…'

'Raúl,' Angela had caught up with them. 'He saw how happy you two were the night before he died.'

'He did not change his will.'

'No, but it was his dream that his two sons would work side by side together.'

'He should have thought about that twenty-five years ago.'

'Raúl…'

But Raúl was having none of it. He strode away from Angela and all too soon they were back in his apartment and rapid decisions were being made.

'I'll sell my share,' he said. 'I will start again.' He would. Raúl had no qualms about starting again. 'And I will sell that vineyard too…'

'Why?'

'Because I don't want it,' he said. 'I don't want anything from *him*. I don't want to build bridges with my brother.' *His* mother's business was being handed over to her husband's illegitimate son—it would kill her if she wasn't dead already.

Raúl was back in the mountains—could hear her furious shouts and screams, the storm raging; he could hear the screech of tyres and the scrape of metal. He was over the cliff again. But that part he could manage—that part he could deal with. It was next part he dreaded.

It was the silence after that, and he would do anything never to hear it again.

'You don't have to make any decisions tonight. We can talk about it—'

'We?' His lips tore into a savage smile. '*We* will talk about *my* future? Estelle, I think *you* are forgetting your place.'

'No.' She refused to deny it any longer. 'The morning your father died, when were talking, we were *both* choosing to forget my place. If you want a relationship you can't pick and choose the times!'

'A relationship?' He stared at her for the longest time.

'Yes,' Estelle said, and she was the bravest she had ever been. 'A relationship. I think that's what you want.'

'Now she tells me what I want? You *love* me, do you? You *care* about me, do you? Have you any idea how boring that is to hear? I *bought* you so we could avoid this very conversation. You'd do well to remember that.'

Estelle just stood there as he stormed out of the apartment. She didn't waste her breath warning him this time.

She refused to be his keeper.

CHAPTER EIGHTEEN

RAÚL SAT IN Sol's with the music pumping and stared at the heaving dance floor.

A vineyard.

A vineyard which, if he sold it, wouldn't even pay for his yacht for a year—would Estelle stick around then?

Yes.

He had never doubted his ability to start again, but he doubted it now—could not bear the thought of letting her down.

'Te odio.' He could hear his five-year-old voice hurling the words at his mother, telling her he hated her for missing his play.

He'd been a child, a five-year-old having a row, yet for most of his life he had thought those words had driven his mother to despair that day.

Could he do it?

Whisk Estelle away from a family that loved her to live in the hills with a man who surely wasn't capable of love?

Except he did love her.

And she loved him.

He had done everything he could think of to ensure it would not happen, had put so many rules in place, and yet here it was—staring at him, wrapping around him like a blanket on a stifling day.

He did not want her love, did not want the weight of it. Did not want to be responsible for another's heart.

She would stand by him, Raúl knew, but the fallout was going to be huge. The empire was divided. He could smell the slash and burn that would take place and he did not want her exposed to it.

His phone buzzed in his pocket but he refused to look at it, because if he saw her name he would weaken.

Raúl looked across the dance floor, saw an upper-class hooker, ordered her a drink and gestured her over.

He took out some money and as she opened her bag made his request.

'Lápiz de labios,' Raúl said, and pointed to his neck.

He did not have to explain himself to her. She delivered his request—put her mouth to his neck and did as he asked.

'Perfume,' he ordered next, and she took out her cheap scent and sprayed him.

'Gracias.'

It was done now.

Raúl stood and headed for home.

CHAPTER NINETEEN

'AMANDA.' ESTELLE ATTEMPTED to sound normal when she answered the landline. She was staring at the picture of them on Donald's wedding night, trying to fathom the man who simply refused to love.

'I tried your mobile.'

'Sorry...' Estelle had started to talk about the charger she'd left in San Sebastian, started to talk about little things that weren't important at all, when she realised that for once Amanda wasn't being upbeat. 'What's happened?'

'I tried to ring Raúl—I wanted him to break the news to you.'

Estelle felt her heart turn to ice.

'We're at the hospital and the doctors say that they're going to operate tomorrow.'

'Has she put on any weight?'

'She's lost some,' Amanda said. 'But if they don't operate we're going to lose her anyway.'

'I'm coming home.'

'Please...'

'How's Andrew?'

'He's with her now. He's actually been really good. He's sure she's going to make it through.'

'She will.'

'I don't think so,' Amanda admitted, and her sister-in-

law who was always so strong, always so positive, finally broke down.

Estelle said everything she could to comfort her, but knew they were only words, that she needed to be there.

'I'm going to hang up now and book a flight,' Estelle told her. 'And I'll try and sort out my phone.'

'Don't worry about the phone,' Amanda said. 'Just get here.'

Estelle grabbed her case and started piling clothes in. Getting to the airport and onto a flight was her aim, but the thought of Cecelia, so small and so weak, undergoing something so major was just too overwhelming and it made Estelle suddenly fold over. She sobbed as she never had before—knew that she had to get the tears out now, so she could be strong for Amanda and Andrew.

Raúl heard her tears as he walked through the apartment and could not stand how much he had hurt her—could not bear that *he* had done this.

'Estelle…' He saw the case and knew that she was leaving.

'Don't worry.' She didn't even look at him. 'The tears aren't for you. Cecelia has been taken back into hospital. They can't wait for the surgery any longer…' She thought of her again, so tiny, and of what would happen to her parents if they lost her. The tears started again. 'I need to get back to them.'

'I'll fix it now.'

He couldn't *not* hold her.

Could not stand the thought of her facing this on her own, not being there beside her.

He held her in his arms and she wept.

And he could not fight it any more for he loved her.

'We'll go now.'

'No.' She was trying to remember that she was angry, but it felt so good to be held.

'Estelle, I've messed up, but I know what I want now. *I know…*'

She smelt it then—the cheap musky scent; she felt it creep into her nostrils. She moved out of his arms and looked at him properly, smelt the whisky on his breath and saw the lipstick on his neck.

'It's not what you think,' Raúl said.

'You're telling me what I think, are you?' Oh, she didn't need him to teach her to cuss in Spanish! 'You win, Raúl!' Her expression revealed her disgust. 'I'm out of here!'

The tears stopped. They weren't for him anyway. She just turned and went on filling her case.

'Estelle—'

'I don't want to hear it, Raúl.' She didn't even raise her voice.

'Okay, not now. We will speak about it on the plane.'

'You're not coming with me, Raúl.'

'Your brother will think it strange if I do not support you.'

'I'm sure my brother has other things on his mind.' She looked at him, dishevelled and unshaven, and scorned him with her eyes. 'Don't make this worse for me, Raúl.'

He went to grab her arm, to stop her.

'Don't touch me!'

He heard her shout, heard the pain—not just for what was going on with her niece, but for the agony of the betrayal she perceived.

'You can't leave like this. You're upset…'

'I'm upset about my niece!' She looked at him. 'I would *never* cry like this over a man who doesn't love me.' She didn't care how much she hurt him now. 'I'm not your mother, Raúl, I'm not going fall apart, or drive over a

cliff-edge because the man I'm married to is a cheat. I'm far stronger than that.'

She was.

'All I want now is to get home to my niece.'

He'd lost her. Raúl knew that. Arguing would be worse than futile, for she needed to be with her family urgently.

'I will call my driver and organise a plane.'

'I can sort out transport myself.' Tears for him were starting now, and she didn't want Raúl to see—love was not quite so black and white.

'If you take my plane it will get you there sooner,' Raúl said.

And it would get her away from him before she broke down—before she told him about the baby…before she weakened.

It was the only reason she said yes.

CHAPTER TWENTY

RAÚL STOOD IN the silence.

It was the sound he hated most in the world.

It was his nightmare.

Only this was one *he* had created.

The scent that filled his nostrils was not leaking fuel and death but the scent of cheap perfume and the absence of *her*.

He wanted to chase Estelle—except he was not foolish enough to get in a car, and he could not follow her as his driver was taking her to the airport.

Raúl called a taxi, but even as he climbed in he knew she would not want him with her on the flight. Knew he would be simply delaying her in getting to where she needed to be. They passed De La Fuente Holdings and he looked up, trying to imagine it without his father and Angela, and with Luka working there. Trying to fathom a future that right now he could not see.

Noticing a light on, he asked the driver to stop…

'Raúl!'

Angela tried not to raise her eyes as a very dishevelled Raúl appeared from the elevator.

He was unshaven, his eyes bloodshot. His hair was a mess, and there was lipstick on his collar…

It was the Raúl she knew well.

'What are you doing here at this time, Raúl?'

'I saw the light on,' Raúl said. 'Estelle's niece is sick.'

'I am sorry to hear that. Where is Estelle?'

'Flying back to London.'

'You should be with her, then.' Angela refused to mince her words. He might not want to hear what she had to say to him—he could leave if that were the case.

'She didn't want me to go.'

'So you hit the clubs and picked up a *puta*?'

'No.'

'Don't lie to me, Raúl,' Angela said. 'Your wife would never wear cheap perfume like that.'

'I wouldn't cheat on her. I couldn't.'

Angela paused. Really, the evidence was clear—and yet she knew Raúl better than most and he did not lie. Raúl never attempted to defend the inexcusable.

'So what happened?' Angela asked.

He closed his eyes in shame.

'You know, when you live as a mistress apparently you lose the right to an opinion on others—but of course you have them.' Harsh was the look she gave Raúl. 'Over and over I question your morals.'

'Over and over I do too,' Raúl admitted. 'She got too close.'

'That's what couples do.'

'I did not cheat. I wanted her to think that I had.'

'So now she does.' Angela looked at him. 'So now she's on her own, dealing with her family.'

Angela watched his eyes fill with tears and she tried not to love him as a son, tried not to forgive when she should not. But when he told her what had happened, told her what he had done, the filthy place his head had been, she believed him.

'You push away everyone who loves you. What are you scared of, Raúl?'

'This,' Raúl admitted. 'Hurting another, being responsible for another…'

'We are responsible for ourselves,' Angela said. 'I have made mistakes. Now I pay for them. Now I have till the morning to clear out my office. Now your aunt and uncle turn their backs on me. I would do it all again, though, for the love I had with your father. Some things I would do differently, of course, but I would do it all again.'

'What would you do differently?'

'I would have insisted you were told far sooner about your father and I. I would have told you about your brother,' she said. 'We were going to before you went to university, but your father decided not to at the last moment. I regret that. I should have stood up to him. I should have told you myself. I did not. And I have to live with that. What would *you* have done differently, Raúl?'

'Not have gone to Sol's.' He gave a small smile. 'And many, many other things. But that is the main one now.'

'You need to go to her. You need to tell her what happened—why you did what you did.'

'She doesn't want to hear it,' Raúl said. 'There are more important things on her mind.'

He could not bring himself to tell Angela that their marriage was a fake. If this was fake, then it hurt too much.

And if it was not fake, then it was real.

'If you are not there for her now, with her niece so ill, then it might be too late.'

Raúl nodded. 'She has my plane.'

'I will book you on a commercial flight,' Angela said. 'You need to freshen up.'

He headed to his office, stared in the mirror and picked

up his razor. He called his thanks as she brought him in coffee and a fresh shirt.

'This is the last time I do this for you.'

'Maybe not,' Raúl said. 'Maybe your sons might have a say in that.'

Angela's eyes welled up for a moment as finally he acknowledged the place she had in his heart. But then she met his eyes and told him, 'I meant this is the last time I help you cover up a mistake. Estelle deserves more.'

'She will get it.'

'Your father was so pleased to see how you two were together,' Angela said. 'He was the most peaceful I have ever seen him. He knew he had not allowed time for you and Luka to sort things out, but you are brothers and he believes that will happen. The morning he passed away we were watching you and Estelle walking in the hills. We saw you stop and kiss.'

Raúl closed his eyes as he remembered that day, when for the first time in his life he had been on the edge of admitting love.

'He knew you were happy. I am so glad that I told him about the baby.'

Raúl froze.

'Baby?'

There was no mistaking his bewilderment.

'She has not told you?'

'No!' Raúl could not take it in. 'She told *you*?'

'No,' Angela said. 'I just knew. She did not have any wine; she was sick in the morning…'

Yes, Estelle was tough.

Yes, she could do this without him.

He did not want her to.

'Book the flight.'

CHAPTER TWENTY-ONE

'RAÚL!'

The only possible advantage to being in the midst of a family crisis was that no one noticed the snap to her voice or the tension on Estelle's features when a clean-shaven, lipstick-free Raúl walked in.

'I'm sorry I couldn't get here sooner.' He shook Andrew's hand.

'No, we're grateful to you for getting Estelle here,' Andrew said. 'We're very sorry about your father.'

It was strange, but in a crisis it was Andrew who was the strong one. Amanda barely looked up.

'Is she in surgery?' Raúl sat down next to Estelle and put his arm around her. He felt her shoulders stiffen.

'An hour ago.' Her words were stilted. 'It could be several hours yet.'

The clock ticked on.

Raúl read every poster on the wall and every pamphlet that was laid out. She could hear the turning of the pages and it only served to irritate her. Why on earth had he come? Why couldn't she attempt to get over him with him still far away?

'Why won't they give us an update?' asked Amanda's mother. 'It's ridiculous that they don't let us know what's going on.'

'They will soon,' Andrew said, and Raúl watched as Andrew put his arm around his wife and comforted her, saw how she leant on him, how much she needed him.

Despite everything.

Because of everything, Raúl realised.

'Why don't you wait in the hotel?' Estelle suggested when she could not stand him being in the room a moment longer. 'I've got a room there.'

'I want to wait with you.'

He headed out to the vending machine and she followed him. 'I need some change,' he said. 'I haven't got any pounds.'

'Why would you make this worse for me?'

'I'm not trying to make it worse for you,' Raúl said. 'I know this is neither the time nor the place, but you need to know that nothing happened except my asking a woman to kiss my neck and spray me with her perfume.' He looked her right in the eye. 'I wanted you gone.'

'Well, it worked.'

'I made a mistake,' Raúl said. 'The most foolish of mistakes. I did not want to put you through what was to come.'

'Shouldn't that be *my* choice?' She looked at him.

'Yes,' he said simply. 'As it should be mine.'

Estelle didn't understand his response, was in no mood for cryptic games, and she shook her head in frustration. She wanted him gone and yet she wanted him here—wanted to forgive, to believe.

'I can't do this now,' Estelle said. 'Right now I have to concentrate on my niece.'

As much as Raúl longed to be there for her, that much he understood. 'Do you want me to wait in the hotel or stay with you here?'

'The hotel,' Estelle said—because she could not think straight with him around, could not keep her thoughts

where they needed to be with Raúl by her side. She wanted his arms around her, wanted the comfort only he could give, and yet she could not stand what he had done.

'Could I get a coffee as well?' Andrew wheeled himself over.

'Of course,' Raúl said as Estelle handed him some change.

'Estelle, could you take Amanda for a walk?' Andrew asked. 'Just get her away from the waiting room. Her parents are driving her crazy, asking how much longer it will be.'

'Sure.'

Estelle's eyes briefly met Raúl's, warning him to be gone by the time she returned, and Raúl knew the fight he had on his hands. He watched as Estelle suggested a walk to Amanda and he saw a family in motion, supporting each other, a family that was there for each other. A family who helped, who fixed—or tried to.

He looked to Andrew. 'You have the best sister in the world.'

'I know,' Andrew said. 'I'd do anything for her.'

As would Estelle for him, Raúl thought. She'd sold her soul to the devil for her family, but now he understood why.

'I am going to wait in the hotel,' Raúl said. 'I didn't sleep at all last night.'

'I know.' Andrew nodded. 'I'm sure Estelle will keep you up to date.'

'What hotel is she staying at?'

'Over the road,' Andrew told him. 'Good luck—I'm sure it's not at all what you're used to.'

'It will be fine.'

'You just wait.' Andrew gave a pale smile. 'I had to wait fifteen minutes just for them to find a ramp.'

They chatted on for a while—Andrew trying to keep

his mind out of the surgery, Raúl simply because Andrew wanted to talk.

'I had my reservations about the two of you at first,' Andrew admitted. 'You're so opposite.'

And then Raúl found out from his wife's brother just how much Estelle hated clubs and bars, found out exactly the lengths she had gone to for her family.

There was one length she would not go to, though. Raúl was certain of that now.

He walked alongside Andrew's chair, down long corridors, past the operating theatres and Intensive Care, and back again a few times over—until he saw Estelle returning and knew it was better for her that he leave.

He paced the small hotel room, waiting for news—because surely it was taking too long. It was now nine p.m., and he was sick to his stomach for a baby he had never met and a family he wanted to be a part of.

'She made it through surgery.'

Raúl could hear both the relief and the strain in Estelle's voice when the door opened.

'When did she get out of Theatre?'

'About six.' She glanced over to him. 'Was I supposed to ring and inform you?'

He could hear the sarcasm in her voice. 'I just thought it was taking too long. I thought…'

'I'm sorry.' Estelle regretted her sarcastic response— she could see the concern on his face was genuine. 'It was just a long wait till they let Andrew and Amanda in to see her. They've only just been allowed.'

'How is she?'

'Still here.' Estelle peeled off her clothes. 'I've lost my phone charger. I gave Andrew your number in case anything happens overnight.'

It was, though she would never admit it, a relief to have him here, to know that if the phone rang in the night he would be the one to answer it. It was a relief, too, to sink into bed and close her eyes, but there was something that needed to be dealt with before the bliss of sleep.

'I'm not going to tell them we're over yet,' Estelle said. 'It would be too much for them to deal with now. But after we visit in the morning can you make your excuses and leave.'

'I want to be here.'

'I don't want you here, though, and given what's happened you don't own me any more.' She stared into the dark. 'Exclusive, remember?'

'I've told you—nothing happened,' Raúl said. 'Which means I do still own you.'

'No,' Estelle said, 'you don't. Because whatever went on I've decided that I don't want your money. It costs too much.'

'Then pay me back.'

'I will…' she attempted, but of course a considerable amount had already been spent. 'I fully intend to pay you back. It just might take some time.'

'Whatever you choose. But it changes nothing now, Estelle…' He reached for her, wanted to speak with her, but she shrugged him off and turned to her side.

'I'd like the night off.'

'Granted.'

She woke in his arms and wriggled away from them, and then rang her brother. Raúl watched as she went to climb out of bed, saw the extra heaviness to her breasts and the darkening pink of her areolae, and he loved her all the more for not telling him, for guarding their child from the contract that had once bound them. It was the only leverage he had.

'You'll leave after visiting?' Estelle checked.

'Why would I leave my wife at a time like this?' Raúl asked. 'I'm not going anywhere, Estelle.'

'I don't want you here.'

'I don't believe you,' Raúl said. 'I believe you love me as much as I love you.'

'Love you!' Estelle said. 'I'd be mad to love you.' She shook her head. 'You might have almost sent me crazy once, Raúl, but if I possibly did love you then it's gone. My love has conditions too, and you didn't adhere to them. I don't care about technicalities, Raúl. Even if you didn't sleep with someone else, what you did was wrong.'

'Then we go back to the contract.' He caught her wrist. 'Which means I dictate the terms.'

'Your father's dead. Surely it's over?'

'We agreed on a suitable pause. You should read things more closely before you sign them, Estelle.' He watched her shoulders rise and fall. 'But I agree it has proved more complicated than either of us could have anticipated. For that reason, I will agree that the contract expires tomorrow.'

'Tomorrow?' Estelle asked. 'Why not now?'

'I just want one more night. And if I have to exercise the terms of the contract to speak with you—believe me, I shall.'

CHAPTER TWENTY-TWO

'SHE'S PINK!'

Estelle couldn't believe the little pink fingers that wrapped around hers. Even Cecelia's nails were pink—it was suddenly her favourite colour in the world.

'That's the first thing we said.' Andrew was holding Cecelia's other hand. 'She's been fighting so much since the day she was born.' Andrew smiled down at his daughter.

All were too entranced by the miracle that was Cecilia to notice how much Raúl was struggling.

Raúl looked down at the infant, who resembled Estelle, and could hardly believe what he had almost turned his back on.

'I have to go and do some work,' Raúl said. 'Do you want to get lunch later?'

Estelle looked up, about to say no, but he was talking to Andrew.

'Just at the canteen,' he added.

'That would be great.' Andrew smiled. 'Estelle, could you take Amanda for some breakfast? She wants one of us with Cecelia all the time but she needs to get out of the unit and get some fresh air.'

'Sure.' Estelle stood.

'I thought we could go for dinner tonight.'

This time Raúl *was* speaking to Estelle.

'I'm here to be with my niece.'

'Andrew and Amanda are with her. As long as she continues to improve I am sure they expect you to eat.'

'Of course we do,' Andrew said. 'Go out tonight, Estelle. You need a break from the hospital too!'

It was a long day. The doctors were in and out with Cecelia, and talked about taking her breathing tube out if she continued to hold her own. Amanda's parents went home, to return at the weekend, and after they had gone Estelle finally persuaded Amanda to have a sleep in one of the parents' rooms.

It was exhausting.

As she closed the door and went to head back to Cecelia she wondered if she had, after all, grown far too used to Raúl's lifestyle—she would have given anything to be back on his yacht, just drifting along, with nothing to think about other than what the next meal might be and how long it would be till they made love again.

Being Raúl's tart hadn't all been bad, Estelle thought with a wry smile as she returned to Cecelia.

It was being his wife that was hell.

'Amanda's asleep,' Estelle said. 'Well, for a little while.'

'Thanks for being here for us,' Andrew said. 'Both of you. Raúl's great. I admit I wasn't sure at first, but you can see how much he cares for you.'

She felt tears prick her eyes,

'Did you ask him to offer me a job?'

'A job?'

She couldn't lie easily to her brother, but instantly he knew that Estelle's surprised response was real, that she'd had no idea.

'Raúl said that when things are sorted with Cecelia there will be a job waiting for me. He wants me to check out his

hotels, work on adjustments for the disabled. There will be a lot of travel, and it will be tough being away at first. But once Cecelia's better he says we can broaden things so it's not just about travelling with disabilities but with a young child as well.'

It was a dream job. She could see it in her brother's eyes. Soon he would be earning, travelling, and more than that his self-respect and confidence would start to return.

'It sounds wonderful.' Estelle gave him a hug, but though she smiled and said the right thing she was furious with Raúl—his company was about to implode, and she and Raúl were soon to divorce quietly.

How dared he enmesh himself further? How dared he involve Andrew in the chaos they had made?

She wanted it to be tomorrow, she wanted Raúl gone so she could sort out how she felt, sort out her life, sort out how to tell him that the temporary contract they had signed would, however tentatively, bind them for life.

There was a note from Raúl waiting for her when she reached the hotel, telling her that he was tied up in a meeting but would see her at the restaurant at eight.

'You signed up for this,' Estelle told herself aloud as she put on her eye make-up. She wondered if it would be just dinner, or perhaps a club after, or...

Estelle closed her eyes so sharply that she almost scratched her eyeball with her mascara wand. He surely wouldn't expect them to sleep together?

He surely wouldn't insist?

Then again, Estelle told herself as she took a taxi to the restaurant, this was Raúl.

Of course he would insist.

Worse, though, she knew she must comply—no matter the toll on heart.

* * *

He turned heads. He just did.

He was waiting for her at the bar, and when they walked into the smartest of restaurants he might as well have being stepping out of a helicopter in a kilt—because everybody was looking at him.

'You look beautiful,' Raúl told her as they sat down.

'Thank you,' she said.

He could feel the anger hissing and spitting inside her, guessed that she must have spoken to Andrew since lunchtime.

'It's a lovely dress,' he commented. 'New?'

'I chose it.'

'It suits you.'

'I know.'

He ordered wine. She declined.

He suggested seafood, which he knew she loved, but he had read in one of the many leaflets he perused in the hospital waiting room that pregnant woman were advised not to eat it.

'I thought you loved seafood?' Raúl commented when she refused it, wondering what her excuse would be.

'I've had enough of it.'

She ordered steak, and he watched her slice it angrily before she voiced one of the many things that were on her mind.

'Did you offer my brother a job?'

'I did.'

'Why would you do that? Why would you do that when you're about to walk away? When you know the company's heading for trouble?'

'We're not heading for trouble,' Raúl said. 'I have been speaking with Luka at length today, and Carlos and Paola too. There is to be a name-change. To Sanchez De La

Fuente… Anyway, if there is trouble ahead it will only be in the office. Your brother will not be dealing with it.'

'What about when we divorce? Will you use him as a pawn then?'

'Never. I tell you this: it is a proper offer, and as long as your brother does well he will have a job.'

'You say that now…'

'I always keep my word.' He looked at her. 'I don't lie,' Raúl said. 'From the start I have only been myself.' He watched the colour spread up her cheeks. 'You get the truth, whether you like or not. I think we both know that much about me.'

Reluctantly she nodded.

'It is only wives that I employ on a whim. I am successful because I choose my employees carefully and I don't give out sympathy jobs. Your brother pointed out a few things that could be changed at the hotel. He would like the menu outside the restaurant to be displayed lower too. He said he would not like to find out about the menu and the prices from a woman he was perhaps dating with.'

Estelle gave a reluctant smile. It was the sort of thing Andrew *would* say.

'He said that a lower table at Reception would be a nice touch, so that anyone in a wheelchair could check in there. That means I do not have to refurbish our reception areas. He has saved me more than his year's wage already.'

'Okay.'

'I don't want my hotels to be good, I want them to be the best—and by the best I mean the best for everyone: businessmen, people with families, the disabled. Your brother, as I told him, will soon be all three.' He looked at her for a long moment, wondering if now she might tell him. 'It is good to see Cecelia improving,' Raúl said. 'It must be a huge relief.'

'It is,' Estelle admitted. 'I think we're only now realising just how scary the last few months have been.'

'Does seeing your niece make you consider ever having a baby?'

She gave a cynical laugh.

'It's just about put me off for life, seeing all that they have had to go through.'

'But they've made it.'

She wasn't going to tell him about the baby, Raúl realised. But, far from angering him, it actually made him smile as he sat opposite the strongest woman he knew.

'Here…' At the end of the meal he smeared cream cheese on a cracker, added a dollop of quince paste and handed it to her.

'No, thanks. I'm full.'

'But remember the night we met…'

'I'd rather not.'

He saw tears prick her eyes and went to take her hand. He could not believe all that they had been through in recent weeks. As she pulled her hand away Raúl wasn't so sure they'd survived it.

'I'm sorry for hurting you. I overreacted—thought I was going to lose everything, thought I might not be able to give you the lifestyle—'

'Like I need your yacht,' Estelle spat. 'Like I need to eat out at posh restaurants seven nights a week, or wear the clothes you chose.'

'So if you don't want all that,' Raúl pointed out, 'what *do* you want?'

'Nothing,' Estelle said. 'I want nothing from you.'

He called for the bill and paid, and as they headed out of the restaurant he took her hand and held it tightly. He turned her to him and kissed her.

It tasted of nothing.

He kissed her harder.

She wanted to spit him out. Not because she loathed his mouth but because she wanted to sink into it for ever—wanted to believe his lies, wanted to think for a moment that she could hold him, that he'd want their baby as much as she did, that he'd want the real her if he knew who she was.

'Where now?' Raúl asked. 'I know…' He held her by the hips. 'You could show me Dario's…'

'I didn't meet Gordon at Dario's,' Estelle said. 'I told you that.'

'We could go anyway,' Raúl said. 'It's our last night together, and it sounds like fun.'

He saw the conflict in her eyes, saw her take a breath to force another lie. He would not put her through it, so he kissed her instead.

'Let's get back to the hotel.'

'Raúl…' She just couldn't go through with it—could not keep up the pretence a moment longer, could not bear to be made love to just to have her heart ripped apart again.

'What?' He took her by the hand again, led her to a taxi.

'Come on, Estelle…' He undressed speedily. 'It's been a hell of a day. I would like to come.'

'You can be *so* romantic.'

'But you keep insisting this is not about romance,' Raúl pointed out.

Her face burnt.

'I don't understand what has suddenly changed. We have been having sex for a couple of months now…' He was undoing her zipper, undressing her. He was down on one knee, removing her shoes. 'Tomorrow we are finished. Tonight we celebrate.'

'I don't want you.'

'So you did the other times?' he checked.

At every exit he blocked her. At every turn he made her see it had never been paid sex for her—not for one single second, not for one shared kiss. She had been lying from the very start. For she had loved him from the start.

'Estelle, after tonight you have the rest of the century off where we are concerned.'

He laid her on the bed and kissed her, felt her cold in his arms. His mouth was on her nipple and he swirled it with his tongue then blew on it, watching it stiffen and ripen. Then he took it deep in his mouth, his fingers intimately stroking her. He filled her mouth with his tongue and she just lay there.

This was what she had signed up for, Estelle reminded herself. She didn't have to enjoy it. Except she was.

It was like a guilty secret—a *filthy* guilty secret. Because she wanted him so—wanted him deep inside her. She turned her cheek away but he turned it back and kissed her. She did not respond—or her mouth did its best not to.

He felt the shift in her…kissed her back to him.

He felt the motion of her tongue on his, felt *her*.

'Tell me to stop and I will,' Raúl said.

She just stared at him.

'Tell me…'

She couldn't

'You can't stop this any more than I can…'

He moved up onto his elbows and she tried not to look at him, looked at his shoulder, which moved back and forth over her.

'Tell me…' he said.

She held on.

'Tell me how you feel…'

In a moment she would. In a moment she'd be sobbing

and begging in his arms. She lifted her hips, and then lifted them again, just so she could hurry him along.

'I'm going to come…' she moaned.

'Liar.'

He pushed deeper within her, hit that spot she would rather tonight he did not, for her face was burning, and her hands were roaming, and her hips were lifting with a life of their own as she let out a low, suppressed moan.

She felt a flood of warmth to her groin, felt the insistence of him inside her, the demand that she match his want.

'You couldn't pay for this…' He was stroking her deep inside and seducing her with his words. 'You could never fake this…'

He slipped into Spanish as she left the planet; he toppled onto her and bucked rapidly inside her as she sobbed out her orgasm. She didn't know where she started or ended, didn't know how to handle the love in her heart and the child in her belly. All belonged to the man holding her in his arms.

'You want me just as much as I want you.'

'So?' She stared back at him. 'What does that prove? That you're good in bed?' She turned away from him and curled up like a ball. 'I think you already knew that.'

'It proves that I am right to trust you. That it is nothing to do with contracts or money. That you *do* love me as much as I love you.'

'You don't know me, though.' She started to cry. 'I've been lying all along.'

'I know you far more than you think,' Raúl said.

'You don't. Your father was right. I like churches and reading…'

'I know that.'

'And I hate clubs.'

'I know that too.'

'I'm nothing like the woman you thought you met.'

'Do you not think I'd long ago worked that out?' Raúl kissed her cheek. 'My virgin hooker.'

He heard her gurgle of laughter, born from exhausted tears.

'I don't get how you're the one with no morals, yet I'm the one who's lied.'

'Because you're complicated,' Raúl said. 'Because you're female.' He kissed her mouth. 'Because you loved me from the start.'

She went to object, but he was telling the truth.

'Do you know when I fell in love with you?' Raúl said. 'When I saw you in those tatty pyjamas and I did not want you in Gordon's bed. It had nothing to do with me paying you. I deserved that slap, but you really did misinterpret my words.'

She was so scared to love him, so scared to tell him about the baby. But if they were to survive, if they were to start to trust, then she had to. It never entered her head that he already knew.

'When were you going to tell me you're pregnant, Estelle?'

She felt his hand move to her stomach, felt his kiss on the back of her neck. All she could be was honest now. 'When I was too pregnant to fly.'

'So the baby would be English?'

'Yes.'

'And you would support it how?'

'The same way that billions of non-billionaires do.'

'Would you have told me?'

'Yes.' She needed the truth from him now and she turned in his arms. 'Are you still here because of the baby?'

'No,' Raúl said. 'I am here because of you.'

She knew he was telling her the truth—not just because he always did, but because of what he said.

'I have had three hellish nights in my life. The first I struggle to speak about, but with you I am starting to. The second was the night after I'd found out about my brother and you were there. I went to bed not thinking about revenge or hate, but about a kiss that went too far and a slap to my cheek. I guess I loved you then, but it felt safer not to admit that.'

'And the third?'

'Finding myself in a nightmare—but not the one I am used to,' Raúl said. 'I was not in a car calling out to my mother. I was not begging her to slow down, and nor was I pleading with her to wake…'

Tears filled her eyes as she imagined it, but she held onto them, knew she would only ever get glimpses of that time and she must piece them together in the quiet of her mind.

'Instead I realised, again, that a woman I loved was gone because of my harsh actions and words. Worse, though. This time it *was* my fault.'

She heard him forgive what his five-year-old self had said as the past was looked at through more mature eyes.

'I went to Angela. She was always the one I went to when I messed up, and I had messed up again. I asked her what to do. I was already on my way to you. It was then that she told me that at least my father had known about the baby… It would seem I was the last to know.'

'I never told her.'

'I'm glad that she guessed. She told my father that morning. I'm glad that he knew, even if I did not.' He looked at her and smiled. 'Opposites attract, Estelle.' He kissed her nose. 'It's law. You can't argue with that.'

'I'm not arguing.'

'Did you hate every dance?' he asked.

She shook her head. 'Of course not.'

'We'll have to get babysitters when we want to go out soon.'

He blew out a breath at the thought of the changes that were to come and she saw that he was smiling.

'Who'd have thought?'

'Not me,' Estelle admitted.

'So, how do you tell your wife you want to marry her all over again?'

'We don't need to get married again,' Estelle said. 'Though a second honeymoon might be nice.'

'Where?'

He was going to make her say it.

'Where?'

'On the yacht.'

Yes, she could get used to that—especially when he made love to her all over again. Especially when he made her laugh about the maid's secret swapping of his DVDs.

No, he had never lied. But he'd never been more honest—and it felt so good.

'Do you think your family will notice a change in us?'

'No.' Estelle smiled. 'They think we met and fell head over heels in love.'

'They were right.' Raúl pulled her to him and then kissed her again. 'We were the only ones who couldn't quite believe it.'

EPILOGUE

It was a beautiful wedding, held on the yacht, which had dropped anchor in Acantilados de Maro-Cerro.

It was Raúl's wedding gift to Gordon for bringing Estelle to him.

The grooms wore white and, contrary to Spanish tradition, there *were* speeches.

'I never thought I'd be standing declaring my love amongst my closest family and friends…' Gordon smiled, and then the dancing started.

Estelle leant against Raúl, feeling the kicks of their baby inside her.

'Is that Gordon's son Ginny is dancing with?' Estelle asked.

'They've been going out for a while.'

'Really?' Estelle smothered a smile. Raúl noticed everything. 'Gordon was once married before—ages ago, apparently.'

'How will they say they met? She can hardly admit she was his father's…' He stopped as Estelle dug him in the ribs. 'Sorry,' Raúl said. 'Sometimes I forget your other life.'

She didn't laugh this time, because the feeling was starting again—like a tight belt pulling around her stomach.

'Do you remember when we stopped here?' Raúl asked.

'When we took out a jet ski and you were scared and trying not to show it.'

'Of course I do.' Estelle attempted to answer normally. 'And I remember when we went snorkeling, and I—'

'Estelle?' He heard her voice break off mid-sentence.

Estelle had been trying to ignore the tightenings, but this one she could not ignore. Raúl's hand moved to her stomach, felt it taut and hard beneath his hands.

'I'll organise a speedboat to take us back to Marbella.'

'It might be ages yet. I don't want to make a fuss.'

'I think it would be a bit more awkward for Gordon if you have the baby here.' He glanced around at the guests and then went to have a word with Alberto, who soon organised transport.

'We are going to head off,' Raúl said when Gordon cornered them. 'Estelle is tired…' But then he couldn't lie—because Estelle was bent over.

'Oh, my!' Gordon was beaming.

'Please,' Estelle begged. 'I don't want everyone to know.'

There was no chance of keeping it quiet as she was helped down to the swimming platform, from where she was guided onto a speedboat. They sped off to the cheers and whistles of the wedding party.

'I wanted to have it in England…'

'I know.' They were supposed to have been flying there the next morning. 'But you wanted to be at the wedding too,' he reminded her.

'I know.'

'You can't have everything,' he teased. 'That's only me.'

She groaned with another pain and buried her face in his neck, wondering how much worse the pains would get, grateful that Raúl was so calm.

He *was* calm—he had everything he wanted right here on this small boat.

He looked up at the cliffs. He had long ago let go of that night, but there was a brief moment of memory just then. It didn't panic him. For a minute he thought of his mother and prayed for her peace.

It was the longest night, and her labour went on well into the next day.

Estelle pushed and dug her nails into his arms, and just when she was sure she could not go on any longer, finally the end was in sight.

'No empujen!'

'Don't push,' Raúl translated.

He had been incredibly composed throughout, but he was starting to worry now, watching the black hair of his infant and realising that soon he would be a father for real.

And then he saw her.

Red, angry, with black hair and fat cheeks.

And as he held her he was more than willing to be completely responsible for this little heart.

The midwife asked if they had a name as she went to write on the wristband and he looked at Estelle. They had chosen a few names, but had opted to wait till the baby was here before they decided. There was one name that had not been suggested till now.

'Gabriella?' Estelle said, and he nodded, unable to speak for a moment. The name that had once meant so much pain was wrapped now in love, and his mother's name would go on.

'Gabriella Sanchez Connolly,' Raúl said.

'She needs a middle name,' Estelle said.

'What about your mother's?' Raúl said, but Estelle al-

ready had her mother's name, and thanks to Spanish tradition Connolly was there, too.

Together they held and gazed at their very new daughter, quietly deciding what her full name would be.

'I want to ring Andrew and tell him he's an uncle,' Estelle said, her eyes filling with selfish tears—because though she could not be happier still she wanted to share the news. She wanted her brother to see Gabriella, as she had held Cecelia the day she was born.

'Why would you ring?' Raúl asked. 'They are waiting outside. I will go and bring them in now.'

Raúl stepped out into the waiting room.

His eyes were bloodshot, his hair unkempt, he was unshaven and there was lipstick on his collar—only this time Angela was smiling.

'It's a girl,' Raúl said. 'Both are doing really well,' he said.

Amanda burst into tears and Andrew shook his hand.

'Baby!' Cecelia said, pointing to her little cousin as Estelle showed off the newest arrival to the Connolly clan and thought that Raúl had somehow made an already perfect day even better.

'Come and see,' Raúl said to Angela, who was standing back at the door.

'She's beautiful.' Angela looked down and smiled at the chubby cheeks, seeing the eyes of Luka and Raúl. 'Just perfect—does she have a name?'

'Gabriella,' Raúl said, and looked at the woman who had been like a mother to him, even if it had been from a distance. 'Gabriella Angela Sanchez Connolly.'

Yes, Spanish names could be complicated at times, but they were very simple too.

It was a perfect day, and later came a blissful night, with

Estelle sharing a drink of champagne with her family till Cecelia was drooping in Andrew's arms.

'We're going to get back to the hotel,' Andrew said, looking down at Gabriella. He gave Estelle's hand a squeeze. 'Mum and Dad would have been really proud.'

'I know.'

And then it was just the two of them, lying in bed together, on their first night with Gabriella here.

'There is a text from Luka.' Raúl gave a brief eye-roll as he read the message. 'I have a feeling Angela may have hijacked his phone and typed it.' Raúl's voice was wry. Things were still terribly strained with Luka, but Raúl, very new to being a brother, was trying to work through it.

Not that Luka wanted to.

'You'll get there,' said Estelle.

'Perhaps,' Raúl said.

'Thank you for today.'

Gabriella, who was snuggled up in her cot beside them, made a small noise, and Raúl thought his heart might burst with pride and love as he gazed at his sleeping daughter.

'Thank *you*,' he said. 'I never thought I could feel so much happiness.'

'I meant for bringing my family over. It means so much to me to have them here.'

'I know it does.' He turned his gaze from his daughter to his wife. 'I know, thanks to you, the importance of family—even a difficult one.' He kissed her tired mouth. 'And no matter what happens I am never going to forget it.'

* * * * *

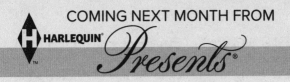

#3189 A DANGEROUS SOLACE
by Lucy Ellis

Gianluca Benedetti might not initially recognize Ava Lord, but the memories soon come rushing back! Exploring their reignited passion, Ava realizes the danger of opening her heart, as the closer he gets, the more cracks in her armor appear....

#3190 SECRETS OF A POWERFUL MAN
The Bond of Brothers
by Chantelle Shaw

Salvatore Castallano is haunted by the accident that left a blank in his memory. His young daughter is the one bright light in his dark existence. He'll do anything for her...even move Darcey Rivers—a delicious temptation—into his castle!

#3191 VISCONTI'S FORGOTTEN HEIR
by Elizabeth Power

Magenta is finally on track after suffering from amnesia. But, meeting Andreas Visconti's familiar gaze, she *knows* he's the father of her child! It's crucial she decipher the scattered puzzle of her mind and recall more than just memories of his touch....

#3192 A TOUCH OF TEMPTATION
The Sensational Stanton Sisters
by Tara Pammi

CEO Kimberly Stanton has rocked the international business world with the announcement of her marriage to outrageous Brazilian bad-boy tycoon Diego Pereira, *and* a pregnancy! If salacious rumors are already spreading, who can say what lies ahead for society's most notorious couple?

REQUEST YOUR
FREE BOOKS!

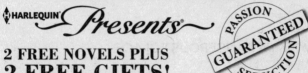

2 FREE NOVELS PLUS
2 FREE GIFTS!

PASSION
GUARANTEED
SEDUCTION

YES! Please send me 2 FREE Harlequin Presents® novels and my 2 FREE gifts (gifts are worth about $10). After receiving them, if I don't wish to receive any more books, I can return the shipping statement marked "cancel." If I don't cancel, I will receive 6 brand-new novels every month and be billed just $4.30 per book in the U.S. or $4.99 per book in Canada. That's a saving of at least 14% off the cover price! It's quite a bargain! Shipping and handling is just 50¢ per book in the U.S. and 75¢ per book in Canada.* I understand that accepting the 2 free books and gifts places me under no obligation to buy anything. I can always return a shipment and cancel at any time. Even if I never buy another book, the two free books and gifts are mine to keep forever.

106/306 HDN FVRK

Name   (PLEASE PRINT)

Address   Apt. #

City   State/Prov.   Zip/Postal Code

Signature (if under 18, a parent or guardian must sign)

Mail to the **Harlequin® Reader Service:**
IN U.S.A.: P.O. Box 1867, Buffalo, NY 14240-1867
IN CANADA: P.O. Box 609, Fort Erie, Ontario L2A 5X3

**Are you a current subscriber to Harlequin Presents books
and want to receive the larger-print edition?
Call 1-800-873-8635 or visit www.ReaderService.com.**

* Terms and prices subject to change without notice. Prices do not include applicable taxes. Sales tax applicable in N.Y. Canadian residents will be charged applicable taxes. Offer not valid in Quebec. This offer is limited to one order per household. Not valid for current subscribers to Harlequin Presents books. All orders subject to credit approval. Credit or debit balances in a customer's account(s) may be offset by any other outstanding balance owed by or to the customer. Please allow 4 to 6 weeks for delivery. Offer available while quantities last.

Your Privacy—The Harlequin® Reader Service is committed to protecting your privacy. Our Privacy Policy is available online at www.ReaderService.com or upon request from the Harlequin Reader Service.

We make a portion of our mailing list available to reputable third parties that offer products we believe may interest you. If you prefer that we not exchange your name with third parties, or if you wish to clarify or modify your communication preferences, please visit us at www.ReaderService.com/consumerschoice or write to us at Harlequin Reader Service Preference Service, P.O. Box 9062, Buffalo, NY 14269. Include your complete name and address.

HP13

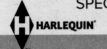
When business tycoon Vincenzo Tomasi needs a wife to
look after his two new small charges, how better to find
the perfect candidate than by interview?
Read on for an exclusive extract from Lucy Monroe's
stunning new story…

* * *

"You're talking about choosing a wife like an employee."

"Exactly." Vincenzo had always done very well choosing
employees.

In the thirteen years since taking over the bank presidency
from his father at the tender age of twenty-three, Enzu had
made exactly four bad hires. He had learned from each
mistake.

"You're not normal, you know that?"

"On the contrary, business arrangements for this sort of
thing are very common in my world."

"And they're amazingly successful, are they?" asked
Audrey.

He let Audrey know with a severe look that he did not
appreciate her levity.

She frowned back. "What if I don't like the idea of going
on a sexual test drive?"

"I'm afraid it's a nonnegotiable."

"But that's not legal. You can't require sex for a job."

"Absolutely, but as much as we are handling this situation
like I'm hiring an employee, I am not actually doing so. You

won't be working for Tomasi Enterprises or the bank. You will be my wife and the children's mother. Your job here is in no way dependent on what happens in this interview, or later between us, for that matter. Should you withdraw from the application process, it will not impact your current or future success with Tomasi Enterprises, or the bank, should you transfer back there."

"By withdraw you mean…"

"Refuse the physical aspect." He would not mince words.

"I… This is insane."

"On the contrary—it is efficient."

Her lovely dark eyes narrowed. "You do realize it is illegal to pay for sex in the state of New York."

Offended, he glared at her, unable to suppress his anger at that particular accusation. "I am not paying for sex."

"It sure sounds like it to me. Two hundred and fifty thousand dollars a year."

* * *

Will Audrey be able to resist the passion that burns between them? Find out in

Million Dollar Christmas Proposal
by Lucy Monroe

November 2013

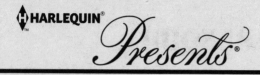